OBSTETRICS
& GYNAECOLOGY
JASON ABBOTT, LUCY BOWYER, MARTHA FINN

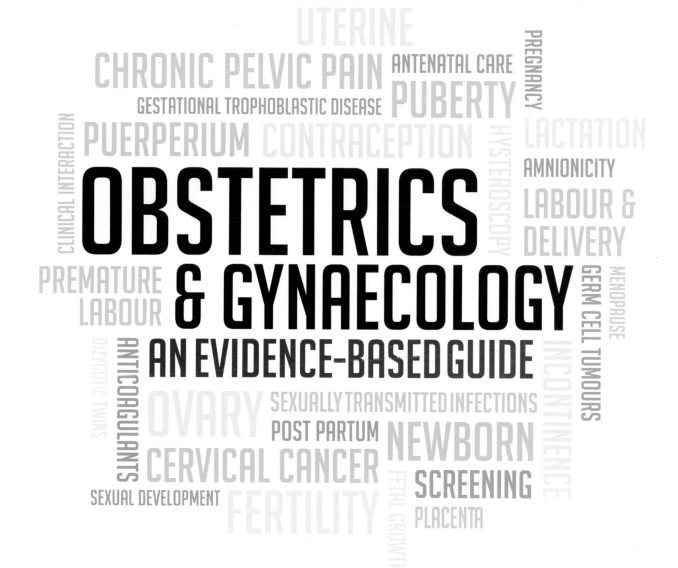

OBSTETRICS & GYNAECOLOGY
AN EVIDENCE-BASED GUIDE

UTERINE

CHRONIC PELVIC PAIN

ANTENATAL CARE

PREGNANCY

GESTATIONAL TROPHOBLASTIC DISEASE

PUBERTY

CLINICAL INTERACTION

PUERPERIUM CONTRACEPTION

HYSTEROSCOPY

LACTATION

AMNIONICITY

LABOUR & DELIVERY

PREMATURE LABOUR

GERM CELL TUMOURS

MENOPAUSE

DIZYGOTIC TWINS

ANTICOAGULANTS

OVARY

SEXUALLY TRANSMITTED INFECTIONS

POST PARTUM

NEWBORN

INCONTINENCE

CERVICAL CANCER

SEXUAL DEVELOPMENT

FERTILITY

FETAL GROWTH

SCREENING

PLACENTA

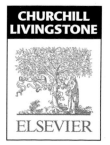

CHURCHILL LIVINGSTONE

ELSEVIER

JASON ABBOTT, LUCY BOWYER, MARTHA FINN

Edinburgh   London   New York   Oxford   Philadelphia   St Louis   Sydney   Toronto

Churchill Livingstone
is an imprint of Elsevier

Elsevier Australia. ACN 001 002 357
(a division of Reed International Books Australia Pty Ltd)
Tower 1, 475 Victoria Avenue, Chatswood, NSW 2067

ELSEVIER

This edition © 2014 Elsevier Australia

First edition © 2005

eISBN: 9780729580731

National Library of Australia Cataloguing-in-Publication Data

---

Obstetrics and gynaecology: an evidence-based guide /
Jason Abbott, Lucy Bowyer, Martha Finn.

2nd ed.
9780729540735 (paperback)
Women's health

Women—Health and hygiene—Textbooks.
Obstetrics—Textbooks.
Gynecology—Textbooks.

Abbott, Jason.
Bowyer, Lucy.
Finn, Martha.

613.042440711

Publishing Director: Luisa Cecotti
Content Strategist: Larissa Norrie
Senior Content Development Specialist: Neli Bryant
Project Managers: Martina Vascotto, Rochelle Deighton and Nayagi Athmanathan
Copy edited by Elaine Cochrane
Proofread by Sue Butterworth
Cover design by Georgette Hall
Internal design by Stan Lamond
Index by Robert Swanson
Typeset by Toppan Best-set Premedia Limited
Printed in China by 1010 Printing Int'l Ltd.

Contents

Chapter 1
The newborn 1
Paul Craven and Nadia Badawi

Chapter 2
Sexual development and puberty 10
Rebecca Deans and Jason Abbott

Chapter 3
Fundamentals of gynaecology: the menstrual cycle and clinical interaction 25
Rebecca Deans and Jason Abbott

Chapter 4
Sexual activity and contraception 35
Terri Foran

Chapter 5
Sexually transmitted infections 49
Terri Foran

Chapter 6
Fertility 60
Neil Johnson and Elizabeth Glanville

Chapter 7
Problems of fertility 70
Neil Johnson and Elizabeth Glanville

Chapter 8
Chronic pelvic pain 79
William Leigh Ledger and Jason Abbott

Preface

Pithy evidenced-based knowledge is desired by both the student and the fully fledged clinician. Dynamic research in any clinical field leads to a proliferation of studies of variable design and quality. It becomes a challenge to interpret the literature and determine what constitutes best evidence that should influence clinical practice. In obstetrics and gynaecology, the learned bodies of international colleges and societies have facilitated this process by incorporation of seminal studies into clinical guidelines. The individual practitioner should continue to critically evaluate the growing body of literature. This text is an evidence-based resource for all healthcare workers in the field of women's health, including medical students, junior doctors, midwives, nurses and general practitioners. We have endeavoured to provide the most up-to-date and relevant knowledge in the field of women's health covering the most common areas of everyday practice, such as taking an obstetric or gynaecological history, the management of abnormal uterine bleeding, and antenatal care. We also address less common issues in obstetrics and gynaecology including the gynaecological malignancies and management of multiple pregnancies — areas that are less frequently seen but remain very important.

Since obstetrics and gynaecology are often divided into two specialties we have sought contributions from experts actively working in these fields. Our authors have sifted through the literature and highlighted the salient evidence in the topic areas covered. This is a first-edition book emerging from the text *Women's Health: A core curriculum*. While initially based on that book, the new text is a focused, evidence-based, medical guide to be used for both everyday problems and as a reference to meet the needs of our broad target audience. We have structured the book as a chronological journey of women's health from conception to old age. For medical students, there are 100 new multiple choice questions (MCQs) and 25 oral structured clinical examination (OSCE) questions to crystallise the information in the preceding chapters, employing a style used in most medical schools nationally and internationally.

We hope that our work will translate into a frequently used guide for many who are interested in applying evidence to the medical care that they provide for women.

Acknowledgements

Each of us is indebted to our co-editors, without whom this book would not have happened. To the many contributors across Australia and New Zealand, thank you for your commitment and expertise in the production of this book.

Foreword

It is an honour to be invited to write the Foreword to a 'state of the art' textbook with potential to appeal to a wide professional readership. Few modern medical textbooks carry a Foreword, yet this tradition has, in the past, allowed an independent individual with a wide experience in the specialty to provide some critical perspective on the potential place and role of the new volume in the available textbook armamentarium.

This book deserves to become a classic. It is a book for all health professionals, and it offers a refreshing approach to a wide range of essential information covering all aspects of obstetrics, gynaecology and women's health. The authors have made a focused effort to ensure that the text is 'evidence-based'; that is, that the clinical recommendations are based on the best level of evidence which has been researched for that particular topic. Not all clinical problems are amenable to testing by randomised, controlled clinical trial.

The authors have also indicated their recognition that women, men and babies are all individuals with greatly varying genetic make-up, and are influenced greatly by varying cultures and environments. Hence, specific conditions present in quite varying ways and may respond unpredictably to specific medical and surgical treatments. Since this is a book for all health professionals, it necessarily emphasises basic concepts and current basic knowledge, the critical starting points for those with limited familiarity with the specialty.

This is actually an essential companion for all those individuals who have a professional health role with women or girls, but are not specialist obstetricians and gynaecologists. It is a very useful resource for those who need fast, efficient access to sound advice on any reasonably common (and many uncommon) aspects of women's health. Readers need to recognise that the evidence presented is based predominantly on the expected presentations and responses of populations living in relatively high resource settings, but much can be translated directly into relevant clinical messages for women living in low resourced settings.

This is an Australian text, with a classical, pragmatic, sound and uncomplicated approach to the understanding and handling of any clinical problem in the specialty. I believe that most readers will relate well to this, and will find the style valuable in rapidly accessing needed guidance. The authors are nationally and internationally recognised in their research fields, are renowned clinicians and are in great demand as teachers. They have launched a valuable new volume, which should find substantial favour among the modern medical student populations, the allied health professionals and many specialists in other fields, as a comprehensive learning resource as well as a quick reference companion.

Ian S. Fraser
Professor in Reproductive Medicine
University of Sydney

List of editors and contributors

Jason Abbott, B Med (Hons), FRCOG, FRANZCOG, PhD
Associate Professor of Gynaecology University of New South Wales and Royal Hospital for Women, Sydney, Australia

Marjorie Atchan, RM, IBCLC, CFHCert, BN, GradCertAdEd (Comm), M/Ed & Wrk
Assistant Professor Midwifery, Faculty of Health, University of Canberra, ACT, Australia

Nadia Badawi, PhD, FRCPI, FRACP
Macquarie Group Foundation Professor of Cerebral Palsy, Medical Director Neonatology, Co-Head Grace Centre for Newborn Care, The Children's Hospital at Westmead, NSW, Australia

Andrew Bisits, MBBS (UNSW), FRANZCOG (RCOG), DipClinEpi (Newcastle), MMedStat (Newcastle)
Director of Obstetrics, Royal Hospital for Women, Randwick, NSW, Australia

Lucy Bowyer, MBBS, MD, CMFM, FRCOG, FRANZCOG
Senior Staff Specialist in Maternal Fetal Medicine, Royal Hospital for Women, NSW and Conjoint Senior Lecturer University of New South Wales, Australia

Jonathan Carter, MBBS, DipRACOG, FACS, FACA, FRANZCOG, MS, MD, CGO
Professor Gynaecological Oncology, The University of Sydney; Head, Sydney Gynaecological Oncology Group, Sydney Cancer Centre, Royal Prince Alfred Hospital; Area Director, Gynaecological Oncology, SLHD, NSW, Australia

Naven Chetty, MBBS, FRANZCOG, CGO
Gynaecological Oncologist, Eve Health, Brisbane, QLD, Australia

Paul Craven, BSc, MBBS, MRCP, FRACP
Acting Director of Neonatal Intensive Care, John Hunter Children's Hospital, Newcastle, NSW, Australia

Amanda Cuss, MBBS (Hons), BMedSci (Hons)
General Surgical Registrar, Central Sydney Network, NSW, Australia

Rebecca Deans, MBBS, FRANZCOG
Gynaecologist and Lecturer, The University of New South Wales, Royal Hospital for Women and Sydney Children's Hospital, NSW, Australia

Paul Duggan, MBChB, Dip Obst, MMedSci, MD, GradCertEd
Head, Discipline of Obstetrics and Gynaecology, The University of Adelaide; Director, Gynaecology Unit, Royal Adelaide Hospital, SA, Australia

Elizabeth Farrell AM, MBBS, HonLLD, FRANZCOG, FRCOG
Head, Menopause Unit, Monash Medical Centre, Clayton; Acting Medical Director, Jean Hailes for Women's Health, Clayton, VIC, Australia

Rhonda Farrell, BAppSc, MBBS, DipRANZCOG, FRANZCOG, CGO
Gynaecological Oncologist, Royal Hospital for Women, Conjoint Lecturer University of New South Wales, Australia

Martha Finn, BSc (Hons), MMedSci, MD, FRCOG, FRANZCOG, DDU
Obstetrician Gynaecologist, Sonologist, Monash Ultrasound for Women, Melbourne, Australia

Terri Foran, MBBS (Syd), MClin Ed (UNSW), FACh, SHM
Sexual Health Physician, Lecturer School of Women's and Children's Health, University of New South Wales, Australia

Kirsty Foster, MBChB, MRCGP, DRCOG, MEd, PhD
Senior Lecturer in Medical Education, Sub Dean (Education) and Sub Dean (International), Sydney Medical School Northern, University of Sydney, NSW, Australia

Elizabeth Glanville
Registrar Obstetrics and Gynaecology, Department of Women's Health, Middlemore Hospital, Auckland, New Zealand

Amanda Henry, BMedSci (Hons), BMed (Hons), FRANZCOG, MPH
Lecturer, School of Women's and Children's Health, UNSW Medicine, NSW, Australia; Clinical Academic, St George Hospital and Royal Hospital for Women, NSW, Australia

Caroline SE Homer, RM, MN, MMedSc (ClinEpi), PhD
Professor of Midwifery, Centre for Midwifery, Child and Family Health, Faculty of Health, University of Technology Sydney, Australia

Jonathan Hyett, MBBS, MD, MRCOG, FRANZCOG
Senior Staff Specialist, Royal Prince Alfred Hospital, NSW, Australia

Neil Johnson, MD, CREI, FRANZCOG, FRCOG, MRCGP
Gynaecologist Auckland Gynaecology Group, Fertility Specialist Repromed Auckland, Honorary Associate Professor University of Auckland, New Zealand

William Leigh Ledger, MA, DPhil, MBChB, FRCOG, FRANZCOG
Professor of Obstetrics and Gynaecology, University of New South Wales, Director of Reproductive Medicine Unit, Royal Hospital for Women, NSW, Australia

Yee Leung, MBBS, FRANZCOG, CGO
Professor, School of Women's and Infants' Health, University of Western Australia, Head of Department, Western Australian Gynaecologic Cancer Service, Lead Clinician (Gynaecologic Oncology), Western Australian Cancer and Palliative Care Network, Director Surgical Education, King Edward Memorial Hospital for Women, WA, Australia

Sandra Lowe, MBBS (Hons), FRACP, MD
VMO Obstetric Physician, Royal Hospital for Women, Conjoint Associate Professor at University of New South Wales, Australia

Jonathan Morris, MBChB, MM, CMFM, DDU, FRANZCOG, PhD, AM
Professor Obstetrics and Gynaecology, University of Sydney, NSW, Australia

Rajit Narayan, MD, FRANZCOG
Fellow in Maternal Fetal Medicine, The Royal Prince Alfred Hospital, Sydney, NSW, Australia

Tanya Nippita, BSc(Med), MBBS (Hons), FRANZCOG
Perinatal and Women's Health Lecturer, The University of Sydney, NSW, Australia

Michael Quinn, MBChB, MGO, MRCP (UK), FRCOG, FRANZCOG, CGO
Professor of Gynaecological Oncology, Royal Women's Hospital and University of Melbourne, VIC, Australia

Thomas G Tait, MBBS, FRANZCOG, FRCOG
Senior Staff Specialist (Retired), Formerly at John Hunter Hospital as Director of Gynaecology and Chairman of the Division of Obstetrics and Gynaecology, NSW, Australia

Alec Welsh, MBBS, MSc, PhD, FRCOG(MFM), FRANZCOG, CMFM, DDU
Head of Department, Maternal-Fetal Medicine, Royal Hospital for Women, Director Australian Centre for Perinatal Science (ACPS), Professor in Maternal-Fetal Medicine School of Women's and Children's Health, University of New South Wales, NSW, Australia

List of reviewers

Academic reviewers

Tony Bushati, MBBS, MRANZCOG, FRANZCOG
Obstetrician and Gynaecologist, Laparoscopic Surgery; Colposcopy and Hysteroscopic Surgery, Hurstville, New South Wales, Australia

Leonie Callaway, MBBS (Hons), FRACP, PhD, GCELead I
Professor of Medicine, Head of the Northern Academic Cluster, Faculty of Health Sciences

Specialist in Obstetric and Internal Medicine, Royal Brisbane and Women's Hospital

School of Medicine, The University of Queensland, Australia

Susan Davis, MBBS, FRACP, PhD
Professor of Women's Health and NHMRC Principal Research Fellow, Monash University, Melbourne, Australia

Caroline de Costa, PhD, MPH, FRANZCOG, FRCOG, FRCS (Glas)
Professor of Obstetrics and Gynaecology, James Cook University School of Medicine, Cairns, Australia

Bronwyn Devine, MBBS, FRANZCOG, Postgraduate Cert Public Health (Sexual Health)
Consultant Gynaecologist, Canberra Fertility Centre, Australia

Medical student reviewers

Michelle Chen, BSc (UQ)
Final year medical student, Flinders University of South Australia, Australia

Kerina Denny, PhD, MBBS, BSc (Hons)
Resident Medical Officer, Royal Brisbane and Women's Hospital, Australia

Preet Gosal, RDN Cadet
Final year B Med, University of New England, New South Wales, Australia

Kathryn Kerr, BA(Hons)/LLB (ANU)
Fifth year medical student, University of Newcastle, New South Wales, Australia

Sarvpreet Pala
Final year medical student, University of New England/University of Newcastle, New South Wales, Australia

Calvin Peng, MBBS, BMedSci
Intern, Royal Melbourne Hospital, Victoria, Australia

Jason Wu
Medical student, University of Western Sydney, New South Wales, Australia

Jordan Young, BPhty (Hons)
Fourth year medical student, Griffith University, Queensland, Australia

Chapter 1

The newborn

Paul Craven and Nadia Badawi

KEY POINTS

A term infant is born between 37 and 41+6 weeks gestation.

Premature infants are born at less than 37 weeks gestation, very premature infants are born at less than 32 weeks gestation.

Apgar scores assess the baby's colour, heart rate, respiratory effort, tone and reflex irritability at birth.

A neonate should usually breastfeed within the first hour of birth.

DEFINITIONS OF PREMATURITY AND GROWTH

Of around 300 000 babies born in Australia each year, the majority are born at term (37–41+6 weeks' gestation). Approximately 7% are born prematurely at less than 37 weeks' gestation[1] and 1.5% at less than 32 weeks' gestation. A baby born at 42 weeks' gestation or more is described as post-term.

The average term baby weighs 3500 g, is 50 cm long and has a head circumference of 35 cm (Figure 1.1). Infants that are small are classified according to their birth weight. Low birth weight infants are those weighing less than 2500 g. Very low and extremely low birth weights are <1500 g and <1000 g respectively.

Babies born smaller than 90% of other babies at the corrected gestation are referred to as being small for gestational age (see chapter 12 on fetal growth). These babies may be symmetrically small or asymmetrically small. Symmetrically growth-restricted babies may be those with genetic defects or those exposed to in-utero viral infections (e.g. TORCH — toxoplasmosis, CMV, herpes, rubella, hepatitis, HIV), while those asymmetrically small babies, that is, their head circumference is spared, are those where there has been placental dysfunction, often secondary to maternal smoking or hypertension.

Although the majority of infants born are normal and full term, complications can occur in the prenatal, perinatal and postnatal periods. Some term babies can be born small or large, and these infants present specific problems. Small for gestational age babies (<10th centile) are likely to become cold (<36.4°C and hypoglycaemic; large for gestational age (>90th centile) babies may become hypoglycaemic if they are macrosomic, as a result of in-utero hyperinsulinaemia.

CHANGES TO THE CARDIORESPIRATORY SYSTEM

During pregnancy, oxygen from the maternal blood diffuses via the placenta to the fetus. Any maternal illness or disease affecting the function of the placenta, such as pregnancy-induced hypertension, may affect the growth of the fetus. The umbilical vein and inferior vena cava transfer oxygenated blood from the placenta to the fetal right atrium. Most of this oxygenated blood bypasses the lungs

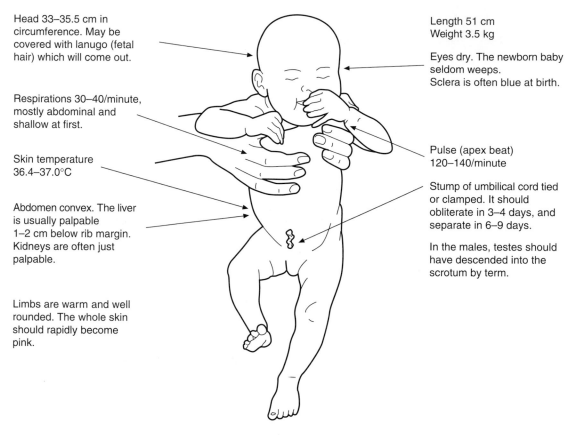

Head 33–35.5 cm in circumference. May be covered with lanugo (fetal hair) which will come out.

Respirations 30–40/minute, mostly abdominal and shallow at first.

Skin temperature 36.4–37.0°C

Abdomen convex. The liver is usually palpable 1–2 cm below rib margin. Kidneys are often just palpable.

Limbs are warm and well rounded. The whole skin should rapidly become pink.

Length 51 cm
Weight 3.5 kg

Eyes dry. The newborn baby seldom weeps. Sclera is often blue at birth.

Pulse (apex beat) 120–140/minute

Stump of umbilical cord tied or clamped. It should obliterate in 3–4 days, and separate in 6–9 days.

In the males, testes should have descended into the scrotum by term.

Figure 1.1
The normal newborn baby.

(Based on Hanretty 2003, p 356, 9780443072673, Obstetrics illustrated.)

and is shunted across the foramen ovale to the left atrium. The small amount of blood entering the right ventricle is pumped into the pulmonary artery and some of this is shunted via the patent ductus arteriosus (PDA) directly to the aorta. A small fraction of blood ejected from the right ventricle supplies the fetal lungs. Oxygenated blood is delivered to fetal tissues, and then de-oxygenated blood is transported by the umbilical arteries to return to the placenta. At birth, the lungs expand, fetal lung fluid is expelled, and the right-to-left circulatory shunts terminate due to a change in the systemic and pulmonary resistance once the placenta is disconnected (Figure 1.2). These complex changes occur around birth and result in the transition from fetal to neonatal circulation. The PDA should constrict and then close over in the first few days of life. The transition is complex, and although the majority of newborn infants manage this without intervention,

up to 10% of infants require resuscitation at birth. If transition does not occur, a condition of persistent fetal circulation exists, requiring resuscitation and intensive care support until the transition to adult circulation finally occurs.

NEONATAL RESUSCITATION

Although the majority of infants are well at birth and stable enough to transfer to the postnatal ward, approximately 10% of otherwise normal newborn infants require some form of resuscitation, and only 50% of these can be predicted from the history. Every delivery, therefore, should be attended by a person skilled in delivery and basic resuscitation.

An indication of the need for neonatal resuscitation is given by assessing all newborn babies after birth, paying attention to heart rate, respiratory effort, muscle tone and oxygen saturations. If the heart rate is below 100 or the baby is not breathing

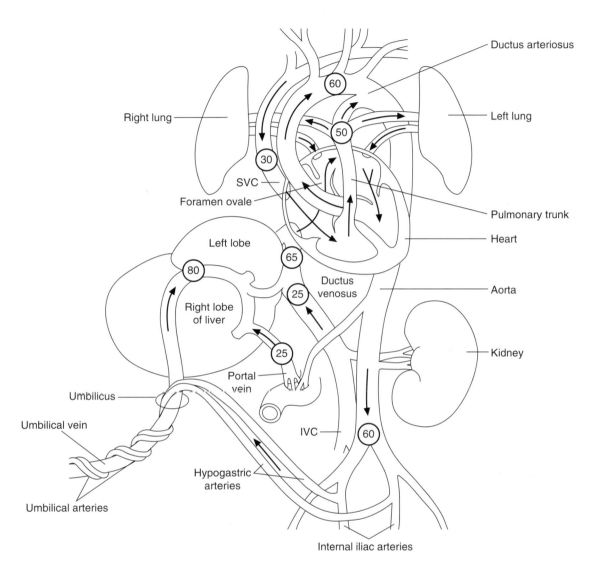

Figure 1.2
Changes in fetal circulation at birth (IVC, inferior vena cava; SVC, superior vena cava; degree of oxygenation shown in circles).

(Based on Llewellyn-Jones 1999, p 29, Fig 4.2; 9780723435099.)

or gasping, support must be given, paying attention to the airway and providing positive pressure ventilation. Once ventilation has been secured fewer than 1% of infants will require cardiopulmonary resuscitation (CPR) or adrenaline.

Clear guidelines have been established for neonatal resuscitation by the International Liaison Committee on Resuscitation (ILCOR) and the Australian Resuscitation Council (ARC): see Figure 1.3. As newborn infants are particularly susceptible to hypoxia, 10–15 minutes of effective advanced life support are required in an asystolic infant before discontinuation is considered and death pronounced.

In addition to assessing the need for resuscitation, the physical condition of every infant born in Australia is evaluated at 1 and 5 minutes after birth and the Apgar score recorded in the notes (Table 1.1). The evaluation is repeated every 5 minutes until the infant achieves a score of 8, with a

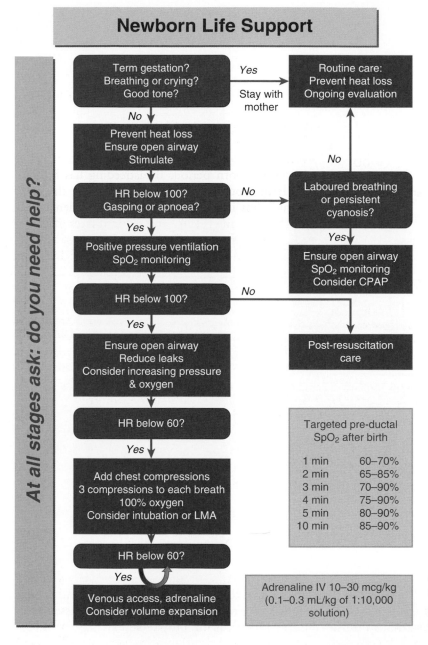

Figure 1.3
Algorithm for neonatal resuscitation.

(ARC — Australian Resuscitation Council.)

maximum possible score of 10. A poor Apgar score at 5 minutes gives some indication of the neurodevelopmental outcome of the infant and may indicate poor fetal adaptation to extrauterine life.

TEMPERATURE CONTROL

Strict attention should be paid to temperature control because newborn infants can rapidly become hypothermic. This especially applies to those babies born prematurely (<37 weeks gestation). Neonates have a large surface area to body mass ratio and only

a little brown fat to generate heat. Infants lose heat from evaporation (wet baby), conduction (warm baby to cold surface), convection (heat removed by air current over the baby) and radiation (warm baby to cool air). Heat is retained by drying infants well, placing them in warm blankets or onto a warm surface (skin to skin with mother) and keeping them out of air currents. There is evidence to support the use of plastic wrap to maintain temperature control in preterm infants, especially those less than 1500 g at birth.

Table 1.1 Apgar scores for neonates[2]			
	Apgar scores		
	0	1	2
Colour	White	Blue	Pink
Heart rate	Absent	<100	>100
Respiratory effort	None	Irregular	Regular
Tone	None	Reduced	Normal
Reflex irritability	None	Reduced	Normal

(Apgar V 1953. A proposal for a new method of evaluation of the newborn infant. Current Researches in Anesthesia and Analgesia 32:261–267.)

Once babies are warm, pink and normoglycaemic, they should be examined and their length, weight and head circumference recorded and plotted on centile charts. They should then be transferred to the postnatal ward or discharged home, depending on parental choice and the medical stability of both the mother and the newborn infant. Some women choose to deliver their babies in their own homes; the same basic care of maintaining warmth and examining these babies thoroughly after birth also applies in these settings.

VITAMIN K AND HEPATITIS B VACCINATION

Vitamin K is offered as prophylaxis against haemorrhagic disease of the newborn and is given within 6 hours of birth, often while still in the delivery suite. Hepatitis B vaccination is offered as prophylaxis within 7 days of birth. Hepatitis B vaccination forms part of the normal childhood vaccination schedule.

FEEDING

Early establishment of feeding after delivery is desirable, and breastfeeding is most successful if mother–infant suckling begins within an hour of birth. Breastfeeding should begin in the delivery suite and then be continued and supported when the mother

is moved to the postnatal ward. Although breastfeeding is optimal for both mother and baby, some mothers choose to feed their infants artificially with formula milk. Feeding should be regulated by demand, that is, as the baby requests it and at a volume that the infant self-regulates. Obviously it is difficult to gauge intake from breastfeeding, but newborn infants normally demand a feed every 2–5 hours. Bottle feeds are normally formula milk and volumes of roughly 100 mL per feed may be offered in the newborn period. Breastfeeding has benefits for both mother and infant. Benefits for the baby include less infection, lower risk of sudden infant death syndrome (SIDS) and reduced rates of diabetes. Benefits for the mother include reduced risk of breast and ovarian cancer and improved bonding between baby and mother.

POSTNATAL CARE

Staff on the postnatal ward care for both the mother and the infant. Any infant with risk factors for congenital infection (e.g. group B streptococcus on low vaginal swab), risk factors for respiratory distress (e.g. birth through meconium-stained liquor), and risk factors for subgaleal haemorrhage (instrumental delivery) should have regular observations for at least 24 hours. Infants at risk of hypoglycaemia (infants of diabetic mothers, small for gestational age infants, macrosomic infants and premature infants 35–36 weeks) should have regular blood sugar monitoring as guided by local policy, and infants of mothers who use opiates in pregnancy should be observed for signs of neonatal abstinence syndrome. Some infants will require longer periods of formal observation in hospital and these observations should be interpreted by someone who is able to interpret these accurately. All infants should have regular feeding assessments. Assessment of an infant's urine output and passage of meconium gives an indication of the general wellbeing of the infant and its ability to maintain adequate hydration. All newborn infants should pass urine within 24 hours and meconium within 48 hours. If urine or meconium has not been passed within this timeframe, pathological causes for this delay should be sought.

The most common conditions requiring admission of an infant to the special care nursery include prematurity, respiratory distress, hypoglycaemia, jaundice, and sepsis. Infants presenting with these conditions require prompt and accurate assessment by nursing and medical staff trained in caring for the neonate.

EXAMINATION OF THE NEONATE

All newborn infants require a thorough postnatal examination. This is routinely performed on day 3 of life and is a baseline measure of growth and wellbeing. It aims to identify common pathologies in the newborn period. Although commonly called the newborn examination, this is a time to interact with the family and take a thorough history including pregnancy, past medical, family, drug and social history. As well as identifying abnormal antenatal scan results, previously inherited conditions or a history of certain medications taken during pregnancy that may have an effect on the newborn baby, this period of history and examination is also an opportunity to counsel parents who smoke, trying to reduce the number of babies going home to a smoking household in Australia (currently 15–30%).

Of major concern in the examination are ductal dependent cardiac lesions, dysplastic hips, spinal anomalies and anogenital anomalies. There are a multitude of other common anomalies that should be identified and managed appropriately. To identify anomalies accurately, a thorough systematic approach to newborn examination should be taken. This includes:

- palpation of the anterior and posterior fontanelles and suture lines
- identification of normal facial features
- direct visualisation of the hard and soft palate
- examination of the chest and cardiovascular, abdominal and genitourinary systems
- examination of the hips for dislocation/relocation upon Ortolani and Barlow manoeuvres (Figure 1.4)
- examination of the limbs, eyes, spine and skin
- palpation of the femoral pulses
- assessment of Moro reflex.

The examination is completed by accurately plotting the weight, head circumference and length of the infant on an appropriate centile chart.

If a number of anomalies are identified in the infant, this raises concern over syndromic or genetic causes of the dysmorphism. Thorough documentation of features is essential for accurate diagnosis and effective communication with genetic specialists.

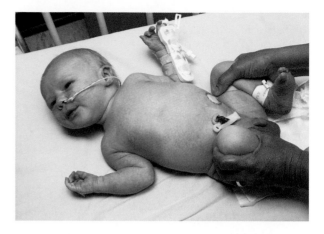

Figure 1.4
Examination of the hips of a newborn infant.
(Pitkin et al. 2003, p. 81, Fig 3; 9780443050350.)

In addition to history, examination and counselling, certain screening tests are often performed prior to discharge. These include:

- Newborn screening of blood for certain metabolic and inherited conditions
- Hearing screening
- Cardiac screening using newborn upper and lower limb oxygen saturations. Both these should be greater than 95% and the difference between the two should be less than 3%. This increases the pick-up of congenital cardiac disease from 50% by accurate examination to 75% by examination and screening.

NEWBORN SCREENING

The newborn screening test is designed to screen for treatable congenital metabolic disorders. Newborn screening tests are free but not compulsory. Each year the Newborn Screening Program tests over 90 000 babies in New South Wales and detects about 90 who need urgent assessment and treatment.

Common conditions that are screened for are phenylketonuria (PKU), congenital hypothyroidism, and cystic fibrosis. PKU is a rare condition. If it is detected by newborn screening and the baby is given a diet low in phenylalanine, normal growth and development will occur. Untreated PKU causes severe neurological impairment. Congenital hypothyroidism affects about 1 in 3500 babies and results in inadequate thyroid hormone, which is essential for normal brain development. If the

Table 1.2 Australian Standard Vaccine schedule (July 2013)	
Age	**Vaccine**
Birth	Hepatitis B
2 months	DTPa-hepatitis B, Hib, IPV, Pneumococcal conjugate (13vPCV), Rotavirus
4 months	DTPa-hepatitis B, Hib, IPV, Pneumococcal conjugate (13vPCV), Rotavirus
6 months	DTPa-hepatitis B, Hib and IPV, Pneumococcal conjugate (13vPCV), Rotavirus
12 months	MMR and Hib, Meningococcal C

DTPa   diphtheria, tetanus, acellular pertussis
IPV   inactivated poliomyelitis
MMR   measles, mumps and rubella
Hib   *Haemophilus influenzae* B

(NHMRC 2002 The Australian Standard Vaccination Schedule 2000–2002. In: The Australian Immunisation Handbook, 7th edn. National Health and Medical Research Council.)

condition is detected early and adequately treated, a child will develop normally. Cystic fibrosis affects 1 in 2500 babies and is characterised principally by pancreatic and respiratory dysfunction. Early diagnosis and treatment are important for the future prognosis of the disease.

In addition to newborn screening, all infants have their hearing formally assessed by audiometry.

All infants are offered immunisation as shown in Table 1.2. The Australian Standard Vaccination Schedule is recommended by the National Health and Medical Research Council (NHMRC), which has sought to reduce the number of injections given at each immunisation session through the use of new combination vaccines.[3] Immunisation is not compulsory, but access to child care benefits and some child care services may be influenced by the immunisation status of the child.

Hepatitis B vaccine should be advised for all infants at birth, and should not be delayed beyond 7 days after birth. Infants whose mothers are hepatitis B surface antigen positive (HbsAg+ve) should also be given hepatitis B immunoglobulin (HBIG) within 12 hours of the birth.

PREMATURE INFANTS

Despite the best efforts to suppress labour, prematurity accounts for many neonatal problems. Preterm infants have a survival rate inversely proportional to their gestational age. At 24 weeks' gestation, 50% of neonates will survive, although a substantial proportion (25%) will suffer from life-altering disabilities. By 29 weeks, this has risen to over 90% survival and a reduced incidence of life-altering disability.[4]

The more premature an infant is, the greater the morbidity and mortality. Infants born premature may develop respiratory distress syndrome, owing to a lack of natural surfactant (a phospholipid released from the type 2 pneumocytes in the fetal lung). The signs of respiratory distress are tachypnoea (RR > 60), expiratory grunt, intercostal and subcostal recession, nasal flaring, cyanosis, and/or increased oxygen requirements. There are many additional causes of respiratory distress in babies, including infection, pneumothorax, meconium aspiration, and retained lung fluid. Non-respiratory causes of respiratory distress may include duct dependent congenital cardiac lesions, such as coarctation, and gastrointestinal lesions, such as diaphragmatic herniae.

Premature infants are at increased risk of a whole host of conditions including:

- hypothermia
  - due to lack of substrate and a large surface area
- hypoglycaemia
  - due to lack of substrate for energy generation
- jaundice
  - due to an increased haematocrit at birth and immature liver function to conjugate the bilirubin produced
- necrotising enterocolitis
  - an inflammatory condition of the gastrointestinal tract with a high mortality and morbidity
- retinopathy of prematurity
  - a vascular proliferative disease that if left unmonitored may result in blindness
- intraventricular haemorrhage (IVH)
  - 30% of infants born less than 32 weeks may develop a bleed in the ventricular or parenchymal region of the brain.

Jaundice

Nearly all babies develop raised bilirubin levels in the first week of life, and this may result in jaundice. Jaundice is especially prominent in preterm infants (60–80% incidence), and the threshold for treatment varies with gestational age. Most jaundice is physiological. Pathological causes of jaundice include Rhesus disease of the newborn and ABO incompatibility. Both of these can cause jaundice within the first 24 hours of life, which requires prompt investigation and early treatment. After 14 days of life, there may be other pathological causes of jaundice, such as extrahepatic biliary atresia, hypothyroidism, and cystic fibrosis. Any infant presenting with persistent jaundice after 14 days of life should be investigated for such causes.

Long-term developmental outcomes

The majority of babies born before 30 weeks' gestation develop normally, but these very premature infants are more likely to have problems with eyesight, hearing, movement and learning. At 24–25 weeks' gestation about 30% of babies will have one or more of these problems, as will 20% of babies born at 26–27 weeks' gestation. Of the babies who do have a problem with their development, about two-thirds will have a mild disability and be able to lead an independent life, for the other one-third their disability will be severe enough that they may never be totally independent.

About 1 in 30 babies born between 28 and 31 weeks will have some degree of cerebral palsy, a permanent muscle tone problem. This incidence may be raised to up to 1 in every 20 babies born at less than 27 weeks' gestation.

TAKING THE BABY HOME

In Australia, some infants are born at home but most are born in hospital settings. Those born in hospitals remain for varying periods, depending on gestation, birth weight and associated morbidities. As a rough guide, parents of preterm infants are told to expect their baby's discharge to coincide roughly with the initial due date. Term babies normally remain in hospital between 6 hours and 1 week.

The arrival of any infant in the home is one of the most profound changes to lifestyle that a family will ever experience. Problems the parents may have to cope with include sleep deprivation, breastfeeding dilemmas and society's attitudes to this, financial constraints as one partner often ceases working, postnatal depression, and sexual difficulties.

A number of services supply support for the family once they have been discharged from hospital. Community midwives, community health centres and general practitioners provide excellent support and primary care facilities for these families. After discharge, it is recommended that the baby be reviewed at the early childhood centre, which will often organise a home visit within the first few weeks following discharge from hospital. The general practitioner provides primary health care for both the mother and the baby. All newly discharged infants require a health check at 6 weeks of age, at which time the health of both mother and child is noted in the parent-held health record. Subsequent consultations, health checks and vaccination schedules are also recorded in the parent-held record.

REFERENCES

1   Beck S, Wojdyla D, Say L, et al. The worldwide incidence of preterm birth: a systematic review of maternal mortality and morbidity. Bull World Health Organ 2010;88:31–8.

2   Apgar V. A proposal for a new method of evaluation of the newborn infant. Curr Res Anesth Analg 1953;32:261–7.

3   NHMRC. The Australian Standard Vaccination Schedule 2000–2002. In: The Australian Immunisation Handbook. 7th ed. Canberra: National Health and Medical Research Council; 2002.

4   NSW Department of Health. New South Wales mothers and babies 2000. Sydney: NSW Department of Health (Public Health Division); 2001.

MCQ

Select the correct answer.

1   Prematurity is a leading cause of morbidity for newborn babies. Which of the following statements is most accurate?

   A   Cerebral palsy affects 30% of infants born at <30 weeks.
   B   Intraventricular haemorrhage occurs in half of babies born at <30 weeks.
   C   Babies born at 29 weeks have a 90% survival rate.
   D   Of babies born <30 weeks, 5% will be blind and 1% are deaf.
   E   Physiological jaundice occurs in half of babies born at <30 weeks.

2   Baby James is born at 39 weeks by vaginal delivery. Which of the following combinations of management is most appropriate for baby James?

   A   He should be dried, fed on demand, have Vitamin K within 6 hours, and be screened for PKU before discharge from hospital.
   B   He should be dried, fed every 2 hours, have his hips checked before discharge, and be offered Hepatitis B vaccine before 1 week of age.
   C   He should be fed on demand, should pass urine within 6 hours of birth, be screened for cystic fibrosis, have auditory testing.
   D   He should be fed every 2 hours, should pass meconium within 48 hours, be screened for hypothyroidism, and have auditory testing.
   E   He should be dried, fed on demand, pass urine within 6 hours of birth, and be screened for ductus closure by day 3.

3   At the time of delivery, 10% of babies will require resuscitation. Which of the following statements is true regarding neonatal resuscitation?

   A   The Apgar score is repeated every 5 minutes until a score of 7 or more is attained.
   B   Preductal SpO_2 should be 90% at 1 minute.
   C   A baby with a heart rate of <80 at 5 minutes requires adrenaline.
   D   The birth history may predict the need for resuscitation in 75% of babies.
   E   The Apgar score gives a maximum of 2 points for pink colour and a heart rate of >100.

Chapter 2

Sexual development and puberty

Rebecca Deans and Jason Abbott

KEY POINTS

Embryological sexual development is dependent on the presence or absence of the Y chromosome.

The genital and urological systems are closely associated and abnormal development in one frequently leads to abnormalities in the other.

Disorders of sexual development require chromosomal assessment.

Müllerian tract abnormalities may present in the neonate or more commonly at puberty.

Pubertal development generally follows a well recognised progression of milestones.

Abnormal sexual or pubertal development may have both substantial physical and psychological issues.

INTRODUCTION

The physiological changes that occur in the neonatal period are the greatest that occur in our lives. The next most dramatic time of change is puberty and sexual development, when both physiological and psychological changes shape our adult lives. Puberty is a time of sexual awareness, a desire for independence, marked physical body changes, and experimentation with peers at a social and sexual level. For girls, the onset of menstruation begins the phase of reproductive life and a range of issues and problems uniquely different from those of pubertal boys.

NORMAL EMBRYOLOGICAL DEVELOPMENT OF THE INTERNAL AND EXTERNAL GENITALIA

From the time of conception, the genetic sex of the developing fetus is determined by the presence or absence of the Y chromosome. Development of all fetuses is the same until week 6, when differentiation into male or female infants commences. During week three, primordial germ cells (the precursors of gametes) can be found in the endoderm of the yolk sac. During weeks 5 and 6 they migrate by amoeboid movement to the genital ridge, an area of mesenchyme medial to the developing mesonephros and Wolffian (mesonephric) duct, which forms the future gonad. During week 6, primitive sex cords form around the germ cells in the indifferent gonad. Two Müllerian (or paramesonephric) ducts also appear lateral to the Wolffian ducts.

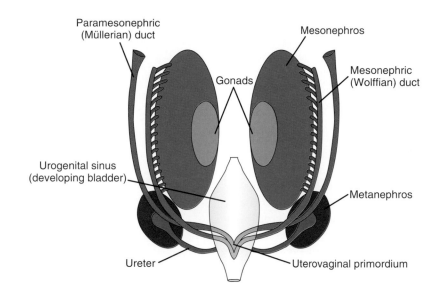

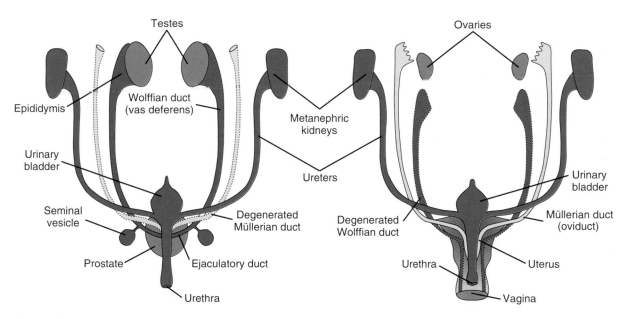

Figure 2.1
Male and female urogenital differentiation.

(Jason Abbott)

Simultaneously, at the caudal end of the fetus, the cloacal membrane folds and is separated into the anterior urogenital and posterior anal parts. The urogenital and the genital tubercle will become the future external genitalia, which by week 7 consists of a genital tubercle, urogenital membrane, urogenital folds and, more laterally, labioscrotal swellings. At the end of week 7, the urogenital membrane has degenerated and the urogenital sinus freely communicates with the amniotic fluid.

After gonadal differentiation has occurred during week 6, the presence or absence of gonadal hormone production and other fetal factors then guides the development of the Müllerian ducts, Wolffian ducts and external genitalia. Figure 2.1 illustrates the developing male and female urogenital systems.

Sertoli cells in the fetal testis secrete anti-Müllerian hormone (AMH), causing active regression of the Müllerian ducts. Leydig cells produce testosterone that acts through the androgen receptor on the Wolffian ducts, leading to the development of the vas deferens, the seminal vesicle and the epididymis.

Testosterone is converted to its active metabolite dihydrotestosterone (DHT). This acts on the target tissues of the perineum, resulting in development and growth of the genital tubercle, urogenital sinus, urogenital folds and labioscrotal swellings into the glans penis, penile shaft, urethral tube and scrotum respectively. The penis is similar in size to the clitoris at 14 weeks and, under the influence of DHT, continues growing until birth. Testicular descent is mediated by the Leydig cells under the influence of the hypothalamus and pituitary hormones; it commences at 12 weeks and is usually complete by week 34.

The fetal ovaries do not secrete either androgen or AMH, and in the absence of these hormones female external genitalia develop. There is growth of the Müllerian ducts and spontaneous regression of the Wolffian ducts from 10 weeks. The paroophoron, epoophoron and Gartner's cysts are all that may remain of the Wolffian ducts in the female. The cranial ends of the Müllerian ducts are independent of the Wolffian ducts, and remain separate as the fallopian tubes. At weeks 8–10, the pelvic Müllerian ducts have fused and subsequent breakdown of their medial walls leads to a single tube, which will become the upper vagina, cervix and the uterine epithelium and glands. The absence of circulating testosterone also leads to an absence of peripheral DHT and directs the genital tubercle, urogenital sinus, urogenital folds and labioscrotal swellings to develop into the clitoris, lower vagina, labia minora and labia majora respectively.

HUMAN SEX DEVELOPMENT

Human sex development is divided into three parts:
1 Chromosomal sex — the presence of X and/or Y chromosomes
2 Gonadal sex — development of the gonad into either testis or ovary
3 Phenotypic or anatomic sex — the appearance of the internal and external genitalia.

It is important to remember that sex development differs from the concept of gender — a more encompassing development that incorporates the individual's gender identity and sexuality.

ABNORMAL EMBRYOLOGICAL DEVELOPMENT — DISORDERS OF SEX DEVELOPMENT
Definition and classification
Disorders of sex development (DSD) conditions are divided into:
1 Sex chromosome DSD
2 46XX DSD
3 46XY DSD

Most DSD conditions occur due to either a genetic or environmental disruption of the fetal sexual development pathway. These disruptions can be to gonadal differentiation or development, sex steroid production, sex steroid conversion, or tissue utilisation of sex steroids.

Sex chromosome DSD
Sex chromosome DSD incorporates numerical chromosomal abnormalities such as 47XXY Klinefelter syndrome and its variants, 45X0 Turner syndrome and its variants, and chromosomal mosaicism such as 45X/46XY and 45XX/46XY chimerism.

Klinefelter syndrome in its classic form is characterised by phenotypic males who are tall and have long arms and legs, with gynaecomastia, small testes, and mental retardation.

Turner syndrome is characterised by patients who are phenotypically female with short stature and congenital anomalies as described later in this chapter.

46XX/46XY DSD is defined by the presence of both ovarian tissue and testicular tissue in the one person. It is said to be the rarest DSD condition, but has a higher prevalence in some geographical areas, such as Africa. Most cases present with ambiguous genitalia, although clinical presentation may be very variable. The degree of genital masculinisation is thought to be a reflection of the amount of functional testicular tissue. The gonads can be any mix of ovary, testes and ovotestes, and the aetiology is unknown.

46XX DSD
46XX DSD incorporates cases of 46XX with abnormal Müllerian tract development, disorder of gonadal development leading to virilisation, and androgen excess.

> ## Box 2.1 Possible presentations of Müllerian anomalies
>
> - Primary amenorrhoea (failure to menstruate)
> - Cyclical abdominal pain (obstruction to menstruation)
> - Severe dysmenorrhoea (painful periods) due to obstruction to menstrual drainage from one Müllerian duct
> - Pelvic mass — haematocolpos (vagina distended with menstrual blood) or haematometra (uterus distended with menstrual blood)
> - Menorrhagia (heavy vaginal bleeding)
> - Malodourous vaginal discharge; infective haematocolpos
> - Dyspareunia (painful intercourse) with transverse or longitudinal vaginal septa
> - Infertility or recurrent miscarriage
> - Ectopic pregnancy
> - Obstetric complications, for example preterm birth, abnormal lie and uterine rupture.

Müllerian anomalies

Müllerian anomalies are characterised by abnormal embryological development of the Müllerian ducts and/or persistence of Wolffian structures.

Congenital Müllerian abnormalities generally fall into one of three groups: normally fused single Müllerian system with agenesis of one or more parts; unicornuate systems due to unilateral hypoplasia or agenesis of one Müllerian duct; or lateral fusion failures including didelphic (uterus didelphis translates to double uterus) and bicornuate (a fused lower uterus with two horns) anomalies. The prevalence of Müllerian anomalies is approximately 1 in 200 women, with subfertile or infertile women having a greater incidence. Septate and bicornuate anomalies are the commonest of these anomalies. Figures 2.2A–C illustrate the normal development of the Müllerian tract and common anomalies. Figures 2.3A and B show hysteroscopic and laparoscopic views of how these anomalies are seen at clinical examinations such as hysteroscopy and laparoscopy.

AETIOLOGY

While the causes of Müllerian anomalies are largely unknown, genetic errors, teratogenic events, or combinations of these may contribute. Rarely is there a family history of similar anomalies. It is assumed that there has been failure of fusion of the two Müllerian ducts, failure of one or both ducts to develop, or failure of resorption of the adjoining areas of Müllerian duct fusion. The causes of transverse vaginal septa are unknown.

PRESENTATION

There is a wide spectrum of anomalous presentations, with 75% of women asymptomatic. The remaining 25% will have variable presentations as summarised in Box 2.1.

Secondary sexual development is normal for all women with a Müllerian anomaly, as ovarian development and function are independent of Müllerian duct and urogenital sinus growth.

INVESTIGATION

Investigation of a suspected Müllerian anomaly must include an assessment of the internal and external uterine contours. Ultrasound, MRI and hysterosalpingogram are often used, and surgery such as laparoscopy and hysteroscopy are used occasionally. Imaging of the renal tract (e.g. by ultrasound) is always indicated, as 30% of women with Müllerian tract anomalies also have urogenital anomalies. Management of these anomalies depends on the type of anomaly and the presenting features. Asymptomatic anomalies require no treatment. Surgery is indicated for symptomatic uterine and longitudinal vaginal septa. Any form of menstrual obstruction requires surgical decompression, which will also prevent pain and endometriosis.

Congenital adrenal hyperplasia

Congenital adrenal hyperplasia (CAH) is a condition that occurs in an XX fetus due to an enzyme deficiency (usually 21 hydroxylase) in the adrenal gland. The XX fetus proceeds down the female development pathway, with ovarian formation and

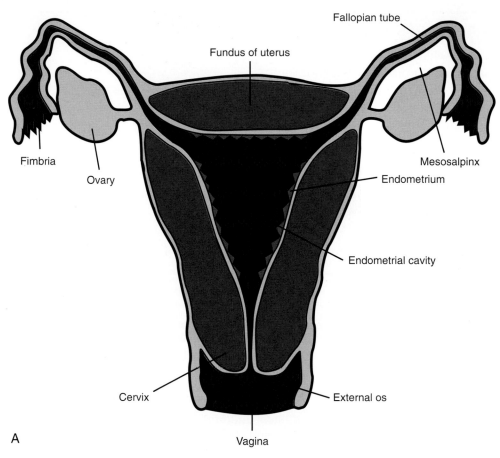

Figure 2.2
A: Normal Müllerian development.

(Jason Abbott)

development of the Müllerian ducts into uterus, cervix and upper vagina. Owing to the adrenal enzyme deficiency, cortisone production is deficient, and so the adrenal gland undergoes hyperplasia to try to produce sufficient cortisol. A byproduct of this survival mechanism is the production of large quantities of androgens. These high circulating androgen levels lead to masculinising effects on the external genitalia, ambiguous genitalia, or normal-looking male genitalia at birth.

CAH is the only DSD condition that can be life-threatening, as unrecognised cortisol deficiency can lead to a salt-wasting crisis in the neonate. Management aims to correct the cortisol deficiency and excess androgen production. Gender assignment at birth is usually female, due to the presence of ovaries and uterus with potential normal female fertility. Where possible, any surgical correction should be deferred until adulthood when consent to any

procedure and the implications of these decisions are better understood.

Other causes of XX fetal virilisation

Other exogenous sources of androgens (e.g. maternal androgen-secreting tumours or the use of virilising drugs such as danazol during pregnancy) may rarely lead to masculinisation of the external genitalia in an XX fetus.

46XY DSD

46XY DSD encompasses 46XY with disorders of gonadal development, and disorders of androgen synthesis or action.

Androgen receptor defects — androgen insensitivity syndrome

Androgen receptor abnormalities result in androgen insensitivity syndrome (AIS) due to an inability of

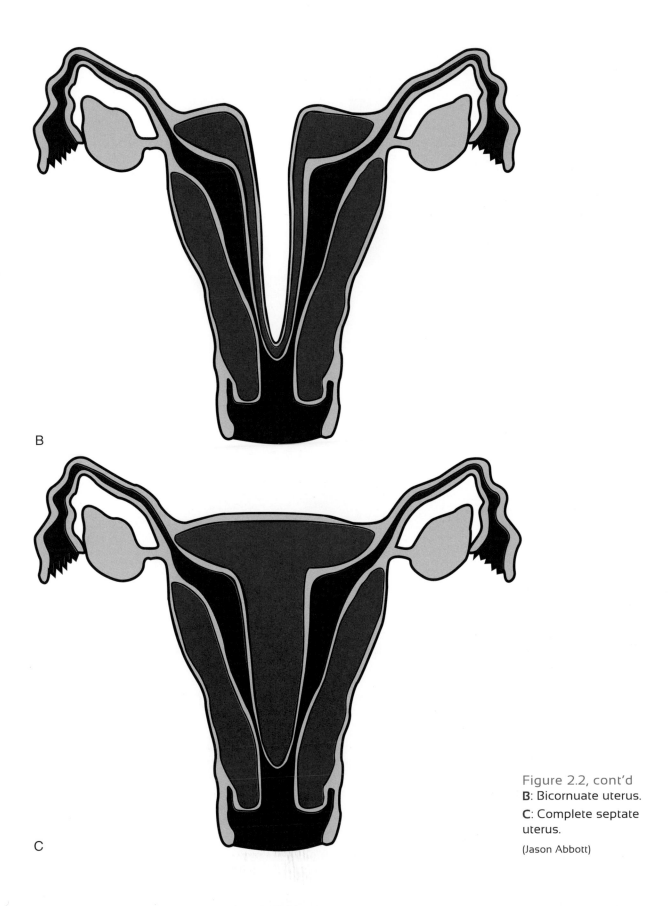

B

C

Figure 2.2, cont'd
B: Bicornuate uterus.
C: Complete septate uterus.

(Jason Abbott)

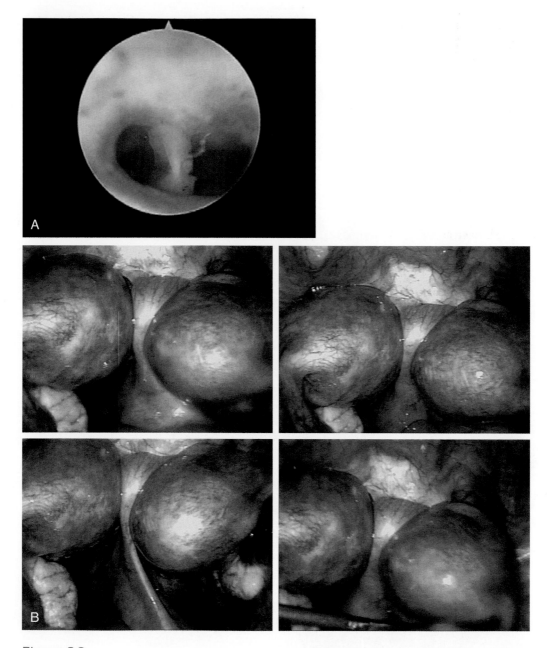

Figure 2.3

A: A hysteroscopic view of a uterine septum showing that the uterine cavity is divided by a central fibrous band of tissue. This can be removed surgically. **B**: The appearance of a bicornuate uterus at laparoscopy. Note the peritoneal band between the two horns.

the body to respond to androgens. This insensitivity may be complete (CAIS), or partial (PAIS). The cause of this syndrome is a disruption of the androgen receptor gene, with an XY fetus initially proceeding down the pathway of male fetal sexual determination with testicular development, and both AMH and testosterone produced normally. The AMH ensures regression of the Müllerian duct; however female external genitalia develop because some cells are insensitive to androgens. In CAIS the result is an XY female with absent Müllerian structures, female genitalia, variable vaginal hypoplasia, absent or sparse pubic and axillary hair, normal breast development, normal female behaviour and gender identity, and intra-abdominal testes that produce high levels of circulating testosterone. In the partial form some response to androgens occurs. Presentation is a spectrum from a normal male phenotype with infertility to ambiguous genitalia. In some cases the diagnosis is not made until puberty, when virilisation occurs.

Gonadal dysgenesis

Gonadal dysgenesis, also known as Swyers syndrome, results from a disruption at the very start of the male sex determination pathway that causes an XY fetus to divert to the female development pathway. The result is dysgenetic (abnormally formed) streak gonads. As these gonads produce neither AMH nor testosterone, the external genital development is female and the Müllerian ducts develop into the vagina, uterus and cervix. Other forms of XY gonadal dysgenesis that can lead to DSD include partial gonadal dysgenesis with some testicular function, and mixed gonadal dysgenesis (a unilateral testis and a contralateral streak gonad), which are conditions that usually present with variable degrees of genital masculinisation or ambiguity.

Androgen biosynthetic defects

Androgen biosynthetic defects may also present with genital ambiguity at birth. The most common are 5 alpha reductase type 2 deficiency and 17 beta hydroxysteroid dehydrogenase type 3 deficiency. Both are autosomal recessive conditions in which an XY fetus initially starts down the male development pathway with normal testicular development. However, there is a deficiency of enzymes involved in androgen synthesis, leading to a variant of female external genital development. If left untreated in childhood, both conditions will result in increasing masculinisation at puberty, and possibly a change in gender identity from female to male for some individuals.

PUBERTY: TIMING AND ITS PROBLEMS
Normal puberty

Puberty is the time at which, under the influence of sex hormones, a child becomes an adult physically, sexually and psychologically. For women, the onset generally varies between 9 and 14 years.

The physical events of puberty tend to follow an ordered sequence in time. Figure 2.4 shows the normal sequence for girls. Although the most obvious changes are within the reproductive system, the first sign is generally a pubertal growth spurt.

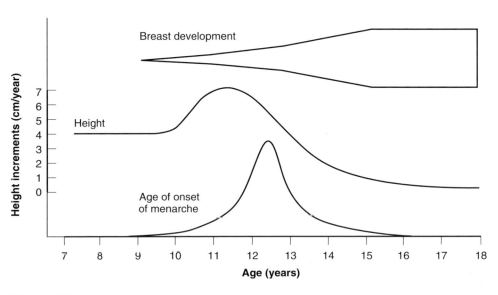

Figure 2.4
The sequence of pubertal events in the female.

(From Llewellyn-Jones D: *Fundamentals of Obstetrics and Gynaecology*, 1999, Fig 9.17 p. 82; 9780723431503.)

Girls tend to go through puberty earlier than boys and therefore until the mid-teens are often taller and heavier than boys of the same age. During later puberty, female growth slows compared to that of males because of earlier epiphyseal closure. The growth spurt is followed by the early development of secondary sexual characteristics. Menarche — the first menstruation — usually occurs between 11 and 14 years. Towards the end of puberty, when secondary sexual development is completed, there is often a further accelerated growth phase.

Central control of puberty: pulsatile GnRH

The initiation of puberty is associated with an increase in gonadotrophin releasing hormone (GnRH) in the hypothalamus, stimulating the hypothalamic–pituitary axis, which has been relatively quiescent since early childhood. GnRH is released in a pulsatile fashion and initially is released only at night. GnRH stimulates the anterior pituitary to secrete the gonadotrophins follicle-stimulating hormone (FSH), which first rises and then plateaus, and is closely followed by luteinising hormone (LH), which has a slow and steady incline. GnRH initially acts as self-primer in the anterior pituitary and is later augmented by gonadotrophin secretion.

FSH causes the ovaries to increase the release of oestradiol, which stimulates breast growth. The ovaries and adrenal glands secrete androgens that instigate the development of sexual hair growth. Towards the end of puberty, the maturation of the hypothalamus is associated with an increased secretion of growth hormone, causing the growth spurt described above.

Stages of puberty

The development of secondary sexual characteristics comprises five changes:
1 The growth spurt
2 Thelarche (breast development)
3 Adrenarche (pubic hair development)
4 Menarche (the onset of menstruation)
5 Urogenital changes.

The growth spurt

The growth spurt — as much as 10 cm per year for 2 years — occurs prior to menarche and is the result of oestrogen and growth hormone release causing stimulation of insulin-like growth factor-1 secretion, principally from the liver. The mean duration of the growth spurt is 4.5 years. Following menarche, growth slows with no more than 6 cm additional height expected after the first period.

Thelarche

The first physical sign of puberty is generally breast development, known as thelarche, followed by growth of sexual hair in the pubic area and then the axillae. Breast development occurs at an average age of 10.3 years and it has five stages, often referred to as Tanner staging. Figure 2.5 demonstrates the Tanner stages of breast and pubic hair development.

Adrenache

The growth of sexual hair is controlled mainly by adrenal androgens and is termed adrenarche. Growth of pubic and axillary hair occurs at a mean age of 10.5 years. Premature adrenarche is pubic or axillary hair before 8 years (6 years in girls of Afro-Caribbean origin) and requires investigation (see discussion of precocious puberty below).

Menarche

The first menstruation occurs at a mean age of 12.7 years (11–14 years) and is considered the final hallmark of puberty. It is often timed approximately with Tanner stage 4–5 of breast development (see Figure 2.5). Initially, menstrual bleeding can be erratic and sometimes heavy, since the initial 'periods' represent the shedding of endometrium from the uterine cavity when oestrogen-stimulated growth outgrows the blood supply, rather than the culmination of an ovulatory hormonal cycle. Menstruation is commonly anovulatory for 12–18 months after menarche, but in 25% of girls anovulatory bleeding may persist for up to 4 years.

Urogenital changes

Deposition of subcutaneous fat in the genitalia occurs and gives both the more rounded female contour and the greater prominence of the labia majora and the mons pubis. The infantile uterus enlarges and its body (corpus) increases in size relative to the cervix. The endometrium changes from cuboidal to columnar and becomes secretory. The vagina lengthens, thickens and begins to secrete mucus. The pelvis acquires the female configuration. All these changes occur under the influence of oestrogen.

The age of pubertal development is commonly genetically determined, however it is also linked to

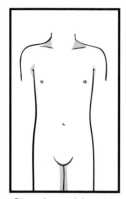 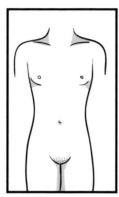 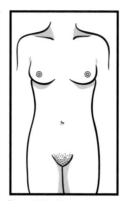 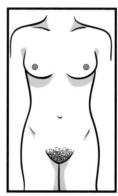 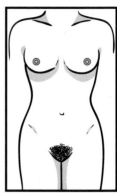

Stage 1, preadolescent: breast elevation of papilla only, and no pubic hair.

Stage 2, breast bud stage: elevation of breast and papilla as a small mound, with enlargement of the areolar region. Pubic hair is present but sparse

Stage 3, further enlargement of breast and areola without separation of their contours. Darker and coarser pubic hair over the mons pubis

Stage 4, projection of areola and papilla to form a secondary mound above the level of the breast. An increased amount of pubic hair over the mons pubis and labia majora

Stage 5, mature stage: projection of papilla only, resulting from recession of the areola to the general contour of the breast. Thickening of pubic hair with extension of pubic hair to the inner thigh

Figure 2.5

The Tanner stages of breast and pubic hair development.

(Image courtesy of Jason Abbott, based on the original description from Tanner.)

a critical body weight or fat content (16–24%). This link is associated with the protein leptin, which is crucial for regulating appetite.

Delayed puberty

Since there is a wide variation in normal development, it is difficult to define the patient with abnormally delayed sexual maturation. Delayed puberty may be defined as the absence of secondary sexual characteristics by the age of 13 years, and absence of menstruation by the age of 15 years in the presence of secondary sexual characteristics. Common causes of delayed puberty can be classified as described in Box 2.2.

History and examination

Past general health, height and weight records are important, along with relevant behaviour such as extreme exercise, abnormal eating habits, and illicit drug use. Physiological delayed puberty tends to be familial and hence it is important to compare the height and pubertal milestones of parents and siblings.

On physical examination, in addition to Tanner staging of any secondary sexual characteristics present (including signs of virilisation), a search for signs of galactorrhoea, hypothyroidism, gonadal dysgenesis and chronic illness should be made. The commonest chromosomal form of delayed puberty is Turner syndrome (45XO). Other signs of this syndrome include short stature, web neck, lymphoedema, coarctation of aorta, and scoliosis.

Patients may present for investigation of primary amenorrhoea, and other diagnoses should be considered. In the patient with primary amenorrhoea, it is important to undertake a neurological examination, looking for signs of intracranial disease such as restricted visual fields or absent sense of smell (anosmia). Anatomical defects of the Müllerian ducts must be sought, especially when a disparity between normal puberty and absent menses is encountered.

Precocious puberty

When pubertal changes occur before 6 years and/or menarche before 8 years of age, investigation as to the causation is required.

Precocious puberty may be divided into two subgroups:

1 GnRH dependent — complete or isosexual (true precocious puberty)
   - idiopathic
   - central nervous system (CNS) causes

Box 2.2 Common causes of delayed puberty

Hypergonadotrophic hypogonadism

- Ovarian failure with abnormal or normal karyotype

Hypogonadotrophic hypogonadism

REVERSIBLE

- Physiological/constitutional delay
- Weight loss/anorexia
- Primary hypothyroidism
- Prolactinomas and other pituitary adenomas
- Congenital adrenal hyperplasia
- Cushings disease

IRREVERSIBLE

- GnRH deficiency
- Hypopituitarism, and congenital central nervous system (CNS) defects
- Craniopharyngioma, and other pituitary tumours

Eugonadism

- Müllerian agenesis
- Discordant karyotype, e.g. 46XY DSD
- Vaginal septum and imperforate hymen
- Inappropriate gonadal hormone feedback

---

2 GnRH independent — heterosexual or incomplete, from a peripheral source of sex steroid secretion including:
   - ovarian cyst or tumour
   - McCune–Albright syndrome (polyostotic fibrous dysplasia) mutation in G protein coupled receptor causing unchecked autonomous sex steroid activity in tissues
   - adrenal feminising or masculinising (CAH)
   - ectopic hormone production.

When infants who were growth restricted, or had extremely low birth weight, reach adolescence, they may have an increased risk of premature adrenarche, often with hyperinsulinism and decreased insulin sensitivity. Follow-up is required since these girls may be predisposed to chronic early polycystic ovarian syndrome and/or metabolic syndrome.

Investigating pubertal abnormalities

When there is an abnormality recognised in the usual pubertal sequence, investigations should include X-rays for bone age, brain imaging, gonadotrophin and prolactin concentrations, adrenal and gonadal steroid measurements, and assessment of thyroid function. Imaging of the brain by MRI should be considered if there are abnormalities on the neurological examination or the prolactin is grossly elevated. Patients with elevated gonadotrophins require a karyotype, pelvic ultrasound and/or pelvic MRI. Very occasionally, an examination under anaesthesia or diagnostic laparoscopy may be required.

Treatment of delayed puberty

In physiological delay, reassurance that the anticipated development will occur is the only management required. Removal or correction of a primary aetiology when detected is important, as in the treatment of hypothyroidism. In hypogonadism, hormone therapy will initiate and sustain maturation and function of secondary sexual characteristics and promote achievement of height potential. Long-term treatment with oestrogen replacement is important to prevent osteoporosis.

Treatment to induce puberty in girls who have not developed secondary sexual characteristics should be initiated with very small doses of ethinyloestradiol 1 mcg daily for approximately 6 months, increasing to 2, 5, 10 and 20 mcg at 6-monthly intervals. Low-dose ethinyloestradiol is not widely available, and referral to a specialist unit is recommended. The low-dose 17β-oestradiol patch can be used as an alternative. Progestogen should be added to the unopposed oestrogen regime after 2 years or when vaginal bleeding occurs.

Traditionally, the OCP, a combination of oestrogen and progestogen, has been the drug of choice for long-term treatment. With the advent of a large variety of hormone therapy (HRT) preparations, a greater choice is available. Regimes with HRT may be superior because the type of oestrogen that these preparations contain and the route of administration (bypassing first pass metabolism) are not associated with an increased incidence of hypertension or unfavourable changes in lipid profiles. The overall oestrogen intake over a long period of time is also increased, as there is no hormone-free week, and this is beneficial in women with Turner syndrome who have no endogenous oestrogen production. Girls on long-term oestrogen supplementation should have their bone mineral density checked at regular intervals.

Specific conditions associated with eugonadism

An imperforate hymen or vaginal septum can lead to obstruction of the flow of menstrual blood (cryptomenorrhoea), whereby girls with a functioning uterus present with cyclical lower abdominal pain. In the advanced stages, a palpable abdominal swelling will be present and separation of the labia will reveal the classic blue-coloured membrane in the case of imperforate hymen. Treatment is surgical, with incision and excision of the thin membrane causing the release of large amounts of tarry, chocolate-coloured fluid. Vaginal septa are more difficult to manage and may need corrective surgery, depending on the location of the septum. If surgery is to be deferred, menstrual suppression with hormonal therapy will be required in the short term to reduce symptoms of cyclical pain.

Vaginal agenesis in the absence of a uterus can be managed by either non-surgical and/or surgical methods. The non-surgical method involves teaching the girl to apply a vaginal dilator to the central dimple in the area of the introitus so that, over time, with progressive dilation and increasing size of dilators, a functional vagina can be produced. Surgical methods include creating a pouch or using a split skin, intestinal, or amnion graft to create a neovagina. When the girl is sexually active, having intercourse will increase the length of the vagina. Surgical formation of a neovagina should only be undertaken when the girl is approaching sexual activity, since ongoing use of dilators or sexual intercourse is important to maintain the newly formed vagina.

Girls with complete androgen insensitivity syndrome have a normal 46XY karyotype but are phenotypically female. The testes are essentially normal and may be found anywhere along the line of testicular descent from the abdomen to the labia. The risk of malignancy in these gonads is between 2 and 15%, and hence they should be removed at the completion of puberty.

For all of the DSDs the diagnosis can be devastating, particularly when a female enters puberty and has a diagnosis of being genetically male. Extensive counselling of the individual and family is required.

Treatment of precocious puberty

Identification of the aetiology, and treatment of reversible causes such as surgery for cranial tumours, or medical management to arrest development, are warranted. An attempt should be made to maximise the final height, as high levels of oestrogen will close the epiphyses in the long bones and cause short stature. This is generally achieved with the use of GnRH agonist therapy, and exogenous growth hormone may also be indicated. Girls with precocious puberty are more likely to suffer from psychological trauma and sexual abuse; therefore support and counselling are indicated and early contraception advice may be required.

FURTHER READING
Embryology
Moore KL, Persaud TVN. Before we are born: essentials of embryology and birth defects / Color atlas of clinical embryology. 8th ed. Philadelphia: Elsevier Saunders; 2013.
Moore KL, Persaud TVN. The developing human: clinically oriented embryology. 9th ed. Philadelphia: Saunders Elsevier; 2012.
Larsen W. Human embryology. 7th ed. Philadelphia: Elsevier; 2003.

Reproductive endocrinology
Speroff L, Fritz M. Clinical gynecologic endocrinology and infertility. Philadelphia: Lippincott Williams and Wilkins; 2011.

DSD consensus statement
Hughes IA, Houk C, Ahmed SF, Lee PA, et al. Consensus statement on management of intersex conditions. Arch Dis Child 2006;91:554–63.
Lee PA, Houk CP, Ahmed SF, et al. Writing Group for the International Intersex Consensus Conference. Pediatrics 2006;118:75.

Other

Deans R, Berra M, Creighton SM. Management of vaginal hypoplasia in disorders of sexual development: surgical and non-surgical options. Sex Dev 2010;4(4–5):292–9.

Saravelos S, Cocksedge KA, Li TC. Prevalence and diagnosis of congenital uterine anomalies in women with reproductive failure: a critical appraisal. Hum Reprod Update 2008;14(5):415–29.

Sloboda DM, Hart R, Doherty DA, et al. Age at menarche: influences of prenatal and postnatal growth. J Clin Endocrinol Metab 2007;92:46–50.

MCQS

Select the correct answer.

1   The embryological structure that is the precursor to the uterus is the:

   A   Wolffian duct.
   B   Müllerian duct.
   C   Gartner duct.
   D   cloaca.
   E   urogenital sinus.

2   The five changes that occur at puberty are:

   A   menarche, sexual differentiation, the growth spurt, axillary and pubic hair growth, breast development.
   B   breast development, ovulation, axillary and pubic hair growth, growth spurt, menstruation.
   C   the growth spurt, axillary and pubic hair growth, breast development, menarche, gender identity.
   D   breast development, axillary and pubic hair growth, the growth spurt, urogenital changes and menarche.
   E   breast development, axillary and pubic hair growth, androgen production, growth spurt, menstruation.

3   The typical karyotype of a patient with Turner syndrome is:

   A   46XY
   B   45XX
   C   45XO
   D   46XO
   E   46XXY

4   The most important reason for identifying and treating precocious puberty is:

   A   to maximise final adult height.
   B   to prevent benign gonads becoming malignant.
   C   stop breast development in young children.
   D   reduce the incidence of sexual abuse.
   E   minimise virilisation.

OSCE

Janelle, a 14-year-old female, presents to the emergency department with an acute abdomen. She has had several months of mild pain that comes and goes but is usually relieved by simple analgesia such as paracetamol and non-steroidal anti-inflammatories. This time the pain is very severe.

What are the important features on history, examination and investigation that would allow you to arrive at a diagnosis? What management would you initiate?

Chapter 3

Fundamentals of gynaecology: the menstrual cycle and clinical interaction

Rebecca Deans and Jason Abbott

KEY POINTS

The hypothalamic–pituitary–ovarian axis regulates menstruation.

The menstrual cycle involves interaction between endocrine and paracrine systems.

The phases of the menstrual cycle are influenced by oestrogen (follicular phases) and progestogen (secretory phase).

There are concurrent actions at the ovary and the endometrium with central nervous system feedback.

Taking a thorough history and performing an appropriate examination in conjunction with a good working knowledge of the menstrual cycle allow many gynaecological issues to be simply addressed.

INTRODUCTION

Gynaecology is the area of medicine that cares for the reproductive health of the non-pregnant woman. In Australia where the number of pregnancies is few — on average just over two for any woman — this means that the woman's reproductive health spans most of her life, and its normal function and problems of menstruation must be appraised and treated as needed. What this requires is an understanding of the normal menstrual cycle; once this is mastered, the problems of menstruation and their treatment are easily understood (on the whole). Importantly, the clinical interaction of history-taking and physical examination are pivotal in taking the knowledge of the menstrual cycle and applying it to the woman that you are caring for. Whether you are in the emergency department of a large teaching hospital, in primary care in a small rural area or a subspecialist gynaecologist, knowledge of these two inextricably linked topics is essential so that you can care for women safely and expertly.

First we examine the heavily physiology focused menstrual cycle. We follow with the essentials of a good history for gynaecology, and the critical findings on examination that help to determine health and variations away from health. In Chapter 18 we will discuss specific problems of menstruation with abnormal uterine bleeding.

THE MENSTRUAL CYCLE

The menstrual cycle is regulated at both endocrine and paracrine levels. There are classical endocrine feedback loops in which ovarian steroids, predominantly androgens, oestrodiol and progesterone, modulate release of hormones from the pituitary. A complex series of paracrine processes that operate within the tissues of the ovary and uterus also impose local regulation on this system.

Physiological events in the endometrium are largely determined by the fluctuating concentrations of ovarian hormones. Prior to ovulation, the endometrium increases in thickness and endometrial glands proliferate (the proliferative phase of the cycle). After ovulation, under the influence of progesterone from the corpus luteum, the endometrium undergoes secretory changes in preparation for reception of the implanting embryo (the secretory phase of the cycle). If a pregnancy does not occur, the decreasing levels of progesterone from the degenerating corpus luteum become insufficient to maintain the endometrial integrity, causing spasm of the spiral arterioles in the basalis layer of the endometrium, and shedding of the superficial endometrial layer (superficialis) occurs at menstruation. The endometrium is shed in patches, rather than synchronously, and the endometrial basalis layer, which allows regeneration of the endometrium in the next cycle, remains.

Typically, the menstrual period lasts 5 days (range 2–6 days) and the length of the cycle is commonly 28 days (range 21–35 days), with a mean blood loss of 30 mL (range 20–60 mL) per cycle. These values vary in different women and from cycle to cycle in the same woman.

Neuroendocrinology
Hypothalamus

Gonadotrophin releasing hormone (GnRH) is a decapeptide released from the hypothalamus in a pulsatile fashion. It is delivered into the portal vasculature via the hypothalamo-hypophyseal portal tract. Its release is affected by various feedback loops of GnRH (autoregulation) and by other neuropeptides, such as kisspeptin, neuropeptide Y, dopamine

and noradrenaline, as well as metabolic hormones such as leptin, opioids, insulin and cortisol. Control of ovulation is complex and may be affected by stress, starvation or satiety, excessive exercise, and chronic disease states.

Pituitary

The anterior pituitary releases two principal gonadotrophins involved in the reproductive cycle: follicle-stimulating hormone (FSH), and luteinising hormone (LH). Both are released in response to pulsatile GnRH, with the amount of each hormone released affected by the pulse frequency and amplitude of GnRH. Therefore through the course of the ovarian cycle, each of the gonadotrophins is released into the circulation at varying concentrations.

Phases of the menstrual cycle

The normal menstrual cycle is further divided into the ovarian cycle and the uterine cycle. The ovarian cycle may be divided into follicular and luteal phases, and the uterine or endometrial cycle denoted by the proliferative and secretory phases.

Follicular phase

Hormonal feedback promotes the orderly development of a single dominant follicle, which should be mature at mid cycle and prepared for ovulation. The mean length of the follicular phase is 14 days (range 10–18 days). Variability of this part of the cycle is usually responsible for variations in the total cycle length, with the rise in oestrogen being a key factor in the variability.

Luteal phase

The luteal phase commences at the time of ovulation and continues to the onset of menses, with a mean length of 14 days. The luteal phase is much more reliably of this duration than is the follicular phase. In the absence of pregnancy, the decline in progesterone is a key trigger to menstruation occurring.

Ovarian follicular development

The human ovarian follicular pool is maximal at approximately five months of fetal life, when the ovaries contain approximately 7 million follicles. At birth, the number is decreased to 1 million primordial follicles, arrested in meiotic division. Follicle depletion continues to occur before and after menarche (the first menstruation); during use of the oral contraceptive pill; during pregnancy; and whether or not regular menstruation occurs. Of the original pool of 7 million primordial follicles, only about 400 will ever ovulate. In addition to the oocyte, two main cell lines exist to support the follicle: theca cells and granulosa cells.

The early stages of follicle development are independent of gonadotrophins and are under the influence of locally acting intra-ovarian paracrine regulators. Once a developing follicle reaches the pre-antral stage of development, further progression to the antral and pre-ovulatory stages are dependent upon the presence of gonadotrophins (FSH and LH). The elevated circulating concentration of FSH in the early follicular phase of the ovarian cycle allows a limited number of pre-antral follicles to reach maturity, creating a group of equally developing follicles. However, only one 'lead' follicle will continue to develop, with support within its granulosa cells, causing an increased local production and secretion of oestradiol. LH stimulates production of precursor androgens, particularly androstenedione, by the theca cell layer and FSH stimulates oestradiol production within the adjacent granulosa cell layer. This is termed the 'two cell, two gonadotrophin' hypothesis.

Once the concentration of serum oestradiol begins to rise in the mid-follicular phase, there is a rapid suppression of pituitary FSH production by both negative feedback and inhibin B, a glycoprotein secreted by the granulosa cells of the developing dominant follicle. The resulting decrease in circulating concentration of FSH withdraws gonadotrophin support from the remaining follicles in the group. The result is regression of all but the dominant follicle, leading to a single ovulation.

Figure 3.1 demonstrates the hormonal changes that accompany the menstrual cycle.

The LH surge and ovulation

Final maturation of the oocyte only occurs after initiation of the LH surge. This ensures that the oocyte is mature and ready for fertilisation after release from the follicle. The LH surge represents a coordinated discharge of LH from the anterior pituitary. This occurs in response to the rapid rise in oestradiol during the late follicular phase of the ovarian cycle. Pulsatile GnRH from the hypothalamus increases in both amplitude and frequency, triggering the LH surge with a rapid release of LH and, to a lesser extent, FSH from the anterior pituitary.

The LH surge initiates final maturation of the oocyte and ovulation about 38 hours after the surge. Ovulation occurs when new blood vessel formation and release of prostaglandins and cytokines cause rupture of the follicle wall and expulsion of the oocyte. At ovulation, a chemotactic effect of ovarian cytokines attracts the fallopian tube to close proximity of the rupturing follicle, and a mucus bridge develops to transit the oocyte into the awaiting fimbrial end of the fallopian tube.

The 'empty' ruptured follicle that results on the ovary rapidly fills with blood. Combined with the theca and granulosa cell layers it forms the corpus luteum (yellow body). A rapid synthesis of progesterone along with oestradiol within the corpus luteum follows. If the oocyte is fertilised and pregnancy ensues, the concentrations of oestrogen and progesterone rise still further, with the corpus luteum being an important source of hormonal support until the placenta develops and takes over this role.

The endometrium

The development of a healthy secretory endometrium is essential for implantation and successful development of pregnancy. In the human, the oocyte is fertilised in the fallopian tube and then travels to enter the uterus on day 3, at the morula stage of development. The blastocyst forms on day 4 and then adheres to the endometrial lining, beginning the process of implantation. Interaction between the maternal cells and fetal cells at implantation is critical to successful pregnancy. An imperative initial interaction is the 'rescue' of the corpus luteum by human chorionic gonadotrophin (hCG) secreted from fetal cells; this prevents the breakdown of the corpus luteum and allows for the continued production of oestrogen and progesterone that is essential for continued pregnancy. Figure 3.2 shows the endometrial changes that are associated with the menstrual cycle.

Menstruation

If implantation and pregnancy does not occur after ovulation, then menstruation follows. This is the process of shedding of the superficial layers of the endometrium, with subsequent repair in preparation for regrowth from the basalis layer. Menstruation is initiated by a fall in the concentration

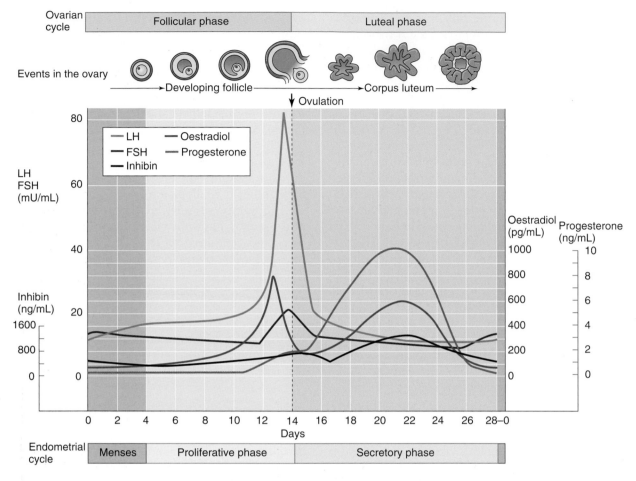

Figure 3.1

Hormonal changes during the menstrual cycle. The menstrual cycle is a cycle of the hypothalamic–pituitary–ovarian axis, as well as a cycle of the targets of the ovarian hormones — the endometrium of the uterus. Therefore, the menstrual cycle includes both an ovarian cycle, which includes the follicular phase, ovulation, and the luteal phase, and an endometrial cycle, which includes the menstrual, the proliferative, and the secretory phases.

(Boron: Medical Physiology, Updated Edition, 2nd ed. Copyright © 2011 Saunders, An Imprint of Elsevier)

of circulating progesterone that follows luteal regression.

In the premenstrual phase, a fall in progesterone activates a complex series of events including:

1. Leucocytes are drawn into the uterus
2. Matrix metalloproteinases are expressed
3. Prostaglandins and other compounds that act on the uterine vessels and smooth muscle are produced.

Prostaglandins are present in high concentrations in the endometrium, and the ovarian steroids regulate their synthesis. Increased production of prostaglandins produces the myometrial contractions and vasoconstriction of the endometrial vessels seen at menstruation, and also leads to pain and tissue oedema. The end result of this cascade of events is constriction of the spiral arterioles with contraction of the uterine muscle, leading to expulsion of the denuded endometrial tissue out of the uterus through the cervix and out of the vaginal orifice.

GYNAECOLOGY HISTORY TAKING AND EXAMINATION

Knowledge of the menstrual cycle and the various changes that occur at various levels (central nervous

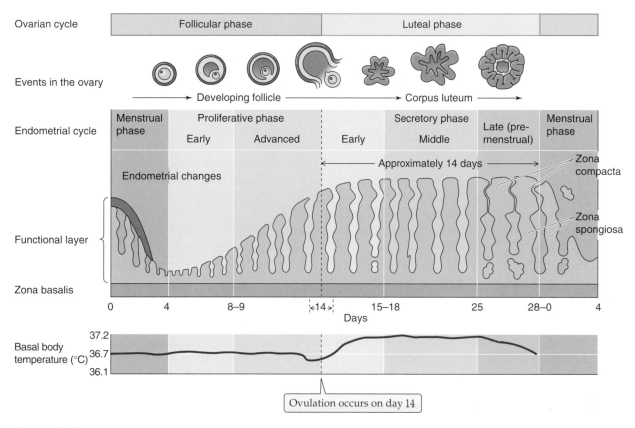

Figure 3.2

The endometrial cycle. The ovarian cycle includes the follicular phase, in which the follicle develops, and the luteal phase, in which the remaining follicular cells develop into the corpus luteum. The endometrial cycle has three phases: the menstrual, the proliferative, and the secretory.

(Boron: Medical Physiology, Updated Edition, 2nd ed. Copyright © 2011 Saunders, An Imprint of Elsevier)

system, ovary and endometrium) is key to the understanding of gynaecological normality and abnormality. It is essential for all doctors to have the capacity to reflect upon this cycle for the woman in front of them and to undertake a tailored history and the appropriate examinations.

Gynaecology history-taking will follow along a similar pathway to any medical history, with the emphasis on specific gynaecological and obstetric conditions and in particular on questioning about the menstrual cycle for post-pubertal women. All relevant subheadings for a medical history will be included, with the order appropriate to the initial presenting issue or problem as summarised in Figure 3.3. Each of the blocks will be utilised for all medical histories, with the blocks shifted depending on the presentation. For a gynaecological history, the importance is placed on the upper blocks, whereas for a medical problem the blocks would be

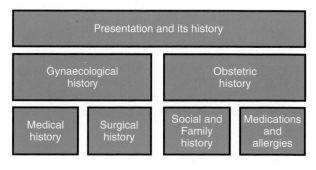

Figure 3.3

Taking a history.

shifted so that gynaecology and obstetrics are less prominent.

The presenting issue

It is imperative that the primary presenting problem be the focus of the consultation and management, since attention to other issues will usually be unsatisfactory for the patient. Occasionally, the presenting issue will not be immediately apparent and only after careful history-taking will the patient's concern become evident. This may be due to sensitive issues — consider the request for termination of pregnancy or discussion of a possible STI — and contrast this with a woman who may have concerns around malignancy and who may not immediately divulge her symptoms. The history should commence with you introducing yourself and asking an open-ended question to give the woman the opportunity to present the information to you. Often you will not need to ask further questions for a few minutes as the patient should be allowed to voice her concerns. Some questions may be required to guide and direct the history. Practising history-taking will refine the skill of judging when to intervene and when to allow the woman to discuss her concerns in her own words.

Since this is the most important issue for the woman, restating the problem as you understand it may help to clarify it for both you and her. Once you have established the primary issue, move methodically through the other components of the history to enlarge the picture. On some occasions, the rest of the history may help to guide further investigations and manage options. Consider how you may take a history in the following common situations:

- a 23-year-old woman presenting for contraceptive advice
- a 46-year-old woman presenting with incontinence whenever she coughs or sneezes
- a 65-year-old woman presenting with vaginal bleeding for the first time in 20 years
- a 28-year-old woman presenting with abdominal pain and vaginal bleeding at 10 weeks of pregnancy by confirmed dates
- a 35-year-old woman presenting with 3 years of primary infertility
- a 24-year-old woman presenting with mid-cycle pain, dysmenorrhoea and pain with intercourse
- a 42-year-old woman with post-coital bleeding who has never had a Pap smear.

Each of these women's concerns are likely to be very different, and the expectations from her health care provider will vary from advice regarding medications, side-effects and reliability of contraceptives to addressing the underlying fear of miscarriage or malignancy. These concerns must be addressed and dealt with in a sensitive manner.

Past gynaecological history

A good gynaecological history starts with a good menstrual history. In the first part of this chapter, the physiology of menstruation was presented in its very scientific form. Understanding the physiology will correlate with an ability to take a good menstrual history and to translate this into practical terms. Knowing that menstruation is due to a decline of progesterone, a rise in prostaglandins and shedding of the endometrium in ischaemic patches, will help to understand the issues of dysmenorrhoea and why non-steroidal anti-inflammatory medications are so helpful in this condition. Recognising the usual range of menstrual cyclicity will aid in understanding of hormonal variations that may lead to subfertility.

In considering the menstrual cycle the following factors will be helpful to note in the history:

1 Menarche
2 Menstrual regularity (cyclicity) and duration. This is frequently annotated to the number of days of bleeding over the number of days in the cycle, so 4–6/28–30 will translate to bleeding for 4–6 days of bleeding with a cycle of 28–30 days. The cycle is counted from the first day of bleeding and finishes on the last non-bleeding day before the next menstrual period.
3 Pain with the cycle. Common types of pain include:
    a dysmenorrhoea (pain with periods)
    b non-menstrual pain (cyclic pain when not having a period)
    c dyspareunia (pain during intercourse)
    d dyschesia (painful bowel motions)
4 Variations in menstruation over time (shortening/lengthening of cycle, or absence of menstruation)
5 Heaviness of menstruation. A useful tip here is to ask the woman how often she changes sanitary protection. Women who change sanitary protection more than 1–2 hourly are likely to be at risk of anaemia, and further investigations are warranted. It is useful to ask women if they change this frequently for hygiene ('I just feel like I need to change') or if sanitary protection is soaked with blood requiring changing — the symptom of flooding describes loss of menstrual fluids over or around sanitary protection and onto clothes, requiring a change of garments. Abnormal uterine bleeding is discussed at length in chapter 18.

6 Associated cyclic symptoms — a change in bladder or bowel function is common with the cycle and is also often prostaglandin-related due to changes in smooth muscle function and action in those organs at the time of menstruation. Cyclic diarrhoea and urinary frequency are not uncommon and may be normal.

Other key areas to cover in the gynaecological history include:

1 A contraceptive history — types, duration of use, reason for stopping (refer to chapter 5)
2 A sexual history — sensitivity and a non-judgmental approach are essential to establish rapport and ensure that you obtain the appropriate and important information.
3 Pap smear and screening history. Consider this an opportunistic time to discuss breast examination and screening as appropriate.

The obstetric history requires a chronological discussion of all pregnancies and their outcomes and whether there is a desire for current or future pregnancy. Again, considerable sensitivity is required, since a history of infertility, recurrent miscarriage and termination often is upsetting for the woman and her support person(s). Is is useful to practise the questions and discussing these issues with colleagues before taking a history in a clinical situation.

The obstetric history is discussed further in chapter 11, but it is always salient to the gynaecological history. For a sound gynaecological history it is imperative to cover issues of perineal trauma at the time of delivery, the type and number of deliveries, postpartum bowel and bladder issues and the desire for further pregnancies.

Other history

The medical, surgical, medication and allergy history are as for any other area of medicine and will not be discussed in detail here. These areas are vital with regards to contribution to gynaecological issues, and may have importance if there is any surgical procedure intended.

A family history is particularly important in obstetrics and gynaecology since heritable disease is a major concern for women planning a pregnancy. It is important to highlight a propensity to malignancy (consider BRCA mutations) or other disease states with known heritable patterns, such as endometriosis.

EXAMINATION

The gynaecological examination requires skill and practice. It is a mainstay of all health practitioners, and every new doctor should be as competent to perform this examination as they would be to examine the heart or limbs.

Examination commences with a general observation of the woman as she walks into the room and during the history, noting posture, gait and use of canes, walking frames or other mobility aids, as well as her affect, interaction with you and with any support persons, and responses to questions. A request for a urine sample will frequently provide useful information. A urinalysis is a mandatory and simple component of the examination and may also be used to exclude pregnancy through a qualitative β hCG.

The physical examination should be undertaken in a private, comfortable area wherever possible. A chaperone may be required. Cultural awareness and sensitivity are required when undertaking a gynaecological examination. Consider the information that you are likely to obtain when performing a gynaecological examination in the middle of a busy emergency department with a curtain drawn around the bed and the woman exposed, often facing into the heavily trafficked area. Moving the woman to a room that can be closed, is warm, and where a door (preferably with a sign signifying 'examination being undertaken: do not enter') will make her more comfortable.

The first place that you touch should not be the genital area. A supine abdominal examination, checking carefully for scars, allodynia (vigorous pain response to light localised pressure), masses and distension is an appropriate first-line step that will aid your examination findings and management.

The genital examination is an integral component of the gynaecological assessment and should be undertaken in every appropriate case. For women who have never been sexually active, you should consider not doing a pelvic examination, referring to someone who has more experience so that it is only done once, or investigating with ultrasound or other modality to complete the examination.

When a vaginal examination is appropriate, and with appropriate consent, chaperone and patient comfort, the woman is best positioned with her legs resting comfortably, allowing adequate access to the genital area but exposed only as needed. A good light source must be immediately available, and all equipment required should be within easy reach during the examination. Discussion of what you are going to do throughout the examination, and interaction with the woman, are essential.

The clinical steps for examination are as follows:

1 The vulva is inspected for irritation, inflammation, lesions, ulcers or discharge. Any prolapse should be noted at this time, and asking the woman to perform a valsalva manoeuvre will help to define any pelvic organ prolapse. Consider the need for vulvovaginal and low vaginal swabs: they should be collected at this time to exclude fungal, bacterial and viral infections as indicated.

2 The vaginal examination commences by inserting one finger only at the skin of the introitus and assessing for both pain and pressure. Ask the patient to both contract and relax her pelvic floor to assess for function in the muscles, her control, and to determine the tone at rest and during a contraction of the pelvic floor. The muscles of the pelvic floor should be gently palpated — they should not be tender — and bony landmarks such as the ischial spine should also be palpated.

3 Palpation of the anterior vaginal wall may elicit tenderness over the urethra and bladder base, indicating possible lower urinary tract infection or other urological issue and directing investigations to this area.

4 The cervix is both palpated and moved, remembering that there is dense innervation of the cervix and too vigorous examination will always be painful. (Note that cervical excitation is a term best avoided since it is non-specific and pain can be induced in many women who have no gynaecological issues.)

5 Supinate the wrist, so that the palm is facing the posterior fourchette, and examine the posterior vaginal wall. Palpate along the uterosacral ligaments for rectovaginal nodularity or localised tenderness that may be indicative of endometriosis. It is rare for malignancy to present with a vaginal mass; however, this may occur. In women with prolapse, bulging pelvic organs may also be felt during this part of the examination.

6 A bimanual examination is performed, as gently as possible, to delineate the surface contour, regularity and size of the uterus and adnexa (if present), determining mobility, eliciting tenderness, and feeling for masses.

7 A speculum examination may be performed if cervical, high vaginal swabs or Pap smear is required. The timing of digital and speculum examinations should be considered. For the woman requiring cervical cytology it is best to take this prior to a digital examination, but for the woman with pelvic pain, a well-performed digital examination is preferred first, since the larger diameter, hard surfaces and the 'foreign' nature of the speculum is more likely to provoke pain and muscle spasms after examination.

8 A rectal examination may be reserved for cases where compressing pathology is suspected or symptoms such as per rectal bleeding are present.

CONCLUSION

The gynaecological basics of history taking and examination are essential components of providing quality clinical care to women. All students should be familiar with both and be able to undertake these in a variety of clinical settings.

FURTHER READING

Diedrich K, Fauser BCJM, Devroey P, et al. The role of the endometrium and embryo in human implantation. Hum Reprod Update 2007;13(4);365–77.

Groome NP, Illingworth PJ, O'Brien M, et al. Measurement of dimeric inhibin B throughout the human menstrual cycle. J Clin Endocrinol Metab 1996;81:1401–5.

Macklon NS, Fauser BCJM. Follicle-stimulating hormone and advanced follicle development in the human. Arch Med Res 2001;32:595–600.

Clifton DK, Steiner RA. Neuroendocrinology of reproduction. In: Straus JF III, Barbieri RL, editors. Yen and Jaffe's Reproductive endocrinology: physiology, pathophysiology, and clinical management. 6th ed. Philadelphia: Saunders; 2009. p. 3–33.

Russell DL, Robker RL. Molecular mechanisms of ovulation: co-ordination through the cumulus complex. Hum Reprod Update 2007;13(3):289–312.

Speroff L, Fritz MA, editors. Clinical gynecologic endocrinology and infertility. Philadelphia: Lippincott, Williams, and Wilkins; 2011.

MCQS

Select the correct answer.

1   A 25-year-old woman presents to you wanting to become pregnant. She has a regular menstrual cycle and asks when ovulation occurs so that she can time intercourse around this. Which of the following combinations of changes best reflects ovulation?

   A   Oestradiol is at its peak, FSH is at its peak, LH has started to rise, progesterone has started to rise.
   B   Oestradiol is at its peak, FSH is declining, LH is at its peak, progesterone is at its peak.
   C   Oestradiol is starting to rise, FSH is at its peak, LH is starting to rise, progesterone is starting to rise.
   D   Oestradiol is at its peak, FSH is at its peak, LH is at its peak, progesterone has started to rise.
   E   Oestradiol is starting to rise, FSH is at its peak, LH is at its peak, progesterone is starting to rise.

2   When pregnancy occurs, the implantation is approximately 4 days after ovulation. Which of the following best describes the physiological events at this time?

   A   The endometrium is thickening under the influence of oestrogen to optimise implantation.
   B   The corpus luteum is producing high levels of progesterone.
   C   The levels of LH are rising to support the pregnancy in its early stages.
   D   Basal body temperature is starting to rise as an indication of implantation.
   E   β hCG secreted from the theca cells maintains support of the corpus luteum.

3   The onset of menstruation is preceded by a number of changes in hormonal function that is followed by endometrial shedding. Which of the following sequential combinations best describes this process?

   A   Leucocytes infiltrate the endometrium, the spiral arterioles contract, the endometrium is shed from fundus to cervix.
   B   Prostaglandin levels rise, inhibin levels rise, FSH levels rise.
   C   Progesterone levels fall, the corpus albicans initiates FSH levels to rise, the endometrium becomes ischaemic.
   D   Matrix metalloproteinases are expressed, FSH levels fall, the endometrial basilis sloughs.
   E   Progesterone levels fall, prostaglandin levels rise, the endometrium is shed in patches.

OSCE

You are teaching a group of first-year medical students how to take a gynaecological history and perform a physical examination. You have 8 minutes to present your mini-tutorial. What are the important areas that you will cover?

Chapter 4

Sexual activity and contraception

Terri Foran

KEY POINTS

The range of contraceptive methods is limited.

Hormonal contraceptives rely on oestrogen and/or progestogen-like activity to interfere with a natural cycle.

Non-hormonal methods of contraception rely on mechanical barriers (such as condoms), prevention of implantation (such as IUDs) or timing (natural family planning) in an attempt to prevent pregnancy.

Permanent male and female contraception involves surgical disruption to the genital system.

No method is 100% reliable.

INTRODUCTION

Humans have long sought to control their fertility, but we have not been particularly effective at this until recently. In 1500 BC, Egyptian physicians recommended the insertion of contraceptive vaginal pessaries made of wool and acacia gum prior to intercourse. Ancient Hebrew texts referred to the use of post-coital douching and contraceptive herbs to ensure that the lesser concubines in the household did not conceive. In a biblical story (Genesis 38), the second son of Judah, Onan, became one of the most famous exponents of the art of coitus interruptus, when he spilt his seed upon the ground in order to avoid impregnating his widowed sister-in-law.

Consider that it has only been since the 1950s, with the development of the oral contraceptive pill and the modern intrauterine device (IUD) that we have had effective forms of fertility control and contraception has moved into the domain of the scientific and medical community. What's more, there is no one ideal method of contraception. A range of different contraceptive devices are displayed in Figure 4.1.

The provision of accurate contraceptive information and advice is critical when assisting couples to make the best choices for their own needs. Consideration should cover such issues as:
- effectiveness of the method
- mode of action
- suitability of that method to the couple's present needs
- risks and benefits
- how the method is used.

If no contraception is used the pregnancy rate per cycle is approximately 15–20%, depending on age of both partners and frequency of intercourse.

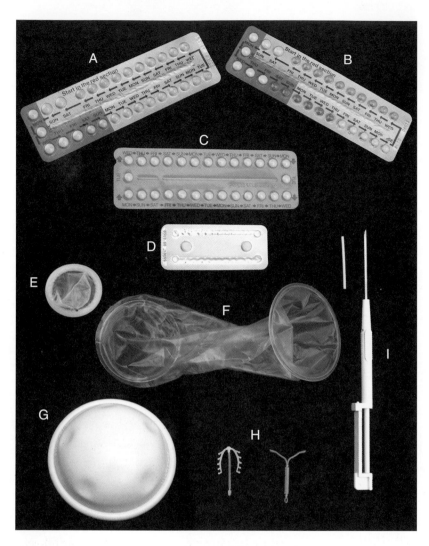

Figure 4.1
Various methods of
contraception: A — monophasic
OCP; B — triphasic OCP;
C — POP (minipill); D —
postcoital contraception;
E — male condom; F — female
condom; G — diaphragm;
H — IUDs; I — Implanon rod
and insertion trocar.

(Photo courtesy Peter Farkas/Royal
Darwin Hospital.)

The 'efficacy' of a contraceptive method refers to its reduction of this monthly probability of conception. The most common way of expressing contraceptive efficacy is the Pearl Index. This figure is determined in contraceptive trials and documents the number of failures per 100 woman-years of exposure (usually based on 1 year of exposure). For example if 100 women used a method of contraception for 5 years and five of them became pregnant, this would give a Pearl Index of 1 per 100 women years for that method. In practical terms this is often quoted as a '99%' efficacy. It is important to recognise that the contraceptive efficacy observed in a clinical trial may not always translate to the real world. This recognition has led to the concept of 'perfect' versus 'typical' use, which can vary greatly depending on the degree of human involvement required. So, when we use contraceptives in the 'real world', our 99% efficacy quoted above may translate to a 92% efficacy in typical use.

HORMONAL CONTRACEPTIVE METHODS
Combined oral contraceptive pill (COCP) — 'The Pill'

The COCP contains both an oestrogen and a progestogen and is taken daily. The progestogen is the primary contraceptive hormone since it effectively suppresses the luteinising hormone (LH) surge and thus prevents ovulation. It also thickens cervical mucus, which impedes sperm penetration and makes the endometrium less suitable for implantation. The oestrogen in the Pill adds to the contraceptive effect by preventing follicular maturation,

---

Box 4.1 Risks and benefits of the combined oral contraceptive pill

Risks

- Adverse side effects from either (or both) active hormones in the preparation
- Increased risk of venous thromboembolism (VTE). This ranges from 2–7 per 10 000 women depending on the preparation and compares to 1 per 10 000 for non-users. (VTE risk during pregnancy/postpartum is 20–30 per 10 000 women)
- Increased risk of stroke — particularly for smokers over 35 years of age and those with pre-existing migraine with aura
- A small increase in breast cancer risk, which returns to background risk by 10 years after cessation of use
- Increased risk of cervical cancer.

Benefits

- Effective reversible contraception
- Positive effects on menstrual cycle and bleeding:
  - Reduction in premenstrual symptoms
  - Less heavy/painful menstrual bleeding
  - Predictable bleeding pattern
  - Control of vasomotor symptoms around menopause
- Fewer functional ovarian cysts
- 50% reduction in the incidence of pelvic inflammatory disease in users
- 50–60% reduction in ovarian and endometrial cancer risk, persisting for at least 10 years.

---

but its main purpose is to stabilise the endometrium so that irregular bleeding occurs less frequently. The COCP has a perfect use efficacy of 99.7% but a typical use efficacy of 92%. The COCP has both risks and benefits for the user, as listed in Box 4.1.

Most of the 'risks' listed in Box 4.1 are related to the oestrogen component. The use of combined contraception is considered an unacceptable risk in women with a number of pre-existing health conditions, such as ischaemic heart disease, previous stroke, VTE, breast cancer, severe liver disease, and migraine with aura. Combined contraception should also not be used by breastfeeding mothers whose infants are less than 6 months of age since it may interfere with the establishment of lactation. The World Health Organization (WHO) e-publishes evidence-based guidelines outlining the eligibility criteria for contraceptive use. The web address is included in your recommended reading material and provides an invaluable guide to the relative and absolute contraindications for all methods, including the COCP.

Types of Pill

COCPs are usually categorised on the basis of their ethinyloestradiol content. Combinations containing 50 micrograms or more are termed 'high dose'. Some newer COCPs contain oestradiol rather than ethinyloestradiol, and for practical purposes these should be regarded as low dose preparations. The qualities and potential side effects of any COCP depend not only on the type and dose of each hormone used in the preparation but also on the relative balance between them. In a 'monophasic' COCP each tablet in the pack has the same dose of oestrogen and progestogen. Other COCPs have variable doses or 'phases' as the user moves through the pack, making the COCP biphasic, triphasic or multiphasic. Box 4.2 lists the common oestrogens and progestogens presently available in contemporary combined Pills.

The choice of oestrogens in Pill preparations is relatively limited and it is largely the progestogen that endows the combination with its particular qualities. Norethisterone-containing Pills, for

Box 4.2 Hormones in oral contraceptive pills

Oestrogens

SYNTHETIC

- Ethinyloestradiol (EE)
- Mestranol (Note: 50 mcg is metabolised to 35 mcg EE)

BIO-IDENTICAL**

- Oestradiol valerate
- Oestradiol

Progestogens

- Norethisterone/Norethisterone acetate* (oldest, introduced 1950s)
- Levonorgestrel
- Desogestrel
- Gestodene
- Cyproterone acetate
- Norgestimate*
- Dienogest
- Drospirenone
- Nomegestrol acetate (most recent)

*Not available in Australia
**'Bio-identical' oestrogens are manufactured, but are identical in chemical structure to those produced by the woman's own ovaries. Although these preparations offer the promise of a lower side effect profile compared with synthetic oestrogens, this will only be determined by post-marketing surveillance.

example, have a particularly suppressive effect on the endometrium, leading to very light or even absent bleeding. Levonorgestrel Pills provide excellent cycle control, but have a slightly higher incidence of side effects such as acne and increased appetite. The newer progestogens (listed below levonorgestrel in Box 4.2) tend to have less effect on mood, appetite and lipid profile, but may confer a slightly higher risk of venous thromboembolism. Cyproterone acetate, dienogest, drospirenone and nomegestrol acetate are specifically anti-androgenic, which may increase their potential for positive effects on skin and excessive hair growth.

In many countries the Pill pack contains only 21 active tablets and the user simply takes a week-long break between packets. In most Australian Pills these active tablets are coupled with seven inactive (placebo) tablets, so that a tablet is taken every day. In some of the newer COCPs the number of active tablets has been increased and there are only 2–4 placebo tablets per month. If a woman starts the COCP with an active tablet on days 1–5 of her menstrual cycle she achieves immediate contraceptive cover. If she starts the COCP later than day 5 she needs additional contraceptive cover (such as a condom or avoidance of penetrative sex) until she has taken seven active tablets. Earlier unprotected sex in that cycle or the prior use of emergency contraception should not preclude a woman starting the COCP, since pre-existing pregnancy can be excluded by means of a urine pregnancy test at the end of the first pill pack. The hormones in the Pill have no adverse effects on such an early pregnancy and should have no bearing on whether the woman decides to continue that pregnancy or not.

During the interval when no active tablets are taken, most women experience menstrual-like bleeding. This is more correctly termed a 'withdrawal bleed', since it is usually shorter and lighter than a natural period. Some women opt not to have a scheduled monthly bleed while taking the COCP. This can be achieved by simply continuing the same dose of active pills for several months at a time. This practice is not dangerous in any way and women may be assured that they are not risking their future fertility with this practice. Such extended cycling is only possible with monophasic Pills, and even then, most women will experience some 'break-through' bleeding over time. Should such bleeding occur for more than 3 days the woman should take a 4-day break from active pills. After the withdrawal bleed that results from that break, it is likely that she can run several more packets together without bleeding. In many parts of the world such extended-use Pills are commercially available, although these are not currently available in Australia.

Missed tablets

If a woman has missed only one tablet, she should simply take it as soon as she remembers (even if it means taking two at once) and can be reassured there is no loss of contraceptive cover. If she has missed two or more tablets (i.e. the last pill was taken more than 48 hours ago), the last two tablets should be taken together — but she must also use additional precautions (condoms or abstinence) for another week in order to maintain her contraceptive cover. The week before the placebo tablet week is a particularly dangerous time to miss tablets, since this effectively extends the time when hormone levels are lowest. Therefore if two or more tablets are missed in the last week of the pack, not only is extra contraceptive cover advised for a week, but the placebo tablets should be skipped and the active tablets continued until the completion of the next pack. Some of the new oestradiol Pills have their own (somewhat complex) missed-tablet advice printed on the packet.

Severe vomiting and diarrhoea can reduce the COCP's absorption and therefore its effectiveness. The efficacy of the COCP can also be affected by a number of drugs that interfere with its hepatic metabolism. These include most of the drugs used to treat epilepsy, tuberculosis, fungal infections and HIV, as well as the herbal antidepressant hypericum (St John's wort). Broad-spectrum antibiotics are no longer believed to affect the COCP's efficacy.

The vaginal ring

The soft, vinyl NuvaRing provides an alternative system for delivering combined hormonal contraception, and has equivalent efficacy to the COCP. The user simply places the 54 mm diameter device within her vagina, and a constant dose of both ethinyloestradiol and etonorgestrel (the systemic equivalent of desogestrel) is delivered to the vessels underlying the vaginal skin. Each ring contains sufficient hormones for 3 weeks' use, after which it is removed for a week before a new ring is inserted. During this 'no-ring' week the woman experiences withdrawal bleeding similar to that which occurs on the COCP. Vaginal hormone delivery offers some advantages over oral since it avoids first-pass metabolism of the hormones by the liver. A daily dose of only 15 mcg EE provides both equivalent contraceptive efficacy to the COCP and excellent cycle control. This low daily hormone dose and the constant delivery system may also result in fewer side effects for the user.

Other combined delivery systems

Contraceptive patches are marketed in some countries. A new patch is applied to the skin every week for 3 weeks. During the fourth week, no patch is applied and the woman experiences a withdrawal bleed before beginning another 3-week cycle. A monthly combined contraceptive injection is also widely used in some countries. Neither of the above methods is presently available in Australia.

Progestogen-only pill (POP) or minipill

Progestogen-only pills contain no oestrogen and only a small dose of progestogen. Their main use in Australia is in women who are breastfeeding since progesterone has no effect on lactation. Women in whom oestrogen is contraindicated may also use this contraceptive. All 28 tablets in available POP formulations in Australia are active (i.e. there are no placebo pills), and contain either 30 mcg levonorgestrel or 350 mcg norethisterone. Both these hormones have variable effects on ovulation and achieve their contraceptive effect primarily through effects on cervical mucus and the endometrium. Maintaining adequate hormone levels is therefore critical for efficacy — if a tablet is taken more than 3 hours late, then additional contraception must be used until two further tablets have been taken. Such strict adherence requirements mean that although the theoretical efficacy of POPs is the same as that of the combined Pill, the typical failure rate tends to be higher. The bleeding pattern is also very unpredictable since there are no scheduled withdrawal bleeds. Some women experience no bleeding at all (most commonly while breastfeeding), while others report almost constant vaginal spotting. An alternative POP containing 75 mcg desogestrel is available in many countries but not currently in Australia. These desogestrel POPs reliably suppress ovulation, making them just as effective as the combined Pill. They also have a 12-hour leeway before additional cover is required.

Injectable progestogen-only contraception

Only one injectable contraceptive method is available in Australia: Depo Provera or depot medroxyprogesterone acetate (DMPA), 150 mg. This formulation provides very effective contraception, with an efficacy of 99.7% in perfect use and 97% in typical use. It is administered by intramuscular injection (into the buttock or upper arm) every 12 weeks (−2 weeks/+4 weeks). A lower dose DMPA injection is available in many countries, although not in Australia. This low-dose formulation contains only 104 mg of DMPA and is delivered by subcutaneous rather than intramuscular injection, allowing users to self-inject after training. DMPA has an identical mode of action to the COCP. It may be a useful option for women in whom oestrogen is contraindicated and for those who have difficulty committing to a daily contraceptive method.

As with all progestogen-only contraceptive methods, irregular bleeding on DMPA is a common problem, although there is a tendency to less bleeding with continuing use. There are presently no evidence-based recommendations for managing this irregular bleeding and an alternative contraceptive method should be considered should it persist. Since there is an average delay of 8 months in the return of ovulation after cessation of DMPA, this method is not really a suitable choice for women planning to achieve a pregnancy in the short term. Weight gain of 2–3 kg is common in the first year of use, possibly because of appetite stimulation. Recent evidence suggests that the relative hypo-oestrogenicity experienced by long-term users of DMPA could adversely affect bone density. The WHO therefore suggests that DMPA use be avoided in those with pre-existing risks for osteoporosis and should be used with care in adolescents and those over 45 years of age. An alternative progestogen injection containing norethisterone enantate is available in some countries though not in Australia. It has similar risks and benefits to DMPA.

Progestogen implants

Only one contraceptive implant, Implanon NXT, is presently available in Australia. This single-rod system releases etonorgestrel over a period of 3 years and is supplied in a pre-loaded inserter. The implant is placed superficially under the skin of the upper, inner, non-dominant arm. Initially 60 mcg of etonorgestrel is released per day but this declines to 30 mcg per day by the third year. The method of action is identical to the COCP but the efficacy is higher, around 99.9%, since user error is virtually eliminated.

In contrast to DMPA, the implant does not completely suppress ovarian follicular activity and oestrogen levels remain adequate for maintenance of bone density. Hormonal side effects such as weight gain, breast tenderness and headache are reported in women using contraceptive implants, but are uncommon due to the relatively low hormone dose released by the implant. However, disruption of the normal menstrual cycle is inevitable, and around 26% of Australian women elect to have the implant removed within 12 months, mainly because of unacceptable bleeding. This can range from amenorrhoea to almost constant light bleeding. By 4–5 months of use, the likely continuing bleeding pattern has usually established and intending users should be encouraged to persist for at least this time. The contraceptive implant may be a useful option in adolescents, who are notoriously poor pill takers, but it is important to recognise they will probably be less tolerant of irregular bleeding.

Implants are rapidly reversible, with most women ovulating within one month of the device being removed.

NON-HORMONAL CONTRACEPTION
Intrauterine devices (IUDs)

There are four types of intrauterine devices:
1 Inert
2 Copper-containing
3 Progesterone-releasing (although this is technically a combined hormonal/non-hormonal method of contraception it is included here for simplicity)
4 Frameless.

Inert IUDs

These plastic or stainless steel devices induce a foreign-body reaction within the uterus that interferes with implantation. They are no longer used in most Western countries since they are associated with a higher rate of menstrual pain and bleeding than the copper or hormone-bearing devices that were developed later. Their main advantage is that they can be left in place indefinitely. They are still widely used in China and Southeast Asia, and some of the more recently developed devices contain anti-inflammatory medications in an attempt to reduce pain and cramping.

Copper IUDs

Adding copper to the plastic backbone enhances the foreign-body effect and permits a significant reduction in the size of the device. Copper ions are also extremely toxic to sperm, preventing fertilisation from occurring in the first place and providing an efficacy of more than 99%. A secondary anti-implantation effect is still utilised when a copper IUD is inserted for emergency contraception. Copper IUDs cause less pain and bleeding than inert devices but there is still an expected 50% increase in menstrual bleeding after insertion. Only two copper IUDs, the Copper-TT380 (effective for 10 years) and the Multiload-Cu375 (effective for 5 years), are available in Australia at present.

Progestogen-releasing IUDs

The plastic backbone of these devices is surrounded by a hormone-containing reservoir that delivers progestogen to the uterine cavity at a constant rate. The progestogen thickens the cervical mucus plug and alters the composition of endometrial fluid, greatly impeding transit of sperm through the uterus. It also thins the endometrium, making it unsuitable for implantation. At 6 months after insertion, approximately 50% of women fitted with a hormonal IUD report no menstrual bleeding, and in almost all wearers bleeding is markedly reduced. Very little of the progestogen finds its way into the general circulation, and systemic side effects are uncommon.

Although a number of progestogen-bearing IUDs are marketed in various countries, only one — Mirena — is available in Australia at the time of writing. This device releases 20 mcg of levonorgestrel daily over 5 years and has a failure rate of approximately 2 in a thousand. Since there is an 80% reduction in menstrual bleeding associated with wearing this device, levonorgestrel IUDs also provide an effective treatment for women with heavy periods (see chapter 18, Abnormal uterine bleeding). They are increasingly used as the progestogen component of hormone replacement therapy for menopausal woman. A smaller 3-year hormonal IUD is also available in some countries, due for release in Australia in 2014.

Frameless IUDs

These devices come in both copper and hormone-releasing varieties but are not presently available in Australia. They dispense with the plastic backbone and instead comprise a series of cylinders strung along a plastic filament, the knotted end of which is embedded within the uterine fundus. These IUDs are said to cause less local discomfort and have a lower rate of expulsion.

Insertion

The insertion of any IUD requires a minor surgical procedure. If care is not taken when placing the device, perforation through the uterine wall may occur, or alternatively the device may be placed too low in the uterus, increasing the risk of expulsion.

A vasovagal reaction as the device is inserted through the cervix may also complicate the insertion procedure. The highest risk of pelvic inflammatory disease (PID) occurs in the first 3 weeks after insertion and then falls to reflect the woman's background risk of sexually transmitted infection. It is however no longer mandatory that the IUD must be removed during treatment for PID, since there is no good evidence that this practice is associated with a better treatment outcome.

Pregnancy

Pregnancy, although rare in IUD users, presents some specific management dilemmas.

If the woman wishes to continue the pregnancy she should be advised that the IUD should be removed as soon as possible, since the enlarging uterus will draw the strings of the device beyond easy reach. Early removal is associated with up to a 30% risk of immediate miscarriage. However, if the IUD is not removed at this early stage, the rate of pregnancy loss increases to 55% and may be further complicated by intrauterine infection. Although copper IUDs do not increase the risk of fetal abnormality, the safety data for hormonal IUDs is currently extremely limited. Last, although the relative risk of ectopic pregnancy is increased in IUD users, this is of little clinical importance since pregnancy prevention of any kind is so high. In other words, a woman has to be pregnant to have an ectopic pregnancy.

Contraindications to IUD use

A complete list of contraindications for IUDs can be accessed through the WHO website referred to earlier in this chapter. The most important contraindications are:

- preexisting pregnancy
- undiagnosed suspicious vaginal bleeding
- cervical cancer awaiting treatment
- endometrial cancer
- marked distortion of the uterine cavity
- current cervicitis or PID.

BARRIER METHODS OF CONTRACEPTION

Barrier contraceptive methods depend on the presence of a physical barrier to prevent fertilisation. Penile sheaths made of linen or sheep intestine were used by the Romans, and in various cultures female barriers have been fashioned from wool, paper, citrus fruits, and even opium resin. Present-day barrier contraceptive methods include condoms and the diaphragm or cap. Condoms have the added benefit of protection against sexually transmitted infections (see chapter 5 for further discussion). They may be used alone or in conjunction with more effective contraceptive methods (such as the COCP) as added protection against STI transmission in addition to pregnancy prevention, a practice known colloquially as 'double-dutching'.

Condoms — male and female

The commonest (and cheapest) condoms are made of latex and come in a variety of shapes and sizes. They are readily available from most pharmacies, supermarkets and vending machines in Australia. Polyurethane male condoms are a more expensive option and may be useful for those with a latex allergy.

Condoms have a perfect efficacy of 98% but this falls to 85% in typical use. For maximal effectiveness the condom should be carefully removed from its cover and applied to the erect penis before there is any genital contact. The rolled edge should be oriented so that it faces upwards, allowing the user to roll the condom smoothly down over the shaft of the penis. If the condom has a teat at the end, this should be pressed together with the fingers just before use so that air is not trapped at the end of the condom. After ejaculation the penis should be withdrawn from the vagina before the erection is lost. The rim of the condom should be held in place at the base of the penis to prevent leakage or slippage. The routine use of a lubricant reduces the risk of friction and condom failure. Only water-based lubricants should be used with latex condoms, since oils may cause the rubber to deteriorate within minutes. Both oil and water-based lubricants are safe to use with polyurethane condoms.

Female condoms can only be purchased in Australia from specialty suppliers or via the internet. Made of polyurethane, they are larger than a male condom and have a flexible ring at each end. The loose ring within the device is used to place the end of the female condom into the upper vagina. The larger, thinner ring at the open end remains outside the vagina during intercourse and partially covers the vulva. Female condoms have a slightly higher failure rate than the male variety, with a typical use efficacy of 80%.

Diaphragms and spermicides

A diaphragm is a dome-shaped cup of silicone attached to a flexible circular spring. Diaphragms must be individually fitted and only a limited number of sizes are now available in Australia. When properly inserted the dome of the device lies in front of the cervix and the vaginal vault, while the spring is held in place by the pelvic muscles. A diaphragm can be inserted any time before intercourse but it must be left in place for at least 6 hours after. Most sperm are prevented from entering the cervical canal and survive only a few hours in the hostile vaginal environment. Although diaphragm efficacy in perfect use is about 94% this falls to 84% in typical use. Spermicides have traditionally been used in conjunction with the diaphragm in an attempt to increase their effectiveness, although there is actually limited evidence for this practice. The efficacy of spermicides when used alone falls to 70%.

Natural family planning

Natural methods of contraception rely on the couple avoiding intercourse during the fertile part of the menstrual cycle. The potential for pregnancy ranges from about 20% for intercourse in the 2–3 days before ovulation to zero in the latter part of the cycle. Various methods have been developed to predict these fertile times.

In the simplest version of the calendar (or 'rhythm') method, day 8 is designated as the beginning if the fertile period and day 19 marks its end. Thus there should be no unprotected sex from day 8 to day 19 inclusive. This calculation is not reliable in women who record two cycles outside the range of 26–32 days in any single year.

The cervical mucus method involves abstaining from intercourse from the time when the typically thin 'fertile' mucus is first noted, and for several days after it disappears. The symptothermal method combines these observations with a daily measurement of basal body temperature, looking for the 0.3°C temperature rise that accompanies ovulation.

If intercourse is reliably avoided at the fertile time, the theoretical efficacy of these methods is high — around 99%. Unfortunately, because these methods are so human-dependent the typical efficacy is significantly lower — more like 75%. In an effort to improve efficacy, hand-held fertility computers have been developed, which detect rising urinary luteinising hormone (LH) from about 6 days before ovulation and build up fertility patterns over time for that woman. Such devices claim an efficacy of 94% in typical use. These devices are not marketed in Australia, but they can be purchased from overseas websites.

EMERGENCY CONTRACEPTION (EC)
Combined emergency contraception
Combined emergency contraception is sometimes called the 'Yuzpe' method after the Canadian gynaecologist who developed it. In the original description, it required that a woman take multiple birth control pills as soon as possible after unprotected intercourse, followed by an identical dose 12 hours later. A minimum of 100 mcg ethinyloestradiol and 0.5 mg of levonorgestrel were required in each dose. This high dose of oestrogen often caused nausea and vomiting for the woman taking it. While this method prevented 75% of expected pregnancies if taken within 3 days, it has largely been superseded by more effective methods.

Progestogen-only EC
This method requires that a single dose of 1.5 mg levonorgestrel be taken as soon as possible after unprotected intercourse. It prevents up to 85% of expected pregnancies and is more effective the earlier it is taken after unprotected sex. Recent studies suggest that this method is markedly less effective when taken more than 4 days after the episode of unprotected intercourse. It is also less effective when taken just before, or right on the day of, ovulation. Progestogen-only EC will not disrupt an established pregnancy, nor have any adverse effects on any pregnancy resulting from its failure. It can be obtained from any pharmacy in Australia without the need of a medical prescription.

Other hormonal methods of emergency contraception
A single 10 mg dose of the selective progesterone receptor modulator mifepristone is used for emergency contraception in some countries, although not Australia. It has few side effects, has a comparable efficacy to progestogen EC, and remains very effective for up to 5 days after unprotected intercourse. Uliprisal acetate 30 mg is a new single-dose progesterone receptor modulator EC that is now widely used in Europe and the United States. It is not only very effective for up to 5 days after unprotected intercourse but also appears to be more effective than progestogen EC when taken immediately prior to ovulation.

Non-hormonal emergency contraception
If a copper IUD is inserted within 5 days of the last unprotected intercourse it acts to prevent implantation and it is an extremely effective method of EC (efficacy 98–99%) up to 5 days after the most likely day of ovulation (i.e. up to day 19 of a 28-day cycle). Hormonal IUDs do not exert their action quickly enough to provide effective emergency contraception and should not be used for this purpose.

PERMANENT CONTRACEPTION
Vasectomy
Vasectomy involves a minor surgical procedure to divide both vas deferens as they transit the scrotum. It has a significantly lower morbidity than female sterilisation and can usually be performed under light sedation. The efficacy is 98.8% provided azoospermia has been established postoperatively. Early complications include pain, bleeding and infection. A small number of men may experience persistent genital discomfort after vasectomy, however this usually settles over time. There is no epidemiological evidence of increased autoimmune disease, atherosclerosis, prostate cancer, impotence or testicular cancer after vasectomy.

While vasectomy reversal is possible, pregnancy cannot be guaranteed even after a successful procedure. Therefore vasectomy should only be performed if the man is convinced that he wants no further children regardless of any future change in circumstances.

Tubal occlusion
Tubal occlusion is a highly effective method of contraception, with a 1 in 200 lifetime failure rate. In Australia it is usually performed laparoscopically, as a day-only procedure. The fallopian tubes are blocked by means of diathermy, clips, rings, or ligation.

As with vasectomy, women undergoing female sterilisation procedures should be carefully counselled regarding the permanence of the method so as to minimise the chances of later regret. The success of reversal varies with the method used, but is around 80% with clips. The critical point is that women should not undergo this procedure while they have any doubts that they have not completed their family.

An alternative to a laparoscopic procedure is transcervical sterilisation via hysteroscopy. This can be performed with IV sedation in an outpatient setting. The procedure involves the insertion of a coiled metal device into the tubes at the point where they enter the uterine cavity; the metal uncoils and the fibres in its core incite a localised inflammatory response. The resulting fibrosis causes complete and permanent closure of the tubes and is extremely difficult to reverse.

TERMINATION OF PREGNANCY

If you are already pregnant, then technically termination of pregnancy is not a method of contraception. It is, however, used as a method of fertility control in many countries.

Termination of pregnancy involves the medical or surgical disruption of a pregnancy after implantation has occurred. There are few topics in medicine that cause so much debate, even leading to the murder of those who perform terminations of pregnancy. Opinions on this topic are polarised, with political, medical, religious, social and economic factions all weighing in on the debate. The discussion (debate, argument or fight — you can insert the most appropriate word) has often centred on the timing of independent life, viability, and conscience of the unborn fetus. Opposing sides quote science, law, religion and morality in their defence of a certain position, and it remains up to the individual to make up their own mind.

In Australia, more than 100 000 terminations of pregnancy are performed every year, and it is estimated that 1 in 4 women will have a termination at some time in her life. Termination of pregnancy is available and legal in this country, although the laws are somewhat complex and vary from state to state. For a full discussion of the laws regarding termination in different states, the reader is directed to: www.racgp.org.au/afp/200611/2006 1103bird.pdf.

Social, economic, medical and psychological factors need to be considered when a request for termination arises. When agreed to, adequate and appropriate counselling prior to the procedure — including a cooling-off period — and a safe and non-threatening environment for the procedure are essential.

The legal implications of termination of pregnancy are important, since in countries where termination is illegal, women simply seek illegal terminations. This may not always be safe. It is important to be aware of the law in your state or territory and to recognise your own responsibilities when advising women around termination or providing services to them when requested.

Surgical termination of pregnancy

Surgical termination of pregnancy can be performed under local anaesthetic, general anaesthetic, or sedation. In Australian termination clinics, 95% of surgical terminations are performed under light intravenous sedation. These agents do not induce complete unconsciousness, but do limit the discomfort and anxiety often associated with termination of pregnancy. Most women undergoing termination of pregnancy under sedation have little recollection of the procedure itself upon recovery.

A number of techniques are used to perform surgical termination of pregnancy.

Vacuum aspiration or curettage

This is the most common method for first-trimester termination of pregnancy in Australia and many other Western countries. The procedure is performed by dilating the cervix with a series of graduated blunt-ended dilators in increments of 1 mm — usually to a dilation of about 6–8 mm — and then the contents of the uterus are evacuated by suction through a small plastic tube inserted into the uterus. This is a simple and safe form of termination. A second instrument called a curette (shaped like a narrow parfait spoon with a sharp edge and no middle) can be used to reach the upper outside areas of the uterus, called the corneal areas, to ensure that the uterus is completely empty.

In pregnancies of 12 weeks or more, a cervical softening agent may be used to aid dilation of the cervix. This may be in the form of a gel or a tablet intravaginally for chemical dilation, or a catheter or a thin wick made from seaweed called laminaria that slowly dilates the cervix, so that a larger suction catheter or instruments may be inserted. As a general rule, the larger the requirement for dilation, the greater the risk of complication. As a guideline, the cervix usually needs to be dilated to the same number of millimetres as the number of weeks pregnancy.

Manual vacuum evacuation

This involves a handheld syringe pump to remove the products and may be undertaken in a patient who has local anaesthesia only. This is a low-tech, low invasive procedure, however it carries a higher chance of patient discomfort and of failure. It is only used for early pregnancies of less than 8 weeks. It is the method most commonly used in the emerging world due to its transportability and low cost, but it is also utilised in Australia for early terminations.

Complications

Complications from an early surgical termination are very rare. Possible vasovagal side effects from parasympathetic stimulation include nausea and vomiting, or hypotension and bradycardia in a severe situation. Other complications included post-procedural bleeding, pelvic infection, anaesthetic issues, and long-term problems such as cervical incompetence (an inability of the cervix to hold a pregnancy, resulting in painless, often midtrimester miscarriages), particularly after repeated late-term terminations. An association between termination of pregnancy and subsequent increased risk of breast cancer, endometriosis and adenomyosis has been hypothesised, but is not established.

Medical termination

Worldwide, the progestogen antagonist mifepristone (RU486) is the agent most commonly used for medical termination. Until 2013 there were fairly restrictive provisions on the prescription of RU486. Since 2013, however, all practitioners who have completed appropriate training may prescribe the drug, which is now listed on the Phamaceutical Benefits Scheme. The recommended dosage regimen varies, with between 200 and 600 mg having reported efficacy with low complications.

Mifepristone is generally used in combination with a prostaglandin such as misoprostol with the woman being involved in the process of administration and completing the miscarriage at home. Using this combination of treatments, 95% will experience a complete termination within a week.

Other medical treatments used for medical termination include methotrexate, either orally or by injection, followed by misoprostol. Methotrexate is an old and inexpensive drug, frequently used for chemotherapy, and may be cheaper and easier to access in many countries than mifepristone. A complete and successful medical termination using this medication generally occurs for 80–85% of women within two weeks of administration.

Medical termination is generally performed at gestations <9 weeks since the failure rate increases with gestational age. Complications and side effects of medications used for termination include nausea, diarrhoea, and unpredictable heavy bleeding. A woman making this choice requires thorough counselling, support, and follow-up in case of complications, as hospital admission for surgical completion or control of bleeding may be required.

Comparative studies of medical versus surgical termination show that medical termination is a safer approach than surgery, even though a small number of women require surgical support through the process. Availability and acceptability varies between areas within a country, and also between countries.

The above discussion relates to early terminations of pregnancy. Later terminations — often for significant fetal abnormality that is demonstrated at midtrimester scanning — may require higher dose medical regimes that will require uterine contractions and expulsion of products just as in labour, or surgical techniques undertaken by skilled specialists within a hospital setting.

FURTHER READING

Guillebaud J. Contraception: your questions answered. 5th ed. London: Churchill Livingstone; 2009. p. 428.

Harvey C, Seib C, Lucke J. Continuation rates and reasons for removal among Implanon users accessing two family planning clinics in Queensland, Australia. Contraception 2009;80(6):527–32.

Piaggio G, Kapp N, von Hertzen H. Effect on pregnancy rates of the delay in the administration of levonorgestrel for emergency contraception: a combined analysis of four WHO trials. Contraception 2011;84(1):35–9.

Read C, McNamee K, Harvey C. An update on contraception. Medicine Today 2009;10(5):46–58.

Richters J, Grulich AE, de Visser RO, et al. Sex in Australia: contraceptive practices among a representative sample of women. Aust N Z J Pub Health 2003;27(2):210–16.

Roumen FJME, Apter D, Mulders TMT, et al. Efficacy, tolerability and acceptability of a novel contraceptive vaginal ring releasing etonogestrel and ethinylestradiol. Hum Reprod 2001;16 (30):469–75.

Sexual Health and Family Planning Australia. Contraception: an Australian clinical practice handbook. 2nd ed. Sexual Health and Family Planning Australia; 2008. Available from State Family Planning websites (e.g. www.fpnsw.org.au).

Trussel J, Vaughan B. Contraceptive failure, method-related discontinuation and resumption of use: results from the 1995 National Survey of Family Growth. Fam Plann Perspect 1999;31(2):64–72.

van Hylckama Vlieg A, Helmerhorst FM, Vandenbroucke JP, et al. The venous thrombotic risk of oral contraceptives, effects of oestrogen dose and progestogen type: results of the MEGA case-control study. BMJ 2009;339:b2921.

World Health Organization. Medical Eligibility Criteria for Contraceptive Use. 4th ed. 2009. Online. www.who.int/reproductivehealth/publications/family_planning/9789241563888/en/index.html; Feb 2011

MCQS

Select the correct answer.

1 Which of the following would be considered an absolute contraindication to the COCP?

   A previous pulmonary embolus
   B migraine without aura in a 30-year-old woman
   C breastfeeding and more than 6 months postpartum
   D past history of cholecystectomy
   E heavy menstrual periods

2 In which of the following methods of contraception is the failure rate with typical use almost identical to that seen with perfect use?

   A the combined oral contraceptive pill
   B the progestogen-only (mini) pill
   C the contraceptive implant — Implanon NXT
   D condoms
   E fertility awareness methods — 'natural family planning'

3 Which of the following contraceptive methods would **not** be recommended for use in mothers who are breastfeeding infants less than 6 months of age?

   A the progestogen-only pill
   B the contraceptive implant — Implanon NXT
   C the vaginal ring
   D the progestogen-bearing IUD
   E depomedroxyprogesterone acetate — DMPA

OSCE

Amanda, a 22-year-old single university student, presents to the Student Health Service complaining of heavier, more painful, menstrual periods over the past 6 months. Amanda has been using condoms for contraception until this time but mentions that she would like to talk about alternative contraceptive methods.

What are the important features on history and examination that would be important in your decision-making? What contraceptive options are available to Amanda and what information would you need to give to her?

Chapter 5

Sexually transmitted infections

Terri Foran

KEY POINTS

Sexually transmitted infections are common.

It is important to note notifiable sexually transmitted infections.

Contact tracing is very important.

Sensitivity is imperative both at diagnosis and throughout management.

Outcomes will depend on the type and possibly severity of infection.

Some sexually transmitted infections may impact fertility.

INTRODUCTION

Sexually transmitted infections (STIs) have been with us as long as sex has. Both the Bible and the Koran contain cautionary tales of terrible plagues and disasters resulting from perceived immorality. Although Christopher Columbus was famously blamed for transporting the 'great pox' (syphilis) from the New World to the Old, the telltale bony lesions of this disease were present in European skeletons long before his journey. Condoms have long been known to reduce the risk of STIs, but no nation has clamoured to claim credit for their invention — in fact, in English they are known colloquially as 'French letters', while on the other side of the Channel, the French refer to them as 'capotes anglaises' — or English hoods!

STIs may present in many ways, but many are asymptomatic. When symptoms are present they may include:

- genital symptoms — discharge, rash, lumps, itching
- general symptoms — rash, fever, skin lesions, lymph node enlargement
- pain on urination
- pelvic pain or pain with intercourse
- irregular vaginal bleeding.

This chapter aims to cover the epidemiology, diagnosis and treatment of the more common STIs.

An important aspect in the effective management of STIs is the need to contact and treat the sexual partner/s of the index case in order to prevent re-infection and further transmission. Some STIs have such profound public health implications that it is a requirement that the infection be reported to the appropriate health authorities — a process known as 'notification'.

PASSENGERS AND PARASITES
Pubic lice

Pubic lice (*Pthirus pubis*) are tiny six-legged insects that most commonly infest the pubic and underarm hair, although they are occasionally seen in the eyebrows and eyelashes. They are usually spread during sexual activity, although transmission is also possible through contact with infested objects such as bed linen, towels or clothes. Pubic lice feed on the blood of their host and the most common symptom is intense itching, which may occur any time up to a month after contact. The diagnosis is made by examining the affected area with a magnifying glass and identifying the adult lice or their eggs (nits).

Treatment

All sexual and household contacts should be notified and treated if necessary. Treatment is usually with an insecticide cream such as permethrin, which may be bought from any pharmacy without a prescription. It should be applied to all coarse-hair-bearing areas from navel to knees, left for 20 minutes, and then washed off. The nits must be carefully removed with a fine comb (the application of vinegar may help) since they are relatively resistant to the insecticide. Petroleum jelly, applied twice a day for 7–10 days, is usually recommended for eyelash and eyebrow infestations. Clothes and bed linen should be washed in hot water and hot tumble-dried. It is not necessary to spray rooms or beds with insecticides since lice can not survive more than 1–2 days off the host. Many authorities recommend repeating the entire process one week after the initial treatment.

Trichomonas

The anaerobic protozoon *Trichomonas vaginalis* is a parasitic STI. Most genital trichomonas infections in males are asymptomatic, though they may cause a non-specific urethritis. Approximately 50% of infected women develop symptoms — typically between 5 and 28 days after transmission. The most common symptom is a malodorous vaginal discharge accompanied by local irritation. In women, identifying the moving protozoa on a freshly prepared light-microscope slide makes the diagnosis, although nucleic acid amplification tests are now available.

Treatment

Trichomoniasis is treated with a single 2 g dose of metronidazole or tinidazole. All sexual partners must be treated concurrently or re-infection will occur.

BACTERIAL SEXUALLY TRANSMITTED INFECTIONS
Chlamydia

The organism that causes this infection, *Chlamydia trachomatis*, must live and grow within the cytoplasm of a host cell in order to transform into its infective form. There are several subtypes that infect humans. Types A–C cause the endemic eye infection trachoma — here the transmission is social rather than sexual. Types D–K are responsible for the common urogenital infections, while types L1 and L3 cause a less common sexually transmitted infection known as lymphogranuloma venereum (LG). Although the incidence of LG is increasing among men who have sex with men in Australia, it remains an extremely rare diagnosis here and therefore will not be covered further.

Urogenital chlamydia is the most common bacterial STI in most industrialised countries, and it is a notifiable disease in all Australian states (Box 5.1). In 2001, there were just over 20 000 chlamydia notifications nation-wide, but by 2008 this figure had nearly tripled. Data suggests that there are probably four or five times more actual chlamydial infections than notifications in Australia, placing the true figure somewhere between 200 000 and 300 000 cases annually.

The risk of chlamydial infection is highest in those under 25 years of age and in those with multiple sexual partners or a recent change of partner. Safer sex may significantly reduce the risk of chlamydia transmission.

Box 5.1 Notifiable sexually transmissible diseases in Australia

- Chlamydia
- Donovanosis
- Gonorrhoea
- Syphilis
- Hepatitis
- HIV

To learn more about STIs and notification go to www.health.gov.au/internet/main/publishing.nsf/content/cda-cdi3502a8.htm

Symptoms and transmission

Urogenital chlamydia is completely asymptomatic in 70–90% of women and perhaps 50% of men. Urogenital chlamydia is completely asymptomatic in as many as 85–90% of those infected. Most of those infected therefore acquire the infection from an asymptomatic partner. Symptoms, when they do occur, usually appear 1–3 weeks after exposure. Urethritis is the most common symptom in males. Women may develop any combination of the following symptoms:

- dysuria
- increased vaginal discharge
- dyspareunia
- post-coital bleeding
- lower abdominal pain.

Untreated chlamydia may lead to pelvic inflammatory disease (PID), ectopic pregnancy and infertility in women, and to chronic epididymitis in males. A rare complication of chlamydial infection, seen more commonly in males, is reactive arthritis. In this condition large-joint arthritis and inflammation of the uvea of the eye accompany the genital symptoms described above. Vertical transmission from mother to infant may also occur during vaginal delivery. Around 25% of infected neonates will present with chlamydial conjunctivitis and 15% will develop respiratory infection.

Investigations

Nucleic acid amplification tests (NAAT) such as polymerase chain reaction (PCR) are now the gold standard for chlamydia diagnosis. These tests are highly specific (99–100%) with a sensitivity of 85–96%. In males a 'first-pass' urine sample (one taken more than 2 hours since the bladder was last emptied) has sensitivity between 90 and 96% and is considered the diagnostic test of choice. A cervical swab provides the most sensitive test in women (85–96%). Urine testing of a first-pass specimen and self-collected vaginal swabs are only slightly less sensitive, however, and since both avoid the need for a speculum examination they are often preferred for screening. In many countries self-testing kits for chlamydia are now made available through pharmacies in an effort to increase the rate of testing. False positives are rare but do occur, particularly in low prevalence populations. Since chlamydia PCR testing has only been validated in urine, cervical and vaginal samples, results from other sites, such as the rectum and pharynx, should always be interpreted with caution. The sexual history may also indicate the need for further STI testing.

Treatment

For uncomplicated infections in both males and females, the recommended treatment is azithromycin 1 g orally as a single dose (use permitted during pregnancy). Doxycycline 100 mg twice a day for 7 days may be used in the rare case of azithromycin allergy, but should not be used in pregnancy. For infections complicated by PID, epididymitis or reactive arthritis, a longer course of antibiotics is required. All current sexual partners of a patient with proven chlamydia should receive standard treatment for chlamydia after appropriate swabs have been obtained, and sexual contact should be avoided for one week after treatment. Patients diagnosed with chlamydia should contact all previous partners over the past 6 months so that they too may seek testing and advice. Although a 'test of cure' is not routinely performed, those who test positive for chlamydia should be advised to have a further test about 2–3 months after treatment since the rate of re-infection may be up to 20%.

Gonorrhoea

The gram-negative diplococcus *Neisseria gonorrhoeae* (NG) is the cause of this infection, which affects mucosal and glandular structures in the genital tract, rectum, oropharynx and conjunctiva. The incubation period is usually 2–7 days but may be longer in some cases. Although the number of notifications is increasing in Australia, gonorrhoea remains relatively uncommon here, except in particular population sub-groups, such as men who have sex with men, and rural and Indigenous communities. In 2010 just over 10 000 Australians were diagnosed with gonorrhoea, a 25% increase from 2009 figures. Safer sex may significantly reduce the risk of gonorrhoea transmission.

Symptoms and transmission

In males, 75% of urethral infections are symptomatic, with the most common symptoms being a purulent urethral discharge and dysuria. Less commonly the infection ascends to the epididymis, testes or prostate gland, causing scrotal pain and swelling. However, in 60% of women gonorrhoea is silent or minimally symptomatic, and it may only be diagnosed if a male partner develops symptoms. The remaining 40% most commonly present with dyspareunia, irregular bleeding or a change in their vaginal discharge. Less commonly a woman may present with a secondary Bartholin's abscess. Ascending infection may lead to PID, tubal factor infertility, ectopic pregnancy and chronic pelvic pain.

Depending on sexual practices, gonorrhoea may also infect the anus and throat. Most infections in these sites are asymptomatic, although patients will occasionally present with rectal discharge/bleeding/pain or with pharyngitis as their primary symptom. Gonococcal conjunctivitis, through autotransmission via the fingers, may also occur, and is usually unilateral. Disseminated infection follows approximately 1–3% of anogenital gonococcal infections. Such patients are often extremely unwell, with symptoms of rash, fever, arthralgia, reactive arthritis, septic arthritis, tendonitis, endocarditis, or meningitis. More rarely, right upper quadrant pain from peri-hepatitis (the 'Fitz-Hugh–Curtis syndrome'), which may cause altered liver function tests, may occur following the spread of organisms upwards along peritoneal planes. Infants may also be infected with gonorrhoea during delivery and may develop conjunctivitis (ophthalmia neonatorum) or less commonly a pharyngeal infection.

Investigations

The diagnosis of gonorrhoea is confirmed by demonstrating the presence of the organism on microscopy and culture. The sexual history should guide the sites from which swabs are taken. Whenever gonorrhoea is suspected the specimens should be transported promptly to the pathology laboratory, since the organism is quite fragile. PCR testing for gonorrhoea is available and is usually performed at the same time as culture, since it provides a much more rapid result. Unfortunately PCR testing does not provide antibiotic sensitivities — an important consideration in a world where multi-resistant gonorrhoea is common.

Treatment

For many years penicillin was the mainstay for gonorrhoea treatment, but resistance to penicillin and other antibiotics is an increasing problem. By 2007 more than half of the gonorrhoea diagnosed in Australian capital cities was penicillin resistant. Throughout the early 2000s oral ciprofloxacin in a single dose of 500 mg was used to treat penicillin-resistant gonorrhoea, and this is still used in some countries/populations. However, with resistance to ciprofloxacin emerging over the last 10 years, a single dose of intramuscular ceftriaxone has become the antibiotic of choice in much of urban Australia. The injection usually incorporates a small amount of local anaesthetic to reduce discomfort. After treatment, patients are advised to abstain from intercourse for a week. The standard Australian dose of ceftriaxone is now 500 mg due to an increasing number of treatment failures. Some NG strains require even higher doses, and unfortunately if this pattern of resistance continues we could be facing the prospect of 'incurable' gonorrhoea within 10 years. Gonorrhoea is a notifiable disease in Australia (see Box 5.1), and contact tracing and treatment of partners is essential. Since the rate of co-infection with chlamydia is high, all patients with suspected gonorrhoea should be treated concurrently for this STI.

Syphilis

Syphilis is caused by the spirochaete *Treponema pallidum*, a corkscrew-shaped bacterium. The Italian physician Girolamo Fracastoro both named the disease and blamed it on the French in a poem published in 1530. However, for centuries, the disease was more commonly called the 'great pox', or simply the 'pox', to distinguish it from gonorrhoea and smallpox.

Until the 1990s, rates of syphilis infection were relatively low in Australia, with the exception of the Indigenous community and those born overseas. An increase in syphilis infections in men who have sex with men saw rates peak in 2007 at 12.1 per 100 000. Since that time notification rates have slowly declined, and by 2010 the figures were 8.9 per 100 000.

Transmission

Syphilis is most commonly spread through sexual contact. Occasionally non-sexual transmission occurs through blood transfusion, or by inoculation (needlestick/scalpel) with material from infected lesions. Syphilis may also spread to the fetus through transplacental transmission from an infected mother.

Routine antenatal screening for syphilis is carried out in Australia despite the low overall incidence since the implications for the infant are dire: if an infected woman is not treated, there is a 40% chance of prematurity and perinatal death. Two-thirds of the surviving infants will be infected with the disease and, of those, 12% will not survive, even with treatment.

Symptoms

The course of an untreated syphilis infection is characterised by a number of different phases, each with its own distinctive set of signs and symptoms.

About 3 weeks after infection, a painless, rubbery, ulcer (chancre) develops at the site of inoculation. This finding is the hallmark of primary syphilis, but if the chancre is located in the vagina, pharynx or anus, it may not be detected by either patient or clinician. The chancre heals completely within weeks, but over the next few months the patient moves into the secondary and most infectious phase of the infection.

The characteristic sign of secondary syphilis is a generalised coppery, maculopapular rash on the face, palms and soles. Other signs include condylomata lata (perianal wart-like growths), patchy hair loss, and painless mouth ulcers that resemble snail tracks. Eventually these too will resolve, and if the infection remains undiagnosed the patient moves into the third phase — latent syphilis.

Patients with latent syphilis may remain asymptomatic for several years, but at a variable time between 3 and 30 years after the initial infection, the effect of multiple organ damage usually becomes apparent. Necrotic inflammatory lesions or 'gummas' that appear in the skin and bone characterise the last phase: tertiary syphilis. Cardiovascular and neurological damage are also common in the final stages of the disease, and in pre-penicillin days these were the major causes of death in these patients.

Diagnosis

Though it is possible to detect spirochaetes using specific microscopic techniques (dark-ground microscopy), a more common practice is to send a specimen from a suspected primary chancre for PCR testing. However, serology remains the mainstay of syphilis diagnosis and management. Treponema-specific enzyme immunc assays (such as Treponemal IgG EIA) have largely replaced non-specific tests for screening. Other treponemal-specific tests may be performed after a positive EIA test to improve the specificity. These include the *Treponema pallidum* particle/haem agglutination (TPPA/TPHA) tests and the fluorescent treponemal antibody absorption (FTA-Abs) tests.

All the treponemal-specific tests remain positive after successful treatment, rendering them useless as a test-of-cure. Other serological tests are therefore required to correctly stage and treat the infection, and it follows that correct interpretation of these tests is dependent on an accurate history of past syphilis infection and treatment. The most commonly used of these tests in Australia is the rapid plasma reagin (RPR) test. This result is reported as a numerical titre, the level of which may be used to indicate both disease activity and response to treatment. Biological false-positives may occur in all the above serological tests.

Treatment

T. pallidum remains exquisitely sensitive to penicillin. Parenteral penicillin is therefore the treatment of choice, with the dose and duration of treatment dependent on the stage of the infection. High-dose doxycycline may be used in those with penicillin sensitivity, except during pregnancy.

VIRAL SEXUALLY TRANSMITTED INFECTIONS

Human papilloma virus (HPV)

Human papilloma virus (HPV) is a double-stranded DNA virus belonging to the family Papillomaviridae. It has an infective inner core surrounded by an outer layer that protects it from its host's immune system attack. Over 200 HPV sub-types are known to infect humans, and about 40 of these are associated with anogenital infection. Nearly 80% of sexually active adults will have been exposed to at least one of the anogenital strains, although most such infections are subclinical and therefore unrecognised. HPV is highly infective, with a 50–80% transmission rate through a single episode of unprotected sexual contact with an infected partner. Condom use reduces the risk of transmission but does not offer complete protection, since the area of viral infection often extends beyond the area covered by a condom.

Clinical HPV

Some HPV subtypes stimulate a local epithelial reaction, which results in a visible papilloma or wart. Genital warts may be single or multiple, and vary greatly in size and colour. Immunosuppression and pregnancy are often associated with persistent, larger and more numerous warts. HPV subtypes 6 and 11 cause 90% of clinical warts in the genital area. These sub-types almost always regress sponta-neously over time and are not associated with neo-plastic change. Treatment of clinical papillomata is usually undertaken for cosmetic reasons, although occasionally they may itch or bleed. Medical therapies include the local application of podophyl-lotoxin, 5-fluorouracil, imiquimod (all contraindi-cated during pregnancy), and trichloroacetic acid. Physical destruction of the warts is also an option. Cryotherapy the most common technique used in Australia, but cautery, laser and excision are also employed, depending on the site and number of lesions. Regardless of the treatment modality, recur-rence rates are high, particularly in the first 3–6 months following treatment.

Subclinical HPV

Some human HPV subtypes are associated with an 'oncogenic' or cancer-inducing potential in the tissues they infect. Types 16 and 18 are responsible for approximately 70% of all cervical, vulval, penile and anal squamous intraepithelial neoplasia, and are an increasing cause of pharyngeal cancer in males. The diagnosis and management of genital intraepi-thelial neoplasia will be covered more fully in chapter 24 in this text.

Genital herpes simplex virus — HSV

Genital herpes infection may result from infection with either HSV-1 (more typically associated with orolabial symptoms) or HSV-2. It is impossible to distinguish HSV-1 from HSV-2 on clinical appear-ance alone. Transmission occurs through genital and orogenital sexual contact. HSV-2 continues to be the most common cause of recurrent genital herpes in Australia. Seroprevalence studies indicate that approximately 8% of men and 16% of women in this country have prior exposure to HSV-2. However, in the last 30 years there has been a sub-stantive increase in genital HSV-1 infections. HSV-1 was responsible for 15.8% of the genital herpes in the patients attending one Melbourne sexual health clinic in 1980, but by 2003 this had increased to 34.9%. This shift in epidemiology was particularly noticeable in younger patients, with 77.3% of genital herpes lesions in those under 20 years attrib-utable to HSV-1.

Symptoms and transmission

Genital herpes is classically described as multiple small blisters that then break down to form shallow ulcers. These ulcers may be acutely painful, particu-larly during the primary episode, which may last up to 4 weeks if not treated. In women the associated dysuria may be so severe that it leads to urinary retention, requiring hospital admission and cathe-terisation. Local lymphadenopathy is common. Sys-temic symptoms during the primary episode include fever, myalgia and, rarely, meningitis. Not everyone experiences a classic primary herpes attack, with cross-sectional studies suggesting that up to 75% of individuals infected have variable periods of latency before clinical symptoms occur. Of those infected with HSV, 90% subsequently shed the virus from the original infection site. This may manifest as recurrent clinical symptoms, although these are usually less frequent and less severe as time passes. Alternatively, the person may remain asymptomatic but still shed the virus intermittently. Unfortunately transmission of the virus to a sexual partner is still possible as a result of such asymptomatic shedding, and around 70% of HSV infections are acquired in this way. Vertical transmission is also an issue, and a woman who is unaware she carries the virus may unwittingly transmit the infection to her newborn. In those with a history of recurrent genital HSV, many obstetricians now recommend the use of HSV-suppressive drugs during the last trimester to reduce the risk of viral shedding at delivery. Because of the risk of herpes encephalopathy, caesarean deliv-ery is usually indicated in women with active HSV infection close to term. However, the highest risk of vertical transmission occurs when a mother acquires her primary herpes infection during pregnancy, par-ticularly when this occurs during the last trimester.

Diagnosis

A polymerase chain reaction (PCR) test performed on swabs from the base of a suspected HSV ulcer has an extremely high sensitivity and may also deter-mine whether the virus responsible is type 1 or type 2. In recurrent attacks, the virus sheds for only a short time and false-negative tests may occur unless the specimen is obtained immediately after symp-toms occur. Self-collected swabs may be very useful in cases where the clinical picture suggests HSV but the diagnosis remains unconfirmed.

Treatment

Drug treatment varies according to whether the infection is primary or recurrent. For a primary infection, acyclovir 200 mg is given five times daily or 400 mg 8-hourly for 5–10 days. Alternatively, valaciclovir 500 mg may be given 12-hourly for 5–10 days. Frequent recurrences may be managed with suppressive regimens of acyclovir 200 mg 8-hourly or 400 mg 12-hourly, valaciclovir 500 mg daily or famciclovir 250 mg 12-hourly. Suppressive therapy reduces both the frequency of attacks and viral shedding. Most authorities recommend a break from treatment every 12 months to assess whether it is still required. For those with less frequent attacks, episodic therapy may be useful. At the first sign of likely symptoms, the patient may commence 2–5 days of therapy, which has been shown to significantly reduce the duration and severity of the attack. Topical lignocaine 5% ointment may also be useful for pain management.

Molluscum contagiosum

Molluscum contagiosum is a pox virus. Infection causes small dome-shaped skin lesions with a typical central indentation. The average incubation period is 2–7 weeks. Transmission in adults is usually sexual, and the lesions are typically clustered around the genital area, lower abdomen and buttocks. Individual molluscum lesions usually resolve without treatment within 2–3 months. However, a high rate of autoinoculation usually means that infections last somewhat longer than this, and it is important then that the lesions not be scratched or shaved in order to limit their spread. This infection responds well to most of the treatments used for genital warts — cryotherapy, podophyllotoxin, imiquimod, and laser.

Hepatitis

The term 'hepatitis' covers a range of non-related viruses (A to E) that infect the liver, leading in some cases to chronic carriage of the virus and significant liver damage. Hepatitis D and E are extremely rare in Australia and will not be covered further.

Hepatitis A (HAV)

Hepatitis A is a piconovirus mainly transmitted by means of contaminated food and water. It may potentially also be sexually transmitted through oro-anal sex or through careless hand hygiene when handling condoms after penetrative anal sex with an infected person. HAV has a mean incubation period of 28 days, and symptoms include nausea, malaise, fever, right upper quadrant pain and jaundice. An effective vaccination is available and should be recommended to high-risk groups and to those recently

exposed to the virus. Human immunoglobulin may also be offered as post-exposure prophylaxis.

Hepatitis B (HBV)

This DNA virus has an inner infective core surrounded by a protective outer capsule. It may be transmitted through blood (IV drug use, contaminated medical equipment), as a sexually transmitted infection, or vertically from mother to child at delivery. The symptom severity and the incubation period of HBV are both extremely variable. A number of serum immune markers allow for categorisation of HBV status. These are outlined in Box 5.2.

Chronic hepatitis B infects over 400 million people worldwide and is responsible for over 1 million deaths annually. Any pregnant woman who is HBsAg positive should have her liver function checked. Her partner/s and any other children should be screened for infection, and vaccinated if they are not already infected. An effective HBV vaccine (which utilises virus-like particles) is now part of the routine infant immunisation schedule in Australia. At-risk newborns are also given passive immunisation following delivery to prevent early transmission.

Hepatitis C (HCV)

This single-stranded flavivirus is most commonly transmitted through IV drug use, although sexually transmitted infection is possible in sexual practices where mucosal trauma or bleeding occurs. Perinatal transmission occurs in approximately 5% of deliveries in Australia; however, routine antenatal screening for HCV remains controversial. Although the acute illness is usually mild, the rate of chronic infection with HCV may be as high as 85%. Around 10–20% of those infected will eventually develop cirrhosis (mean 30 years), and 1–5% will die of hepatocellular carcinoma. In 2009, around 291 000 Australians were estimated to have been infected with HCV, of whom around 217 000 (75%) were living with chronic hepatitis C. There is no vaccine for HCV, and public health messages remain the major prevention strategy. Patients with abnormal liver function tests are usually treated with antiviral drugs.

Human immunodeficiency virus

The human immunodeficiency virus (HIV) is a retrovirus seen in the blood, vaginal fluids and semen of infected people. HIV infects cells vital to the

---

Box 5.2 Serological markers for hepatitis B

HB surface antibody

Present in both immune and immunised individuals since the immunisation contains viral-like particles that replicate the virus's outer capsule.

HB core antibody

Only seen following natural infection.

HB surface antigen

Indicates the presence of the virus. When it persists in the serum for more than 6 months the person is said to be a carrier. This occurs in about 5% of those infected as adults but in about 90% of those infected as infants. Carriers are at risk of chronic liver failure, cirrhosis and liver cancer, and may require treatment with interferon and other drugs designed to reduce viral replication. Carriers may also potentially infect sexual partners and household contacts.

HBe antigen

The presence of this marker indicates a highly infectious carrier.

---

maintenance of the immune system, notably helper T lymphocytes (CD4 cells) and, to a lesser extent, macrophages and dendritic cells. The decline of infected CD4 cells is accelerated since other lymphocytes are recruited by the immune system to destroy them. Once the CD4 cell count falls below a critical level (around 350 per microlitre), cell-mediated immunity is severely compromised and the patient becomes progressively more susceptible to opportunistic infections. The term AIDS, which stands for 'acquired immune deficiency syndrome', is reserved for those with advanced immunodeficiency, opportunistic infections, and/or malignancies such as Kaposi's sarcoma.

Transmission

HIV may be transmitted during sex, through needle sharing, through contaminated blood products, and by vertical transmission during childbirth or breast-feeding. In Australia HIV infection occurs most commonly in men who have sex with men. In 2009 there were, however, 2301 women living with HIV in Australia, representing about 7% of the total number of cases in this country. Thankfully the spread of HIV in the Australian IV drug-using population has largely been contained through easy access to clean injecting equipment. Very occasionally healthcare workers are infected through occupational exposure.

Symptoms

Approximately 50% of those infected with HIV experience a seroconversion illness between 2–4 weeks post transmission. The clinical symptoms are similar to infectious mononucleosis, with headaches, fever, nausea, myalgia, swollen glands, mouth ulcers, and a maculopapular rash common. These early symptoms resolve over 2–3 months, and a variable dormant phase follows. Once the immune system is compromised a wide range of clinical symptoms may follow, including generalised lymphadenopathy, fever, weight loss, chronic diarrhoea, anaemia, oral thrush, and recurrent shingles. Most Australian patients are diagnosed during this phase of the illness, and respond extremely well to treatment. Unfortunately, a small number of those infected in this country still present with an AIDS-defining illness as the first sign of a previously undiagnosed HIV infection.

Investigations and treatment

The diagnosis of HIV is made by means of testing for HIV antibodies in the serum. These are detectable 2–3 months after infection and remain positive for life. Seroconversion may take longer if the person had been treated with post-exposure medications, such as following an occupational needlestick injury. Informed consent, by means of pre-test counselling, should always occur before HIV testing is performed. Although definitive HIV testing is currently performed in reference laboratories in Australia, point-of-care tests have recently become available. While not as accurate as laboratory testing, these new tests offer the advantage of an almost instant answer, particularly where infection is strongly suspected. Confirmatory testing may then proceed while support and referral of the patient is undertaken.

Confidentiality and privacy issues remain important, as there is still a degree of stigma attached to the diagnosis of HIV. A positive result may also have profound implications with regard to overseas travel, employment options, and life insurance. All current and past partners who may be at risk of HIV must be identified and contacted.

A rising viral load and falling CD4 count indicates progression of the infection, in which case antiretroviral therapy may be initiated. At least three agents are now used to ensure adequate potency of the regimen. The field of HIV therapy is a rapidly evolving one, and management usually requires a team approach involving both specialist and general practice care.

Antenatal screening for HIV

Australian authorities recommend that screening should be offered to all pregnant women in this country after appropriate counselling. Ideally the HIV-positive pregnant woman should be co-managed by an infectious diseases specialist and should continue on her usual antiretroviral therapy (excluding the drug efavirenz, which may be teratogenic). The aim is to achieve an undetectable viral load, since a higher viral load increases the risk of vertical transmission. The use of combination antiretrovirals, elective caesarean delivery and the avoidance of breastfeeding in any woman known to be HIV positive has reduced fetal transmission in developed countries to less than 2%. Even in developing countries, a short course of the single agent AZT in late pregnancy has dramatically decreased maternal–infant transmission.

FURTHER READING

AVERT. Australian HIV and AIDs Statistics. Online. Available: www.avert.org/aids-hiv-australia.htm. December 2011.

Cook RL, Hutchison SL, Ostergaard L, et al. Systematic review: noninvasive testing for Chlamydia trachomatis and Neisseria gonorrhoeae. Ann Intern Med 2005;142:914–25.

Cunningham AL, Taylor R, Taylor J, et al. Prevalence of infection with herpes simplex virus types 1 and 2 in Australia: a nationwide population based survey. Sex Transm Infect 2006;82:164–8.

Department of Health and Ageing. Notifiable diseases sexually transmissible. Online. Available: www.health.gov.au/internet/main/publishing.nsf/content/cda-cdi3502a8.htm.

Fairley CK, Gurrin L, Walker J, et al. 'Doctor, how long has my chlamydia been there? Answer — Years.' Sexually Transm Dis 2007;34(9):727–8.

National Centre in HIV Epidemiology and Clinical Research. HIV/AIDS, viral hepatitis and sexually transmissible infections in Australia. Annual Surveillance Report. National Centre in HIV Epidemiology and Clinical Research 2010;128. Online. Available: www.nchecr.unsw.edu.au/NCHECRweb.nsf/resources/SurvRep07/$file/ASR2010-rev1.pdf. 28 Jan 2011.

Hosenfeld CB, Workowski KA, Berman S, et al. Repeat infection with Chlamydia and Gonorrhea among females: a systematic review of the literature. Sex Transm Dis 2009;36:478–89.

Johnson VJ. The management of sexually transmitted infections by Australian general practitioners. Sex Transm Inf 2004;80:212–15.

Kirby Institute. HIV, viral hepatitis and sexually transmissible infections in Australia. Annual Surveillance Report 2011. Online. Available: www.med.unsw.edu.au/NCHECRweb.nsf/resources/2011/$file/KIRBY_ASR2011.pdf. Dec 2011.

Peeling RW, Ye H. Diagnostic tools for preventing and managing maternal and congenital syphilis: an overview. Bull World Health Organ 2004;82:439–46.

Russell D, Bradford D, Fairley C, editors. Sexual health medicine. 2nd ed. Melbourne: IP Communications; 2011.

Sexual Health Society of Victoria. National management guidelines for sexually transmissible infections. 7th ed. Victoria: Sexual Health Society of Victoria; 2008. Online. Available: http://mshc.org.au/Portals/6/NMGFSTI.pdf.

World Health Organization. Sexually transmitted and other reproductive tract infections: a guide to essential practice. Online. Available: www.who.int/reproductivehealth/publications/rtis/9241592656/en/index.html.

MCQS

Select the correct answer.

1   Which of the following sexually transmitted infections may lead to infertility if untreated?

   A   syphilis
   B   genital herpes
   C   HIV
   D   trichomoniasis
   E   gonorrhoea

2   A 24-year-old single mother screens positive for *Chlamydia* at her first antenatal visit in her second pregnancy. Which one of the following would **not** be considered appropriate management?

   A   abstinence from intercourse for one week after antibiotic treatment is completed
   B   notification and treatment of all sexual partners in the past 6 months
   C   rescreening for *Chlamydia* 2 months later
   D   treatment with doxycycline 100 mg BD for 7 days
   E   advice about safer sex in order to prevent re-infection

3   Which of the following statements is true with regard to hepatitis B?

   A   It is a double-stranded flavivirus.
   B   Hepatitis B vaccine contains live attenuated virus.
   C   Chronic carriage is more common when infection occurs during childhood.
   D   The persistent presence of hepatitis B surface antibody indicates carrier status.
   E   Vertical transmission occurs most commonly through the transplacental route.

OSCE

You are working in a sexual health clinic in an Australian capital city where Sarah, a 20-year-old sales assistant, attends with a history of intermittent vaginal bleeding after sex for the past month.

What are the important points on history, examination and investigation for Sarah?

Chapter 6

Fertility

Neil Johnson and Elizabeth Glanville

KEY POINTS

The average monthly chance of conceiving in normal fertile couples is 20%.

Within 12 months, in a woman under the age of 35, the chance of conception is more than 80%.

The key processes to achieve a pregnancy include ovulation, normal spermatogenesis, fertilisation of the egg, and implantation of the embryo.

When attempting pregnancy women should be advised to take folic acid and iodine supplementation.

NATURAL FERTILITY, THE FERTILE PHASE OF THE CYCLE AND SEXUAL FUNCTION

Fecundity is the capacity to conceive and is measured as the monthly probability of conception. The average monthly chance of conceiving in normal fertile couples is only 20%, but it is higher in the first 3 months of trying to conceive. Within 12 months, the natural rate of conception in a woman under the age of 35 years is more than 80%. During the next 36 months, 50% of the remaining couples will conceive spontaneously. In each subsequent year, the chance of success declines.

The ability to become pregnant naturally depends not only on ovulation, sperm production, fertilisation and implantation, but crucially on the ability of the couple to have sexual intercourse at the key time of the cycle.

Some, but not all, ovulatory women experience a mid-cycle mucus change. The high levels of oestrogen towards the latter part of the follicular phase of the cycle are reflected in their vaginal secretions, which may become more copious, watery and 'stretchy'. 'Preovulatory mucus' is often said to resemble egg white. Such cervical mucus changes typically last 1–3 days, and the time of maximal mucus change is usually considered a woman's most fertile time of the cycle. Women who do not recognise mucus changes may be able to calculate when they are likely to ovulate, based on the observation that the luteal phase of the cycle is of consistent length, typically 13–14 days — thus ovulation is anticipated 13–14 days before their expected next menstrual period. Some couples find ovulation test kits that detect the LH hormone surge in a urinary sample helpful towards their timing of sexual activity.

The most fertile approach is for couples to have sex approximately daily for 5 days prior to, and including, the day of ovulation. The rationale for this is the short survival of the egg after ovulation, the recognition that sperm may survive a number of days in the female genital tract, and the improvement in sperm quality (with reduced sperm DNA damage) seen with frequent (daily) ejaculation. Alternate-day sexual activity in this fertile phase is almost as effective and may be more attainable by couples, within the constraints of busy lifestyles and the stress associated with the need to have very frequent sex.

It is important to acknowledge that sexual dysfunction, to a greater or lesser extent, is a normal accompaniment to fertility problems for all couples. It is important to give couples the chance to ask questions about this, and it is reassuring to them to understand that this is a very common experience.

LIFESTYLE FACTORS

Understanding of the importance of lifestyle factors, and their impact on both female and male reproductive health, is emerging.[1] Couples maximise their fertility chances by not smoking, minimising or abstaining from alcohol, abstaining from recreational drugs, maintaining an ideal body weight, maintaining healthy (but not unduly excessive) exercise levels, eating a healthy diet, and minimising caffeine consumption to two or fewer cups of coffee (or its equivalent) per day.

Women must also be advised of the need to take folic acid and iodine supplementation when attempting pregnancy. Folic acid is not known to improve fertility, but it lowers the chance of neural tube defects in offspring when taken before conception and in early pregnancy. Iodine supplementation minimises the risk of subclinical hypothyroidism, which has been associated with a lower intellectual quotient (IQ) in the offspring.

OVULATION

The hypothalamic–pituitary–ovarian axis regulates follicular development and steroidogenesis in the ovary (Figure 6.1). At the beginning of each menstrual cycle, low levels of oestrogen allow release of gonadotrophin-releasing hormone (GnRH) from the hypothalamus. The pulsatile release of GnRH stimulates the anterior pituitary gland to release gonadotrophins: follicle-stimulating hormone (FSH) and luteinising hormone (LH). FSH and LH act on the ovary to initiate recruitment and growth of several follicles, each containing an ovum. The follicles will produce oestradiol, which has a negative feedback effect on the pituitary gland, leading to reduction in the release of gonadotrophins. Usually only one dominant follicle will continue to grow, through acquisition of unique FSH receptors that the non-dominant follicles do not possess, and it

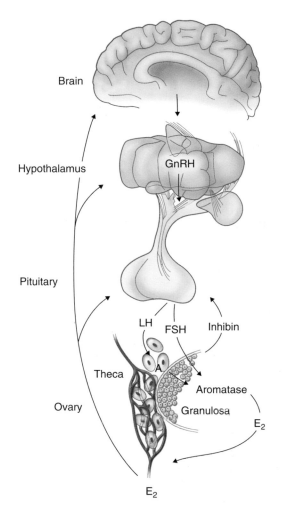

Figure 6.1
The hypothalamic–pituitary–ovarian axis in the regulation of follicular maturation and steroidogenesis. A = androgens, E2 = oestradiol, FSH = follicle-stimulating hormone, GnRH = gonadotrophin-releasing hormone, LH = luteinising hormone.

(Goldman: Goldman's Cecil Medicine 24e; 2011 Saunders; FIGURE 244-2 The hypothalamic-pituitary-ovarian axis in the regulation of follicular maturation and steroidogenesis. A = androgens; E2 = estradiol; FSH = follicle-stimulating hormone; GnRH = gonadotropin-releasing hormone; LH = lutenizing hormone. Modified from Endocrine and Metabolism Continuing Education Quality Control Program, 1982. Copyright American Asociation for Clinical Chemistry, Inc.)

will produce a mature oocyte for release. This follicle produces increasing levels of oestradiol, and these high levels result in a switch to a positive feedback effect on the pituitary, which responds by producing high levels of LH and FSH. The surge

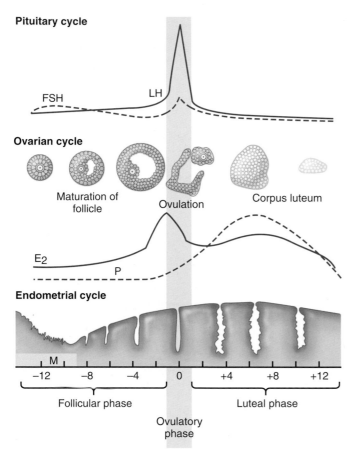

Pituitary cycle

FSH   LH

Ovarian cycle

Maturation of
follicle   Ovulation   Corpus luteum

E₂

P

Endometrial cycle

M

−12   −8   −4   0   +4   +8   +12

Follicular phase   Luteal phase

Ovulatory
phase

Figure 6.2
The menstrual cycle showing hormonal, ovarian and endometrial changes.

(Goldman: Goldman's Cecil Medicine 24e; 2011 Saunders; FIGURE 244-1 The idealized cyclic changes observed in gonadotropins, estradiol (E2), progesterone (P), and uterine endometrium during the normal menstrual cycle. The data are centered on the day of the luteinizing hormone (LH) surge (day 0). Days of menstrual bleeding are indicated by M. FSH = follicle-stimulating hormone; LH = luteinizing hormone. From Endocrine and Metabolism Continuing Education Quality Control Program, 1982. Copyright American Association for Clinical Chemistry, Inc.)

in LH will trigger ovulation (Figure 6.2). Once released, the oocyte will survive for 12–24 hours unless fertilisation occurs.

The delay of childbearing until later in women's lives has meant that diminished ovarian reserve is taking on ever greater importance as a cause of infertility, because a woman's egg supply depletes progressively over time. As many as 10% of women in their early thirties can have fertility delay on the basis of diminished ovarian reserve. While there will be some women who will continue to be fertile well into their forties, the average age at which female fertility ceases on the basis of diminishing ovarian reserve is 40–41 years.

Disorders of ovulation contribute to approximately 30% of cases of subfertility. The more common causes of anovulation include:

- polycystic ovarian syndrome (PCOS)
- hypothalamic hypogonadism
- thyroid dysfunction
- hyperprolactinaemia
- premature ovarian failure.

Polycystic ovarian syndrome is a complex endocrine disorder that affects 12–21% of Australian women of reproductive age and is more common among those who are overweight or of Indigenous background. Although reproductive features are prominent, PCOS is also associated with major metabolic consequences, including obesity, type 2 diabetes mellitus and cardiovascular disease. Increased androgens and/or hyperinsulinaemia secondary to insulin resistance lead to hormonal imbalance and ovulatory dysfunction.

Hypothalamic hypogonadism or secondary hypogonadism may arise from disorders of the hypothalamus or pituitary resulting in low output of gonadotrophic hormones. Reversible causes may be associated with anorexia, stress or excessive exercise. Sheehan's syndrome of hypopituitarism is irreversible and due to the rare pituitary infarction associated with severe postpartum haemorrhage.

Hypothyroidism or hyperthyroidism may lead to ovulatory dysfunction, which responds to correction of the underlying thyroid disorder.

Premature ovarian insufficiency (premature ovarian failure) occurs in about 1% of women. In the majority of women the cause is unknown, but an increasing number of women experience ovarian failure following treatment for pelvic cancer (bilateral oophorectomy, chemotherapy and radiotherapy). Oophorectomy may also be necessary in the management of endometriosis and severe chronic pelvic inflammatory disease. Women born with gonadal dysgenesis (e.g. Turner's syndrome) generally have severe ovarian dysfunction.

Treatment of anovulation is explored further in chapter 7, Problems of fertility.

SPERM PRODUCTION

The hypothalamic–pituitary–testicular axis controls sperm production and steroidogenesis (Figure 6.3). Gonadotrophin-releasing hormone is released from the hypothalamus to stimulate LH and FSH release from the pituitary. LH acts on the Leydig cells in the testis, which produce testosterone. Sertoli cells in the testis are responsible for spermatogenesis and are controlled by FSH and testosterone. FSH secretion is under negative feedback control via inhibin B, which is produced by the Sertoli cells. Sperm production is continuous, and it takes approximately 70 days for each sperm to complete development (Figure 6.4). Adequacy of sperm is assessed by semen analysis. The WHO lower reference limits for normal semen analysis, which were derived from a large population-based study of men whose partners conceived within 12 months, are given in Table 6.1.

A male factor is solely responsible in about 20% of infertile couples and contributory in another 30–40%. Not only does semen need to have optimal characteristics on a routine semen analysis, it needs to be largely free from sperm DNA fragmentation (also sometimes called 'sperm DNA damage'). Sperm DNA damage is more common in older men and those with the adverse lifestyle factors mentioned above. Sperm DNA damage levels can be reduced by frequent (even daily) ejaculation, since much of this damage is believed to occur in the collecting system after the sperm has been released from the testis but prior to ejaculation.

The more common causes of male factor infertility include genetic, environmental and infectious factors. Genetic factors may include abnormal karyotype such as Klinefelter's syndrome (XXY) and microdeletions of the Y chromosome. Cystic fibrosis may be associated with a gene-related congenital

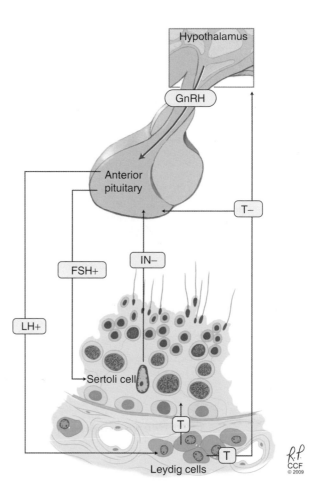

Figure 6.3

The hypothalamic–pituitary–testicular axis. Gonadotrophin-releasing hormone (GnRH) is released from the hypothalamus, stimulating release of luteinising hormone (LH) and follicle-stimulating hormone (FSH). FSH stimulates germ cell epithelium and LH induces testosterone production by the Leydig cells. Both testosterone (T) and inhibin (IN) downregulate gonadotrophin release.

(Wein: Campbell-Walsh Urology 10e; 2011 Saunders; 978-1416069119 Figure 21.1)

bilateral absence of vas deferens. As men age there is a consistent decline in semen quality and damage to sperm DNA has been implicated. Impotence also increases with advancing age.

A wide range of environmental factors may influence sperm production. There is increasing evidence of the adverse effect of tobacco smoking on sperm, attested by the fact that male smokers are

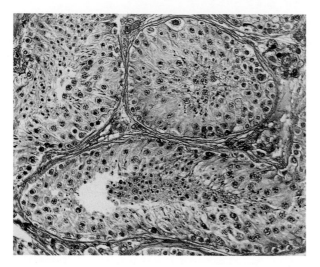

Figure 6.4

Three seminiferous tubules undergoing active spermatogenesis. Elongate spermatids are present along the luminal border of each tubule.

(Zhou & Magi-Galluzzi: Genitourinary Pathology, 1st ed. 2006 Churchill Livingstone 9780443066771; Figure 9.25)

Table 6.1 WHO lower reference limits for normal semen analysis[2]	
Parameter	Lower reference limit
Volume	1.5 mL
Sperm concentration	15 million spermatozoa/mL
Progressive motility	32%
Total motility	40%
Morphology	4% normal forms

30% more likely to be infertile than non-smoking men. Obesity increases the risk of hypogonadotrophic hypogonadism. Animal models have implicated leptin insensitivity in the hypothalamus leading to altered release of gonadotrophins. Moderate alcohol use does not affect male fertility, but excessive alcohol use may cause associated liver dysfunction and nutritional deficiencies, which are also detrimental for sperm production. Recreational drugs such as marijuana and cocaine reduce both sperm count and motility.

Medications that may affect spermatogenesis include chemotherapy and anabolic steroids, the latter having a reversible effect. Sperm motility may be reduced by the antibiotics tetracycline and nitrofurantoin. Sulfalazine, which is used in the treatment of ulcerative colitis and rheumatoid arthritis, has a similar effect. The antihypertensive spironolactone affects the hypothalamic–pituitary–gonadal (HPG) axis, resulting in reduced output of gonadotrophins. Calcium channel blockers have been shown to block fertilisation by interfering with calcium-sensitive receptors on sperm cells. Beta-blockers interfere with fertility by decreasing libido and negatively affecting sexual function. Alpha-adrenergic blockers and thiazide diuretics can cause erectile dysfunction.

An increase in scrotal temperature, such as occurs in cryptorchidism or varicocele, negatively influences sperm production. Performing certain prolonged activities such as bicycling or horseback riding, especially on a hard seat or poorly adjusted bicycle, may also be detrimental.

Viral and bacterial infections of the reproductive tract, including prostatitis, epididymitis and orchitis, may lead to postinflammatory scarring and damage to the sperm ducts and testis. Adolescent mumps orchitis may cause irreversible testicular failure.

Excessive exercise, as in women, may affect hypothalamic function, and long-distance runners (men who run more than 160 km per week) and distance cyclers (men who ride more than 80 km per week) have decreased spermatogenesis. These activities should be moderated when a couple is planning conception.

Most vaginal lubricants are toxic to sperm. Couples wishing to conceive should avoid their use during the fertile time of a woman's cycle.

Unexplained oligospermia accounts for 30% of male infertility.

FERTILISATION

Once the oocyte is released, it is picked up from the surface of the ovary by the fimbrial ends of the fallopian tube and carried along through the fallopian tube by the cilia lining it. The sperm released into the vagina are required to travel through the cervix, uterus and into the tube to meet the oocyte. Cervical mucus is present to provide a suitable environment for the sperm to navigate the cervical canal. In good conditions, sperm may survive for up to 5 days in the female genital tract while awaiting ovulation.

Barriers to the gamete transport that leads to fertilisation include problems with sexual intercourse, impaired penetration and survival of sperm in cervical mucus, and damage to the fallopian tubes.

Problems with sexual intercourse may be of psychological or organic aetiology. Counselling, a key component of fertility management, is particularly important here. Organic causes may include deep dyspareunia associated with endometriosis or chronic pelvic inflammatory disease.

The micofibrillar architecture of cervical mucus is designed to prevent penetration of sperm (and infectious organisms) at times other than close to ovulation. Cervical infection, and the anti-oestrogenic effects of clomiphene citrate, an ovulation-induction agent, may alter this environment and prevent sperm penetration. Cervical anti-sperm antibodies may contribute to poor survival of sperm in the ovulatory mucus.

Damage to the delicate cilia of the fallopian tubes may occur following pelvic infection with organisms such as *Chlamydia*. Blockage of the tube due to damage of the fimbrial end may occur as a consequence of endometriosis or of adhesions from previous pelvic surgery. Tubal transport plays an important role in fertility, with tubal factors accounting for 30% of causes of infertility.

IMPLANTATION

Once the sperm fertilises the egg in the fallopian tube, the zygote divides and the resulting cluster of cells (the morula) travels towards the uterus. By the time it has reached the endometrial cavity it has attained the blastocyst stage, containing an inner cell mass — the embryoblast — and the trophoblast, which will form the placenta. The blastocyst needs to lose the outer zona pellucida and 'hatch' before it can implant.

In the follicular phase of the menstrual cycle, oestrogen produced by the dominant follicle leads to thickening of the stratum functionale of the endometrium. This proliferative phase of endometrial development has a distinctive appearance in ultrasound imaging, which plays an essential role in assessment of fertility. The hypoechoic endometrium represents the relatively sparse glands in a thickened stroma (Figure 6.5).

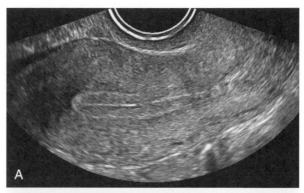
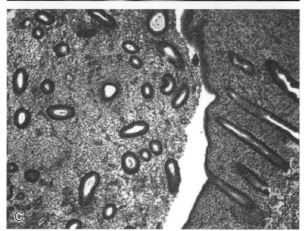
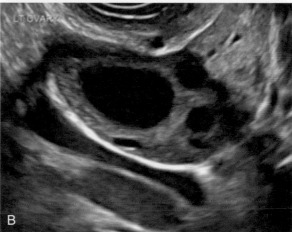

Figure 6.5
The endometrium in the follicular phase of the cycle. A: Ultrasound appearance of proliferative phase; B: Dominant 20 mm follicle in the ovary; C: Histology of proliferative phase endometrium.

(Ultrasound images provided courtesy of D Sutton, Monash Ultrasound for Women.)

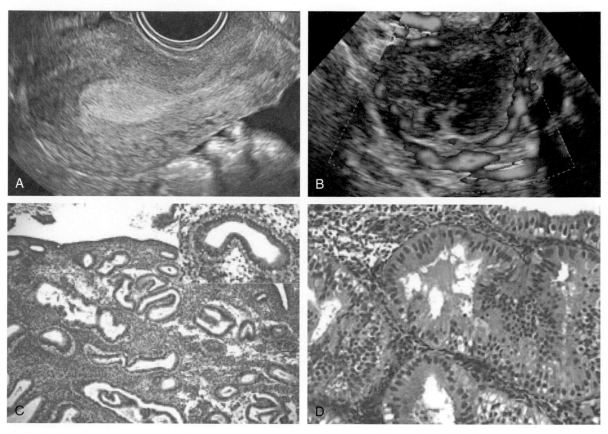

Figure 6.6
The endometrium in the secretory phase of the cycle. **A**: Ultrasound appearance of mid-secretory phase; **B**: Corpus luteum in the ovary with peripheral vascular 'ring of fire'; **C**: Histology of mid-secretory phase endometrium low power and **D**: High power.

(Ultrasound images provided courtesy of S Atkinson, Monash Ultrasound for Women.)

The corpus luteum formed in the ovary following ovulation releases progesterone, which prepares the endometrium for implantation of the blastocyst. The endometrium is enhanced by glandular enlargement and secretion of gylcogen-rich fluid. Together with increased tortuosity of the spiral arteries, the marked glandular development presents multiple interfaces for insonation and hence a highly echogenic endometrium (Figure 6.6). The period of time during which the endometrium becomes receptive to implantation is known as the implantation window, and is surprisingly short, usually occurring on one particular day around 6–7 days after ovulation.

Embryo implantation, which follows hatching of the blastocyst, involves adherence, apposition and invasion stages. The chance of successful implantation is influenced by embryo quality and by endometrial receptivity. Endometrial receptivity might be reduced by endometrial or uterine pathology, such as endometrial polyps or submucosal fibroids. The endometrium of women with endometriosis is now recognised to be generally less receptive (endometriosis contributes to at least 20% of all cases of infertility). However there are also more subtle endometrial factors affecting implantation receptivity, often only apparent at a molecular level. Molecules that appear to be important for the endometrium to express are known as integrins, a family of cell-surface receptors important in cell-to-cell communication. These receptors influence many aspects of cell behaviour, including cell

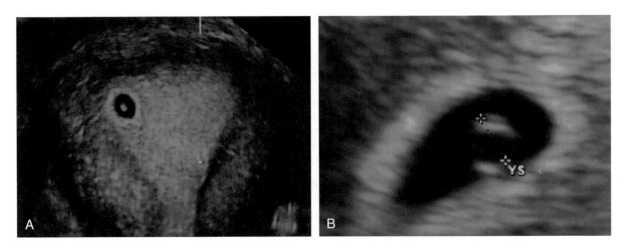

Figure 6.7

Three-dimensional representation of early intrauterine pregnancy at 5 weeks 3 days. A: Coronal view of 6 mm gestation sac in the right fundal region of the endometrial cavity; B: Magnified image of the gestation sac shows 3 mm yolk sac. No embryo is yet visible. The strong endometrial decidual reaction around the gestation sac indicates successful implantation.

(Ultrasound images provided courtesy of K Ransome, Monash Ultrasound for Women.)

migration, growth, survival and proliferation, angiogenesis, invasion and neoplasia. Alteration of gene expression and differentiation of these molecules is likely to affect the complex events of fertilisation, embryogenesis, embryo–endometrial interaction and implantation.

The earliest sonographic confirmation of early pregnancy, at approximately 4 weeks and 2 days, is visualisation of a 2–3 mm gestation sac on trans-vaginal ultrasound examination. A yolk sac appears at 5 weeks' gestation (Figure 6.7). A live embryo may be visualised at 6 weeks' gestation.

REFERENCES

1   Anderson K, Normal RJ, Middleton P. Preconception lifestyle advice for people with subfertility. Cochrane Database Syst Rev 2010;CD008189.
2   Cooper TG, Nonnan E, von Eckardstein S, et al. World Health Organization reference values for human semen characteristics. Hum Reprod Update 2010;16:231.

Chapter 7

Problems of fertility

Neil Johnson and Elizabeth Glanville

KEY POINTS

Infertility is defined by the failure to achieve a clinical pregnancy after 12 months or more of regular unprotected intercourse.

One in six couples seeks specialist help because of difficulty in conceiving.

In 15–30% of these couples, infertility will remain unexplained.

A thorough history and examination of both partners may reveal an underlying explanation for infertility.

The emotional impact of infertility on a couple should not be underestimated.

The most technically advanced form of ART is IVF/ICSI, which is associated with a 25–35% chance of success per cycle.

EPIDEMIOLOGY

The World Health Organization (WHO) defines infertility as 'a disease of the reproductive system defined by the failure to achieve a clinical pregnancy after 12 months or more of regular unprotected sexual intercourse'. Infertility is divided into primary (no previous pregnancy) and secondary (previous pregnancies). One in six couples seeks specialist help because of difficulty in conceiving. There is no evidence that there has been a marked rise in the prevalence of infertility but, because many effective treatments are now available, there has been a large increase in the number of couples seeking help.

PATHOPHYSIOLOGY

Causes contributing to infertility include:
- male factors (50%)
- ovulatory disorders (30%)
- fallopian tube disease (30%)
- endometriosis (20%)
- coital problems (5%)
- cervical factors (<5%).

In many couples more than one cause contributes to the infertility. No obvious cause is found in 15–30% of couples — so called unexplained infertility.

HISTORY AND EXAMINATION

A detailed history from both partners can reveal potential problems. Infertility is a stressful situation and so a full social history including occupation, family issues and the impact of the failure to conceive is worthwhile. Frequency of sexual intercourse, timing, and other problems involving intercourse should be explored with both partners.

In the male, specific features in the history should be sought, including sexually transmitted disease; mumps as an adult; operations such as repair of inguinal hernias and orchidopexy; drugs such as antimitotic agents, beta blockers; excess alcohol, smoking history, history of recreational drug use; and occupational or leisure pursuits that could compromise fertility, such as intense exercise training. Examination should include general appearance, noting any signs of hypoandrogenism, such as loss of secondary sex characteristics. Genitalia should be examined to assess the size and consistency of the testicles, as well as the presence of the vas deferens and/or varicocele.

In the female, features associated with normal ovulation include a regular menstrual cycle, mid-cycle pain, changes in vaginal discharge, premenstrual symptoms, and primary dysmenorrhoea. The reproductive history should be documented. There may be predisposing factors for pelvic infection, such as sexually transmitted infections, the use of an intrauterine device, or previous pelvic surgery. Symptoms suggestive of endometriosis should also be explored, such as secondary dysmenorrhoea, dyspareunia, and bowel symptoms including dyschesia. Examination should identify secondary sexual development, evidence of pelvic inflammatory disease (PID), or endometriosis. Pelvic examination should exclude fibroids, ovarian masses, nodules, or reduced mobility of pelvic organs that could suggest endometriosis. This examination is an opportunity to take genital tract swabs to exclude active infection or carriage of agents such as *Chlamydia*.

INVESTIGATIONS

The standard investigation of infertility includes semen analysis in the male. In the female, investigations include blood serum samples to test early follicular FSH level (ideally combined with an oestradiol level), midluteal progesterone level, and antenatal screen tests including rubella immunity, in addition to routine genital tract swab tests.

Other investigations may need to be undertaken if the standard investigations are abnormal.

Male

Semen should be analysed after at least 48 hours' abstinence from ejaculation. The sample must be brought promptly (within 1 hour) to the laboratory. The standard criteria for normal semen analysis are listed in chapter 6, Fertility.

If the specimen is suboptimal, the test should be repeated after 4–6 weeks before a final assessment of quality is made.

For consistently abnormal semen analysis results, it is important to evaluate serum follicle-stimulating hormone (FSH), luteinising hormone (LH), testosterone and prolactin levels to determine if the

aetiology is primary or secondary testicular dysfunction. In cases of severe oligospermia (<5 M/mL), chromosomal analysis should be considered, as gonadal dysgenesis may be associated with abnormal karyotype, such as Klinefelter's syndrome (XXY).

Fructose concentration in the semen helps determine the origin of the azoospermia. A fructose-negative semen may indicate absence of the seminal vesicles, or absence of or obstruction of the vas deferens at the level of the seminal vesicles. If azoospermia is found in association with absent vas deferens on examination, mutations of the cystic fibrosis conductance regulator (CFTR) gene should be tested for. Identifying genetic abnormalities is important prior to potential fertility treatment, as genetic counselling may be necessary.

Testicular biopsy is rarely required for diagnostic purposes. Men with azoospermia and elevated FSH levels (>7.5 mIU/mL) or testicular long axis length less than 4.6 cm may be considered to have non-obstructive azoospermia and accordingly counselled. Therapeutic testicular biopsy and sperm extraction may be offered for use in in-vitro fertilisation. Causes of non-obstructive azoospermia include spermatozoan maturation arrest or Sertoli cell only development (Figure 7.1). Men with FSH levels of 7.6 mIU/mL or less or testicular long axis length greater than 4.6 cm may be offered reconstructive surgery, with or without testicular biopsy and sperm extraction.

Tests for sperm DNA fragmentation are also now available, but there is no consensus on how relevant the results are, or the precise place of this investigation.

Female
Ovulation

It should be established that ovulation is occurring regularly.

The easiest single test for ovulation is measurement of serum progesterone taken around 7 days following ovulation (midluteal). If the cycle is irregular and the timing of ovulation is difficult, serial samples should be taken. Values greater than 25 nmol/L indicate ovulation.

If ovulation cannot be confirmed, it is important to exclude endocrine causes such as thyroid dysfunction, hyperprolactinaemia, polycystic ovarian syndrome (PCOS) and premature ovarian insufficiency.

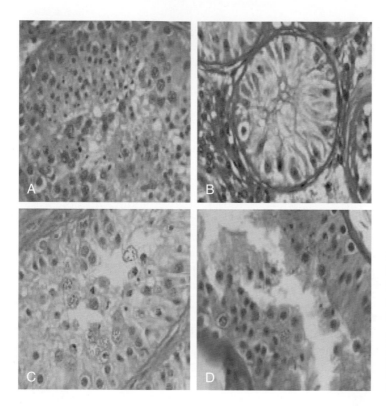

Figure 7.1
Diagnostic testicular biopsies. **A**: Normal testis; **B**: Maturation arrest of spermatogenesis; **C**: Sertoli cell only; **D**: Hypospermatogenesis.

(Bieber: Clinical Gynecology, 1st ed. Copyright © 2006 Churchill Livingstone, An Imprint of Elsevier; 9780443066917. Courtesy of Dr Thomas Wheeler, Department of Pathology, Baylor College of Medicine, Houston)

Measurement of serum TSH and thyroid hormones identify clinical and subclinical thyroid dysfunction. Elevated serum prolactin should prompt further investigation to exclude pituitary adenoma. Elevated follicular phase LH, FSH and abnormal androgen screen (serum testosterone, sex hormone binding globulin, free testosterone index and androstenedione) indicate biochemical PCOS. Measurement of the anti-Müllerian hormone (AMH) may be useful as it is usually elevated in PCOS and is a reliable marker of diminished ovarian reserve if low. Elevated serum FSH in the presence of low serum oestradiol is suggestive of ovarian failure.

Transvaginal pelvic ultrasound scan may assess the antral follicle count and identify polycystic ovaries, where at least 12 follicles of 2–9 mm are present (Figure 7.2).

The clinical disorder of PCOS, a common cause of oligo- or anovulation, is diagnosed by the presence of two of the following:

- ultrasound evidence of polycystic ovaries
- clinical and/or biochemical evidence of hyperandrogenism
- oligo- or anovulation.

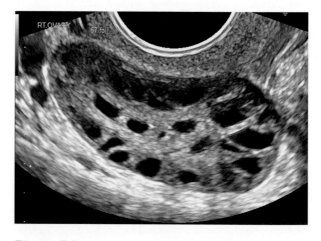

Figure 7.2
Transvaginal ultrasound image of polycystic ovary. This ovary contained in excess of 60 antral follicles of 2–9 mm.

(Image courtesy of D Sutton, Monash Ultrasound for Women.)

Obesity worsens the severity of PCOS-related symptoms, including anovulation.

Tubal patency

Tubal patency needs to be established if a woman is ovulatory and no other cause of infertility is apparent.

Hysterosalpingography involves the introduction of radio-opaque material through the cervix into the uterus and the fallopian tubes. An abdominal X-ray is then taken. Intrauterine anatomy and tubal patency can be documented. Hysterosalpingography has the advantage of being an outpatient procedure, and is usually well tolerated. It provides no information about problems occurring elsewhere in the pelvis, such as adhesions or endometriosis, and there is a small risk of introducing or reactivating pelvic inflammatory disease. A similar outpatient procedure, sonohysterography, utilises contrast material introduced through the cervix and ultrasound visualisation of fill and spill of the material through the fallopian tubes, into the pelvis and around the ovaries (Figure 7.3).

Laparoscopy with dye instillation is performed under general anaesthesia. A laparoscope is introduced through an umbilical incision to visualise the anatomy of the pelvis and reveal pathology, such as adhesions, endometriosis, and ovarian disease. Tubal patency is assessed by observation of the flow of fluid (typically methylene blue dye) through the fallopian tubes, after instillation of this fluid through the cervix. Laparoscopy is often performed together with hysteroscopy, which may show intrauterine pathology such as adhesions, polyps or fibroids.

Cervical factors

The postcoital test, which evaluated sperm survival in ovulatory cervical mucus, is no longer recommended as a means to assess possible cervical factors in infertility, as its results are poorly correlated with the chance of natural conception and tend not to alter management.

TREATMENT
Male

General advice should be given regarding modification of alcohol consumption, smoking cessation, and wearing loose underwear to enable autoregulation of testicular temperature.

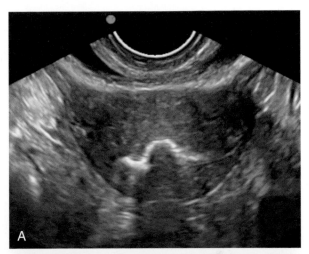
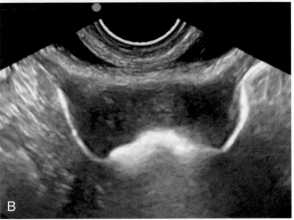

Figure 7.3

Ultrasound tubal patency test. A: Transvaginal transverse view of the uterus showing balloon of catheter in the upper endometrial cavity prior to injection of contrast material; B: Filling of both fallopian tubes with contrast material. Subsequent identification of free contrast in the pelvis confirmed tubal patency.

(Image courtesy of M Finn, Monash Ultrasound for Women.)

Newer evidence suggests that not only does varicocele ligation improve spermatogenesis, but also it could improve fertility outcomes through natural conception in male factor infertility.

Intrauterine insemination (best employed with controlled ovarian stimulation) improves outcomes with mild oligospermia.

The development of intracytoplasmic sperm injection (ICSI) in conjunction with in-vitro fertilisation (IVF) has transformed the prognosis, enabling successful treatment in severe cases of male factor infertility.

There is preliminary evidence of the benefit of a multivitamin/antioxidant approach for men with male factor infertility when the couple has experienced repeated ICSI failure.

Female
Anovulation

In women with PCOS or hypothalamic amenorrhoea, induction of ovulation improves the chance of conception to almost normal rates, provided the couple persists for 6–12 months. Lifestyle intervention should be first line for obese women with anovulation related to PCOS. The evidence-based approach to PCOS involves first-line ovulation induction treatment with either metformin or clomiphene, which have similar effectiveness for non-obese women with PCOS. Women with polycystic ovaries, however, have increased sensitivity to ovulation-induction agents and a lower initial dose is commenced to minimise the risk of ovarian hyperstimulation and multiple birth.

Metformin, an insulin sensitiser, is taken continuously and the woman's response monitored by midluteal serum progesterone measurement or documentation of improved regularity of cycles. Clomiphene is used for 5 days in the early follicular phase of the menstrual cycle. It increases FSH production by acting as an anti-oestrogen at the pituitary level. Metformin has some advantages over clomiphene as response to the latter treatment should be monitored in the fertility clinic setting through follicular phase oestradiol measurements and ovarian follicle scanning to avoid higher order multiple pregnancies. Later midluteal serum progesterone results may confirm ovulation. If neither treatment is effective, combination therapy with both could be considered. Next line, laparoscopic ovarian drilling can be used (working through destruction of androgenic ovarian tissue); evidence shows that ovarian drilling is as effective as daily FSH injections and has some advantages, including patient preference, avoidance of multiple pregnancy, and the ability of women to establish long-term regular ovulation and thus to have more than one baby. IVF is used for women with PCOS who have been unsuccessful with various other treatment options.

Evidence points to the specific first-line treatments for other causes of anovulation. Gonadotrophin induction of ovulation for hypothalamic anovulation should only be prescribed in specialist units and must be monitored closely, as complications include multiple pregnancy and ovarian hyperstimulation. The dopamine agonist bromocriptine or cabergoline is the appropriate treatment for hyperprolactinaemia, thyroxine or antithyroid drugs to correct hypo- or hyperthyroidism respectively, and ovum donation for premature ovarian failure.

Tubal factor infertility

Tubal surgery is now rarely undertaken, since its success rates of only 20–30% compare unfavourably with the success rates of IVF. Reversal of clip sterilisation remains the one area in which tubal surgery is worthwhile, and it is now sometimes possible for such tubal reanastomoses to be undertaken laparoscopically in the context of high-expertise advanced laparoscopic surgery.

IVF has now been used for more than 30 years and results in pregnancy rates higher than 25–35% per cycle, according to patient selection. With more severe tubal disease that results in a hydrosalpinx, a salpingectomy (removal of the tube) or clipping of such a tube to prevent spill of hydrosalpinx fluid into the uterus has been shown to significantly improve the chance of IVF success.

Endometriosis

Endometriosis, which is growth of endometrial tissue outside of the uterine cavity, may lead to pelvic adhesions and tubal occlusion. The evidence-based approach to fertility treatment with endometriosis is determined by whether a woman's fallopian tubes are normal or not. If they are not, IVF is the only realistic option. If a woman's fallopian tubes are normal and patent, treatment options shown to significantly enhance fertility include laparoscopic removal of endometriosis, use of an oil-soluble contrast medium such as lipiodol to bathe the endometrium and flush the fallopian tubes (a simple low-cost minimally invasive procedure that carries a low risk of complications and no increased risk of multiple pregnancy), intrauterine insemination (IUI) with controlled ovarian stimulation, and IVF.

Unexplained infertility

Treatment of unexplained infertility is influenced by the age of the woman, the duration of infertility, results of tests of ovarian reserve (usually an early follicular FSH and oestradiol level, an anti-Müllerian hormone (AMH) level on blood testing, and sometimes an ovarian antral follicle count on ultrasound), and the urgency felt by the couple. The wisest option might be a 'wait and see' approach ('expectant management'), while lifestyle factors are optimised and attention is given to optimising timing of sexual activity, as many couples with unexplained infertility will ultimately become pregnant naturally. Use of empirical clomiphene alone, formerly given to secure an ovulatory boost, has been shown to be unhelpful for couples with unexplained infertility, presumably owing to negative effects on cervical mucus and endometrial receptivity in some cases.

The range of evidence-based treatment options for unexplained infertility includes lipiodol flushing of the fallopian tubes, IUI with controlled ovarian stimulation (with either clomiphene or FSH injections), typically achieving success rates of 10–15% per cycle for women under 35 years, and IVF.

IVF/ICSI

IVF/ICSI is the most technically advanced form of assisted reproductive treatment (ART) available (Figure 7.4). As a single-cycle treatment, its results also tend to be associated with the highest chance of success, now in the range of 25–35% per cycle or higher. Success rates decline with age, with success rates under 10% in women aged 40 years

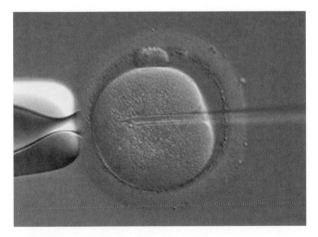

Figure 7.4
Intracytoplasmic sperm injection. The egg is held by a suction pipette (left) and the sperm injected into the cytoplasm.

(From Pitkin et al 2003, p. 133 Figure 5)

and older. It is rare for women to have a successful live birth over age 45 years.

The procedure was primarily developed to bypass tubal disease, but its application has broadened substantially with the evolution of ICSI and its use in unexplained infertility. IVF involves induction of multiple follicles with subcutaneous FSH injections and the collection of multiple oocytes under ultrasound control. Fertilisation with the partner's sperm then occurs in the laboratory. One or two embryos are replaced transcervically into the uterine cavity after 48–72 hours. The major complication of IVF is severe ovarian hyperstimulation syndrome, which occurs in <1% of cases.

MEDICOLEGAL AND ETHICAL ISSUES

As reproductive medicine adopts the latest technological advances in cell biology and molecular genetics, the potential for treatment with manipulation of gametes and their genetic makeup opens a Pandora's box of ethical and medicolegal dilemmas. The possibilities become endless and complex. The options of gamete (egg or sperm) donation, and embryo donation (where a couple who have frozen embryos from IVF/ICSI have completed their family and have no further wish to have embryos replaced), have become established in most settings. Surrogacy (gestational carrier), where a woman carries a pregnancy of a replaced embryo for which she has not typically provided gametes, is established in many settings. The emergence of reproductive possibilities for single women, same-sex couples (both female and male), and transgender individuals — along with a growing expectation of the availability of reproductive treatments among these groups — has led to a need to balance progressive and complex ART with what society deems to be reasonable. It is, after all, barely 30 years since society was shocked at the birth of the world's first 'test tube baby'!

In general, most countries with the technology to be able to undertake advanced ART have developed laws governing these procedures. Most countries in which advanced ART is possible also have formal ethics approval processes for treatments deemed to be close to the borderline of what may be approved in law. The ethical approval processes endeavour to balance ethical principles of justice (equitable access), reproductive autonomy and non-malificence, but the overarching key principle is always to protect the future interest of the, as yet unborn, child.

The type of treatments governed by these laws and ethics approval processes include surrogacy, gamete donation for single women, pregnancies for older women through egg donation (particularly for women aged 50 years and older), posthumous use of a man's sperm or of frozen embryos in the context of death of one of the intended parents, and sex selection (now possible through embryo biopsy and pre-implantation genetic diagnosis) for gender balancing of families. Newer technologies such as somatic cell nuclear transfer (so-called 'cloning'), for research and possible clinical application — always tightly controlled through ethical guidelines — must always be for therapeutic and non-reproductive purposes.

Many of these issues pose personal questions that clinicians have to deal with individually, notwithstanding the laws and ethics approval processes involved. Each jurisdiction (country or state) has subtly different laws at the borderlines of what are considered to be morally and ethically acceptable; some highly conservative, some liberal. This leads to patients seeking treatment outside of their own jurisdictions, a phenomenon that has become known as 'reproductive tourism'.

FURTHER READING

National Institute of Clinical Excellence (NICE). Fertility: Assessment and treatment for people with fertility problems. Clinical Guideline 11. February 2004. Online. Available from: www.nice.org.uk.

The Cochrane Library. www.thecochranelibrary.com. The Menstrual Disorders and Subfertility Group publish up-to-date reviews and protocols covering all the treatments described here.

Teede HJ, Misso ML, Deeks AA, et al. Assessment and management of polycystic ovary syndrome: summary of an evidence-based guideline. Med J Aust 2011;195(6):65–83.

MCQS

Select the correct answer.

1 Which of the following is **not** a test routinely requested in a woman with anovulation?

   A   TSH
   B   FSH
   C   testosterone
   D   prolactin
   E   cortisol

2 Of the following, which is **not** a useful treatment for unexplained infertility?

   A   IVF
   B   IUI
   C   lipiodol
   D   clomiphene
   E   conservative management

3 Natural fertility can be aided by all of the following except which?

   A   reducing caffeine intake in the female partner
   B   smoking cessation by both partners
   C   reducing female BMI to a healthy range
   D   restricting intercourse to one or two well-timed attempts per month in the fertile phase
   E   minimising alcohol intake in the female partner

OSCE

Polly is a 28-year-old woman who comes to see you as she is trying to conceive. She has a cycle that is variable with bleeding that lasts 4–7 days and recurs at an interval of 28–90 days. What are the further important features on history and examination that you need to collect? What investigations may be helpful in this setting?

Chapter 8

Chronic pelvic pain

William Leigh Ledger and Jason Abbott

KEY POINTS

Chronic pelvic pain is a common issue for women of reproductive age.

Differentiation from pain associated with the normal menstrual cycle is challenging.

A thorough history, physical examination and simple investigations such as ultrasound are very helpful in understanding chronic pelvic pain.

Common problems such as endometriosis should be considered.

Simple analgesia and hormonal treatments should be considered for most women with chronic pelvic pain prior to embarking on surgery.

Consideration of desire for fertility is important.

Other systems such as the urological, gastroenterological and musculoskeletal systems may contribute substantially to chronic pelvic pain.

INTRODUCTION

'A riddle wrapped in a mystery inside an enigma.' Winston Churchill's description of Russia could equally be applied to chronic pelvic pain (CPP). Just like Russia, the problem of pelvic pain is vast — in fact up to 25% of women will have chronic pelvic pain at some time of their life — and 90% will have dysmenorrhoea with their menstruation. Research into pelvic pain has been largely absent despite its prevalence, palmed off as too difficult or too tricky to approach. Yet unlocking some of those mysteries can bring great joy to your patient and is rewarding for you as her carer — all it takes is knowledge, time and careful interaction with your patient. And just like Russia — the key is the history …

Although causes of acute lower abdominal or pelvic pain are often obvious, for example acute PID with profuse vaginal discharge, or a ruptured ectopic pregnancy, many of the chronic forms of pelvic pain are less obvious. CPP affects 4–25% of women of reproductive age, and despite being a common gynaecological presentation, there are limited high quality data on its identification and management. Dysmenorrhoea (painful periods) is very common, with up to 90% of women experiencing pain with some menstrual cycles and nearly 60% of women having varying levels of pain with most cycles. This is a major issue for the diagnosis and management of CPP, since there is no other system in the body where pain is a part of normal homeostasis. A woman presenting to her doctor with 3–4 days of pelvic pain in each month requiring multiple analgesics will frequently be told that this is normal and will rarely be investigated — certainly not immediately. A female presenting with chest pain for 3–4 days each month requiring multiple analgesics would almost certainly be considered to have a pathological process and be investigated.

Differentiating between the 'normal' component of menstrual pain and pathological pain is a marked problem and one that requires time, sensitivity, and knowledge of how chronic pain may present. The most common pathological cause of CPP is endometriosis, with chronic PID, adenomyosis, uterine fibroids and pelvic floor myalgia also contributing. Non-gynaecological systems may also contribute, and disease such as irritable bowel syndrome or interstitial cystitis may be responsible, or be diagnosed instead of or in conjunction with other causes of pain.

A multidisciplinary approach is vital, with input from gynaecological, colorectal and urological surgeons, physicians, anaesthetists and pain specialists, radiologists, specialist nurses, counsellors and pharmacists, among others. A long-term strategy has to be offered and accepted by the patient, her partner, her family and her employer. Management for patients with CPP ranges from simple medical treatment such as the combined oral contraceptive pill (COCP) or analgesics to surgery. The COCP and analgesics may be used as a first-line treatment prior to invasive investigations and management such as surgery. This is a complex area of reproductive medicine, and a structured approach to the patient who presents with CPP is vital for long-term successful care.

DEFINITION AND EPIDEMIOLOGY

Given that pain may occur with a 'normal' menstrual cycle and be considered physiological, it is important to define CPP.

CPP is said to occur when pelvic pain persists for at least 6 months, has sufficient intensity to interrupt normal activities of daily life, and requires medical or surgical treatment. CPP may be either cyclic or non-cyclic, and does not always have to be associated with the menstrual cycle.

It is difficult to identify the prevalence of CPP clearly because of its multiple pathologies, modes of presentation, and variation in definition. Given that 5–10% of women will be affected during their lifetime with persistent CCP, and many more with transient CCP, the problem is as common as asthma, diabetes and breast cancer.

ASSESSMENT OF PELVIC PAIN
Clinical history

The most important part of the assessment for CPP is accurate and meticulous history-taking (Box 8.1).

Box 8.1 Clinical history for acute pelvic pain

The clinical history for acute pelvic pain should include:
- character, site, intensity, duration, periodicity, radiation, onset
- aggravating and relieving features
- effects of micturition, defecation, vomiting, coughing
- features of nausea, vomiting, sweating, urge to pass urine or faeces
- effect of any pain relief administered previously for this pain
- relationship to last menstrual period (LMP), movement, coitus
- previous pregnancy or surgical procedures
- past obstetric and gynaecological history
- past medical, surgical and psychiatric history
- social history, including marital, sexual and occupational history
- history of physical or mental abuse, including domestic violence
- orthopaedic and postural problems
- medication and allergies.

A detailed, chronological history of pain must be obtained. History should include results of previous investigation and treatments, both successful and unsuccessful, current medications, and limitations on quality of life. The menstrual and obstetric history needs to be covered early in the assessment, with particular attention to pain in relation to menstruation. Any associated symptoms, such as dyspareunia (painful intercourse), dyschesia (pain when passing a bowel motion), dysuria (pain when passing urine), or non-menstrual pelvic pain are important. A woman should be asked about obstetric trauma such as instrumental delivery or episiotomy. Knowledge of her plans for immediate or future fertility is crucial to determine what investigations and management options are appropriate. A detailed sexual history may reveal risk factors for pelvic inflammatory disease (see chapter 5) and the presence of superficial or deep dyspareunia.

> ### Box 8.2 Examination for the woman with CPP
>
> - General appearance of the patient? Is she shocked, distressed, tense, anxious, moving about, or lying still with her pain?
> - What can you tell from her gait?
> - Check vital signs.
> - General examination, including abdominal and musculoskeletal examination. Include the abdomen and make sure that the genital examination is not the first time that you touch the patient.
> - Pelvic examination: start with the external genitalia, observe for signs of irritation or localised trauma, discharge, bleeding.
> - Take appropriate specimens for pathology if indicated.
> - Bimanual pelvic examination, checking for uterine size, consistency, tenderness, mobility, shape and consistency. Palpate the uterosacral ligaments and posterior compartment and each of the fornices and the adnexa, for masses, tenderness and fixity.
> - Consider the indication for a speculum examination and the increased diagnostic capacity over a bimanual examination.
> - If bowel pathology or endometriosis affecting the rectovaginal space is suspected, consider a combined rectal and vaginal examination that may identify blood, mucus or tender nodularity of the rectovaginal septum, signs often associated with infiltrative endometriosis.

Physical examination

The physical examination of a patient with pelvic pain should be thorough (Box 8.2). Sensitivity is required when performing vaginal or rectal examinations, and verbal consent should always be obtained. It is important to remember that a woman with CPP must be examined as a whole, rather than just feeling the uterus and cervix. The use of the term 'cervical excitation' at physical examination should be avoided, whether in the emergency department or in clinical consultation. If there is pain with movement of the pelvic organs, a more focused description of pain location and the presence of pathology that may be leading to pain should be substituted.

Examination commences with general inspection of the patient as she walks into the room and during history, looking at posture, gait, and use of canes, walking frames or other mobility aids. A urinalysis is a mandatory and simple component of the examination. A supine abdominal examination, checking carefully for scars, allodynia (vigorous pain response to light localised pressure), masses and distension follows. The presence of allodynia may be a warning factor for psychologically driven pain, but it is also present in an advanced chronic pain

syndrome. A pelvic examination is also mandatory and should follow the principles of gynaecological examination in chapter 3 of this text.

Investigations

Investigations should be guided by the physical signs and should commence with those that are simple, inexpensive and widely available, such as urinalysis, midstream urine specimen for microscopy, culture and sensitivity, vaginal swabs, and serological investigation such as full blood count, C-reactive protein or CA 125. CA 125 may be used in conjunction with ultrasound to determine a risk-of-malignancy index (RMI) for a patient with a pelvic mass. (See chapter 27 for further information on RMI.) CA 125 on its own has poor sensitivity and specificity. Pregnancy should always be considered if the patient is less than 60 years of age and a β hCG should be performed to include or exclude this possibility.

Diagnostic imaging is more expensive than pathology and judicious use is appropriate. Transvaginal and transabdominal ultrasound offer a readily available, inexpensive and moderately invasive investigation with excellent capacity to evaluate the female genital tract. Using ultrasound, normal

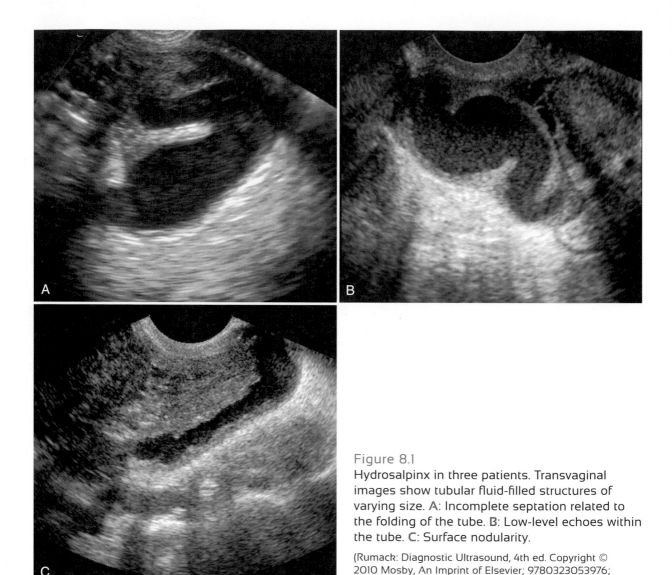

Figure 8.1
Hydrosalpinx in three patients. Transvaginal images show tubular fluid-filled structures of varying size. **A**: Incomplete septation related to the folding of the tube. **B**: Low-level echoes within the tube. **C**: Surface nodularity.

(Rumack: Diagnostic Ultrasound, 4th ed. Copyright © 2010 Mosby, An Imprint of Elsevier; 9780323053976; Figure 15.47)

structures may be clearly identified and structural abnormalities such as myomas, adenomyosis and ovarian cysts, hydrosalpinges (fluid-filled, blocked fallopian tubes) or pelvic fluid collections may be demonstrated. Figure 8.1 shows ultrasound images of hydrosalpinges in various presentations. Ultrasound is effective in distinguishing cystic from solid lesions, and allows information on vascular characteristics of the uterus and any pathological findings that may be present. Using the ultrasound transducer may aid in the identification of tender areas in the pelvis, such as over cystic ovarian lesions. For women with endometriosis as a cause of their CPP,

it is important to remember that pelvic ultrasound will only diagnose ovarian involvement with cystic disease (ovarian chocolate cysts), a finding that occurs in fewer than 20% of patients with endometriosis. Figure 8.2 shows the laparoscopic view of a patient with a right-sided ovarian endometrioma. Ultrasound is not helpful in diagnosing small volume peritoneal disease.

Other imaging modalities such as computed tomography (CT) or magnetic resonance imaging (MRI) have a more limited role in imaging the female genital organs but may be considered if involvement of the gastrointestinal tract, urinary

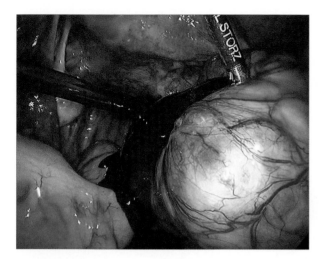

Figure 8.2
Laparoscopic view of a pelvis with severe endometriosis. Note the right ovarian endometrioma with the chocolate material that is typical for severe ovarian disease. The normal left ovary is seen to the left of the image; the uterus is anterior and the sigmoid is to the left and inferior.

(Image courtesy of Jason Abbott)

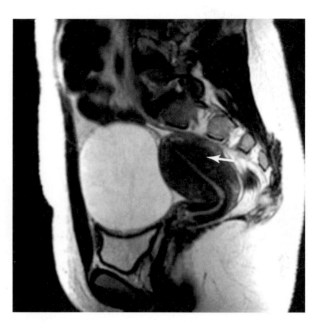

Figure 8.3
Adenomyosis on MRI. The junctional zone (*arrow*) in this patient measures 16 mm, indicating diffuse adenomyosis. Also note the cystic lesion anterior to the uterus and superior to the bladder, which is a pathologically proven serous cystadenoma.

(Pretorius: Radiology Secrets Plus, 3rd ed. Copyright © 2010 Mosby, An Imprint of Elsevier; 9780323067942; Figure 26.6)

tract or retroperitoneal structures is suspected. MRI may have some role in diagnosing adenomyosis (see Figure 8.3), deep endometriosis and neuromuscular problems that cause CPP, but its use is limited by high cost and limited availability.

Laparoscopy is an invasive investigation in which a telescope is placed into the abdomen through the umbilicus to visualise the contents of the pelvis and abdomen. This investigation is indicated in patients with CPP where pelvic pathology is suspected but cannot be diagnosed by noninvasive means. Laparoscopy may also be used as a treatment modality and is considered gold standard to diagnose pathology such as endometriosis or adhesions. Since all surgical investigations carry morbidity, thorough clinical assessment and pragmatic management including symptomatic treatment may lead to avoidance of unnecessary surgical procedures. A link to a patient information sheet on laparoscopy can be found in the Further reading list. Figure 8.4 shows the laparoscopic view of a normal pelvis with a corpus luteal cyst on the left ovary.

PATHOPHYSIOLOGY

CPP is frequently hormonally driven and gynaecological causes of pain should always be considered

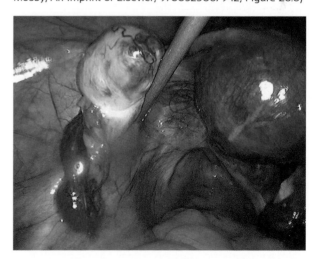

Figure 8.4
Laparoscopic view of a normal pelvis. Note the left-sided corpus luteal cyst with the surface vascular markings. The Pouch of Douglas can be seen easily and the uterus is a normal size and shape. There is no evidence of peritoneal disease or other abnormality.

(Image courtesy of Jason Abbott)

primarily when the pain cycle is synchronous with the menstrual cycle. There are certainly physiological causes such as Mittelschmerz and primary dysmenorrhoea, with the most common gynaecological pathology being endometriosis. Other gynaecological causes include adenomyosis, myomas, premenstrual pelvic vascular congestion and retrograde menstruation. Less common causes include cervical stenosis, or an obstructive abnormality due to Müllerian tract abnormality (see chapter 2).

CPP may also originate from the bowel, urinary bladder, the musculoskeletal system, or other intraabdominal structures higher up in the abdomen. There is an overlap between pelvic organs and muscles that share the same nerve supply, and a variety of contributing factors often coexist. Rarely is the pain psychosomatic; however, CNS involvement is common as with many chronic pain states. An underlying depression, anxiety state, sexual problem or domestic violence should always be kept in mind as a primary or secondary component of the pain. Broaching these issues with patients requires rapport, time, and considerable sensitivity.

One useful approach in trying to understand the pathogenesis and consequences of pelvic pain is to separate the phenomena into 'acute' and 'chronic'. While not altogether satisfactory — acute pelvic inflammatory disease may progress to chronic pain and inflammation, and inflammatory bowel disease can spontaneously improve even though it is seen as a chronic disease — this separates the common infective and acute inflammatory disorders from the chronic disease associated with endometriosis and adenomyosis. The third category of pain — that without a demonstrable cause — is particularly difficult for both patient and physician to accept and understand, and can lead to years of repeated medical and surgical interventions and long-term use of strong painkillers, including opiates.

Box 8.3 lists common causes of chronic pain.

Primary dysmenorrhoea

Primary dysmenorrhoea is a diagnosis of exclusion and is defined as menstrual pain without pelvic pathology. It is caused by vasoactive eicosanoids producing abnormal uterine contractions and decreasing uterine blood flow, with subsequent ischaemia similar to what may be seen in angina. The intensity of menstrual cramps and associated symptoms, such as nausea, fatigue and bloating, are directly proportional to the amount of eicosanoid

---

Box 8.3 Common causes of CCP

Gynaecological
- Physiological
  - Primary dysmenorrhoea
  - Mittelschmerz
- Pathological
  - Endometriosis
  - Adenomyosis
  - Uterine myoma
  - Cervical stenosis or obstructive abnormality
  - Pelvic venous congestion syndrome
  - Ovarian remnant/residual ovary syndrome
  - Pelvic adhesions
  - Post-pelvic inflammatory disease
  - Endosalpingiosis

Gastrointestinal tract
- Irritable bowel syndrome
- Inflammatory bowel disease
- Chronic constipation

Urinary tract
- Interstitial cystitis

Nervous system
- Pudendal neuralgia
- Provoked vestibulodynia

Musculoskeletal
- Pelvic floor myalgia
- Myofascial pain

Psychosocial
- Depression
- Physical and/or sexual abuse
- Drug-seeking behaviour

Physiological causes

---

produced, which is the reason that nonsteroidal anti-inflammatory drugs (NSAIDs) are effective treatment.

Primary dysmenorrhoea is the most common CPP for women of reproductive age, occurring in 60% of women and 70% of adolescents, with colicky, cramping pain occurring during menses. It may last for 1–5 days, resolving with or before the end of menstruation. Pain may be localised to the pelvis or radiate to the lower back and particularly to the upper and inner thighs.

NSAIDs and the COCP are the mainstay of treatments for primary dysmenorrhoea. There are no data to support an individual NSAID as the most effective and safe, and any medication at the lowest dose to control symptoms is reasonable. The COCP acts via ovulation suppression and endometrial thinning, which reduces production of eicosanoid prostaglandin.

Mittelschmerz pain

Mittelschmerz (German for 'middle pain') is said to occur in ovulatory women due to normal pre-ovulatory follicular enlargement, or normal follicular rupture with subsequent intraperitoneal spillage of follicular fluid and blood. As its name suggests, it occurs in the midpart of the cycle, in time with folliculogenesis (see chapter 3). Typically the pain is mild and unilateral, lasting for a few hours to a few days, and is seldom severe enough to distress women. If severe or persistent it may be treated with NSAIDs or the COCP.

Pathological gynaecological causes
Endometriosis

Endometriosis is the finding of endometrial-like tissue outside of the endometrium. Its diagnosis is a histological one, requiring two of the following three findings:

1 endometrial glands
2 endometrial stroma
3 haemosiderin-laden macrophages.

Endometriosis is the most common gynaecological pathology causing CPP, with 10% of women affected. It accounts for up to one-third of reproductive-age women undergoing laparoscopy for pelvic pain, and more than 50% in the adolescent population. Given this high prevalence, endometriosis is a significant public health problem. It is the third leading cause of gynaecological hospitalisations in the United States and a leading cause of hysterectomy.

The main theories of causation include retrograde menstruation, coelomic metaplasia, altered immune function, or some combination of these. It is considered an epigenetic disease. Oestrogen is important in maintaining the presence and proliferation of abnormal tissue, since endometriosis is rarely seen before adolescence and it usually settles after menopause. Medical treatments that suppress oestrogen secretion or activity often improve symptoms. The two cardinal symptoms of endometriosis are pain and infertility. Women with endometriosis may be asymptomatic. Pain symptoms may include dysmenorrhoea, deep dyspareunia, dyschesia and abnormal menstrual bleeding, and may reflect the site and depth of endometriotic infiltration. In particular, deep dyspareunia and dyschesia are suggestive of posterior deep infiltrating endometriosis at the rectovaginal septum. It is important to note that the severity of symptoms (pain or infertility) does not correlate with the severity of endometriosis.

Physical examination in endometriosis is important, since the finding of nodularity, tenderness or induration, particularly in the posterior compartment, may alter management. It is also possible to find full-thickness vaginal disease that may not be demonstrated by ultrasound, a finding that has significant impact on management. At the current time, only laparoscopy and biopsy with histological evidence of endometrial glands and stroma can confirm a diagnosis of endometriosis. New research that demonstrated certain types and density of nerve fibres in the endometrium may in future offer a low-invasive diagnostic investigation.

Managing a woman with endometriosis is dependent on her desire for current and future fertility, side effect profile of medications, and personal preference. The best medical treatments for endometriosis include the COCP and progestogens in their various forms, since they may be used in the long term, have acceptable side effect profiles, and are inexpensive. Many other treatments are used, including androgenic agents (danazol) and centrally acting drugs like gonadotrophin-releasing hormone analogues (GnRHa), but these are limited by significant and occasionally irreversible side effects, cost, or short duration of symptom relief. In addition, these drugs may not offer significantly greater benefits than the COCP. Using the COCP in a continuous manner (that is not taking the placebo or sugar pills) will prevent menstruation and prevent dysmenorrhoea, although a plan is needed to manage side effects, particularly breakthrough bleeding. Progestogens have multiple mechanisms of action including suppression of ovarian activity, and many different forms have been demonstrated to be effective for treating CPP. Side effects including breakthrough and irregular menstrual bleeding, weight gain, mood swings and decreased libido are reported, and are the most significant limiting factor with these medications.

Androgenic medications often induce amenorrhoea for women with endometriosis, although side effects such as central weight gain, acne, clitoromegaly and deepening of the voice (both irreversible) are often unacceptable to patients. GnRHa suppresses ovarian activity, oestrogen production and hence the pain symptoms of endometriosis, but side effects including bone density loss and menopausal symptoms such as hot flushes and vaginal dryness limit its long-term use.

The surgical management of endometriosis aims to remove all abnormal endometrial tissue and retain all normal tissues for future fertility. A key feature of endometriosis is the presence of fibrosis and adhesions that may affect fertility, and surgical management should aim to remove these abnormal tissues and reduce the chance of recurrence as far as possible. Surgical management is the preferred option for women wanting a pregnancy, since medical managements will prevent pregnancy in most circumstances. Ovarian endometriomas will not respond to medical treatments, although their size may be controlled medically. Only surgical management will remove these and other deeply invasive pelvic disease in the rectovaginal space and uterosacral ligaments. Any symptomatic patients are likely to benefit most with surgical excision, with reduction of dysmenorrhoea, as well as dyspareunia and non-menstrual pelvic pain. Randomised controlled trials comparing the effect of surgery to conservative management have shown that surgery and excision of endometriosis results in symptomatic improvement in CPP regardless of the stage of endometriosis.

Other techniques to control pelvic pain in conjunction with endometriosis involve the interruption of nerve pathways. Two techniques have been studied: laparoscopic uterine nerve ablation (LUNA), which involves the transection of the uterosacral ligaments at their insertion into the cervix, and presacral neurectomy (PSN), which involves the total removal of the presacral nerves. Results from randomised controlled trials demonstrate that LUNA has no place in the management of chronic pelvic pain, while PSN may have some benefit. The downside to PSN includes the considerable risk of side effects such as long-term bowel and bladder dysfunction, and it should be reserved for selected patients and performed by expert surgeons.

Uterine leiomyomas

Uterine leiomyomas (myomas or fibroids) may cause one of four cardinal symptoms, including pain, abnormal vaginal bleeding, mass effects, and subfertility. They are the most common pelvic tumour in females. Nearly 50% of women are likely to have a myoma at some time during her life, and 50% of these women come to clinical attention because of it. While abnormal uterine bleeding does occur (see chapter 18), pelvic pain may arise from uterine contraction and heavy menstrual flow. Myomas, particularly anterior and fundal fibroids, may also lead to dyspareunia.

The diagnosis may be made clinically and confirmed with transvaginal ultrasound (TVUS) as the preferred imaging modality. Management is dependent on symptoms, size and myoma location. Medical treatments include the COCP, progestogens, levonorgestrel-releasing intrauterine system, or GnRH analogues, although there is a high rate of persistence or recurrence of symptoms in the long term with medical management. Conservative surgical treatments include hysteroscopic resection of submucous myomas, with laparoscopy or laparotomy possible for large myomas or those outside the cavity. Hysterectomy is a definitive surgery, while uterine artery embolisation and surgical uterine artery ligation are alternative treatment options. Figure 8.5 shows a hysteroscopic view of a submucous myoma and the commencement of its removal.

Adenomyosis

Adenomyosis is a histological diagnosis where endometrial glands and stroma are present within the uterine myometrium. It is often considered to be on the continuum of endometriosis because of this histology, the similar presenting symptoms, and the subsequent management options. Both pain and menorrhagia are common presenting symptoms of adenomyosis, with pain often attributed to bleeding and swelling of endometrial islands confined by myometrial fibres. This may cause subsequent myometrial hypertrophy and hyperplasia, resulting in a clinically evident and diffusely enlarged uterus. Ultrasound is the most common imaging modality; MRI may be used with greater sensitivity and

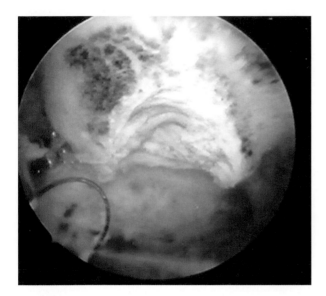

Figure 8.5
A hysteroscopic image of a submucous myoma. Note the exophytic growth into the uterine cavity. There are gas bubbles on the left, since fluid is used as a distention medium for the uterine cavity. There is an electrosurgical loop to the left and inferiorly. The first pass of a resection procedure has been performed, with the white myoma fibres exposed in the centre of the image.

(Image courtesy of Jason Abbott)

specificity but also greater cost (Figure 8.3). Management options are limited to progestogens (commonly Mirena is used), and the COCP may relieve dysmenorrhoea and menorrhagia. Symptoms usually reoccur with cessation of treatment, making hysterectomy the only definitive treatment. Conservative surgical treatments include endometrial ablation or resection and laparoscopic removal of myometrium affected, although there are technical difficulties with both of these options.

Pelvic venous congestion syndrome

Pelvic venous congestion is a controversial entity, proposed as a cause of pelvic pain. The syndrome is said to occur with a variety of pelvic pains and the imaging findings of pelvic varicosities that display reduced blood flow, although dilated ovarian veins are frequently seen on imaging in asymptomatic parous women. There is no pathognomonic test. Management options include medical treatment by progesterone; surgery is often unsuccessful.

Ovarian remnant and residual ovary syndrome

Ovarian remnant syndrome occurs in women who have had both ovaries removed surgically, but where an amount of ovarian tissue has been inadvertently missed and remains functional. Residual ovary syndrome occurs in women who have had ovarian conservation but who present with pathology subsequently. A key feature of the chronic pain in these patients is that there is expansion of the ovarian tissue, which is frequently trapped in adhesions or a confined area, and this engages mechanoreceptors to cause pain. A mass or cystic space may be demonstrated clinically, by ultrasound or other imaging technique. Of women having hysterectomy with ovarian conservation for benign indications, 2–3% present with residual ovary syndrome requiring further surgical procedures, where most pain can be attributed to functional cysts and benign tumours. Malignancy of the ovary is responsible for symptoms in 12% of cases. Management is frequently surgical.

Other gynaecological causes

Pelvic adhesions may be the result of previous surgery, infection, inflammation (endometriosis) or assisted reproductive technology procedures. Debate is intense as to the mechanism of pain in the presence of adhesions and whether their division or removal is helpful. A definite correlation between adhesion presence and pain is uncertain. For patients with chronic pelvic pain and adhesions as the only demonstrable pathology, a multidisciplinary team approach is frequently required.

Pelvic inflammatory disease (PID) can be complicated by chronic pelvic pain in 18% to 33% of women, regardless of antibiotic therapy. The exact mechanism for chronic PID is unclear, however both pelvic adhesions and neurological priming are considered to be factors and surgical treatments are rarely helpful in the long term. Figure 8.6 shows adhesions around the liver, typical in women who have had PID. This is Fitz-Hugh–Curtis syndrome, and may account for chronic pain.

Endosalpingiosis is the finding of ciliated tubal epithelium outside of the fallopian tubes. Once the diagnosis is confirmed histologically management is symptomatic, and medical or surgical treatments are often ineffective. This condition is not responsive to hormonal treatments but is not implicated in subfertility.

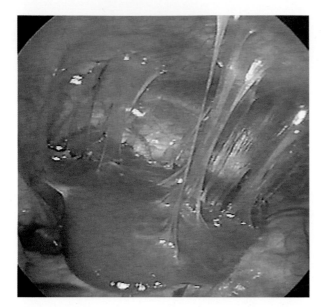

Figure 8.6
Liver adhesions typical of Fitz-Hugh–Curtis syndrome.

(Image courtesy of Jason Abbott)

> ### Box 8.4 Differential diagnosis for acute pelvic pain
>
> Gynaecological
> - Miscarriage variant
> - Ectopic pregnancy
> - Pelvic infection
>   - PID
>   - Salpingitis
>   - Endometritis
> - Ovarian cyst accident
>   - Rupture
>   - Haemorrhage
>   - Torsion
>
> Non-gynaecological
> - Urological
>   - Cystitis (UTI)
>   - Renal calculus being passed (ureter or bladder)
>
> Gastrointestinal
> - Acute appendicitis
> - Diverticular disease/abscess
> - Bowel obstruction
> - Mesenteric thrombosis
>
> Musculoskeletal injury

Ovarian cysts rarely cause chronic pelvic pain, and are more likely to lead to an acute pain presentation due to haemorrhage, rupture or torsion. Box 8.4 lists ovarian cyst accidents and other causes of acute pelvic pain.

Non-gynaecological causes of chronic pelvic pain

Gastrointestinal tract

Irritable bowel syndrome (IBS) is a common diagnosis that is said to affect 10–20% of adults in developed countries. This functional disorder is characterised by abdominal pain and bowel symptoms such as bloating, urgency, diarrhoea, and constipation. Cross-sectional studies have shown that approximately one-third of women with chronic pelvic pain have irritable bowel syndrome, and there is frequently crossover with other common problems such as endometriosis. Treatment is symptomatic and medical, involving dietary modifications, fibre supplements, and antispasmodic agents. Women with inflammatory bowel disease may have similar presenting features, with intermittent cramping abdominal pain along with fatigue, diarrhoea, weight loss, and/or rectal bleeding. Where suspected, endoscopy with biopsy is required to make a diagnosis.

Urinary tract

Interstitial cystitis (IC) is a non-infectious chronic inflammatory condition of the bladder that has poorly understood aetiology and pathophysiology. IC often presents with CPP and frequency, dysuria, urgency or nocturia that is variable and fluctuant and often worse during or after intercourse. As for IBS, there is a large overlap between IC and chronic pelvic pain. Urinalysis and a midstream urine sample must be obtained to exclude infection. Cystoscopy with hydrodistension of the bladder may aid in diagnosis, demonstrating glomerulation and submucosal haemorrhage, as well as being therapeutic, giving symptomatic relief in 20–30% of cases for several months. Management is symptomatic and may include simple analgesics, physiotherapy, and dietary modification to exclude acidic foods. Figure 8.7 shows the cystoscopic view of a patient with chronic pain who has interstitial cystitis.

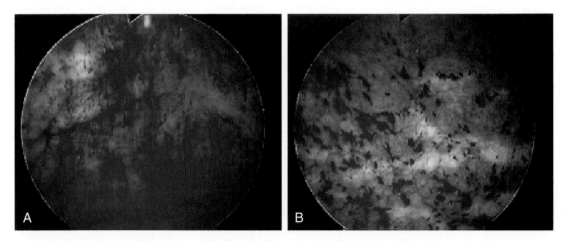

Figure 8.7

Glomerulations with cystoscopic hydrodistension in a patient with interstitial cystitis. A: Mucosal haemorrhages during emptying phase after hydrodistension. B: Glomerulations after refilling the bladder.

(Bieber: Clinical Gynecology, 1st ed. Copyright © 2006 Churchill Livingstone, An Imprint of Elsevier; 9780443066917; Figure 4.3)

Musculoskeletal system

CPP may occur due to pelvic floor dysfunction as well as problems with muscles of the abdominal wall, back, hips and upper thighs. There is increasing recognition that spasms of these muscles can be primary or secondary causes of pelvic pain. Up to 85% of patients with chronic pelvic pain have musculoskeletal dysfunction, such as muscular spasm of the pelvic floor or postural changes such as scoliosis and pelvic rotation. Abnormal postures from such musculoskeletal dysfunction increase muscular tensions and spasm, with consequent muscle shortening that then exacerbates or prolongs pain. As part of the examination, consideration of posture, scoliosis, pelvic asymmetry, and vaginal examination of the pelvic floor muscles is necessary.

Pelvic floor myalgia is usually associated with involuntary spasm of the pelvic floor muscles. This pain can be either continuous or episodic, and may manifest as a sense of aching, heaviness, or burning. It is not associated with the menstrual cycle, although menses may exacerbate the pain. Sexual intercourse or certain activities may trigger pain symptoms, and dyspareunia is the most common symptom of this condition. Treatment should be with physiotherapy initially, with consideration of long-term muscle relaxants such as botulinum toxin type A for refractory cases.

Neurological

Patients with pudendal neuralgia (PN) present with severe sharp pain along the anatomical territory of the pudendal nerve (vagina, vulva, labia, perineum, and anorectal region). Dyspareunia is the most common presentation. It is exacerbated by prolonged sitting, and relieved by standing. The pathophysiology of PN is not clear, but is believed that a neuronal insult from stretching and compression is a significant contributor. Treatment options range from conservative physical therapy to nerve blockade, surgical decompression, and neuromodulation, with referral to specialist centres appropriate.

Provoked vestibulodynia is pain in the vaginal vestibule evoked by any kind of stimulation such as intercourse and light touch. It is reported to affect up to 12–15% of women of reproductive age at some time of their life. It is one of the diagnoses that may be considered under the term 'vulvodynia' — a group of problems, rather than a specific diagnostic category. Treatment options include physiotherapy, medical treatment with tricyclic antidepressants, topical anaesthetics, local steroid injections, and, rarely, surgery such as vestibulectomy. Again, specialist treatment is recommended.

Psychosocial

Consideration of physical or sexual abuse is important for the patient with CPP. While the trauma

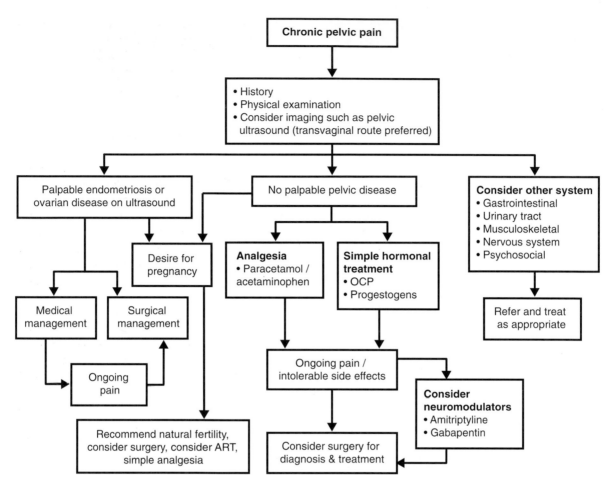

Figure 8.8
Potential management options for premenopausal women with CPP.

(Diagram by Jason Abbott and Haryun Won)

is usually not the cause of pain, the impact of any pain may be exacerbated for women experiencing abuse. This history may not be given readily by a patient, and may be kept hidden for many years, even when the history is directly sought. Considerable sensitivity, capacity to deal appropriately when the history is revealed, and an empathic approach are essential.

Depression is the most common psychological sequela of CPP of any type, and its presence should be sought and addressed for this group of patients. Medical treatments, counselling and cognitive behavioural therapy by an appropriate healthcare professional may all be considered in affected women.

MANAGING CHRONIC PELVIC PAIN

Management of CPP is often complex and must be undertaken depending on the list of differential diagnoses and the desire of the patient for specific treatments, requirement of diagnosis, and fertility desire. A thorough history and examination will often help to guide management in conjunction with the woman's wishes. In Figure 8.8, a flowchart of potential management options is suggested for the premenopausal woman with CPP. This flowchart should be considered as a guide only, as other variables such as the patient's age and treatment preference or previous surgery may influence the choice of managements.

First-line treatment without having a diagnosis may be appropriate and cost effective utilising simple treatments such as the OCP and NSAIDs, since the majority of gynaecological causes of CPP are hormonally driven. Treatment with the OCP is appropriate in women with a normal physical examination who do not want to conceive, if there are no contraindications to its use. A monophasic preparation with a monthly cycle for three months can be trialled initially. If the woman has a good response to this treatment, then she could trial a continuous program of the OCP with a plan for common issues such as breakthrough bleeding. Simple analgesics such as NSAIDs or paracetamol should be used in conjunction with the OCP as additional management options. Other hormonal treatments such as progestogens (medroxyprogesterone acetate, norethindrone acetate) or the levonorgestrel-releasing intrauterine system may be considered as alternative second-line medical treatment or when there are contraindications to the OCP. GnRH analogues have a very limited role in CPP and should be used under expert guidance, with a clearly defined plan about the impact of this treatment to long-term health.

The use of opioid medication in a young woman for a long period of time has many disadvantages and these medications should be used sparingly, only under long-term team care with frequent review and observation for side effects (e.g. constipation) and reassessment for other analgesic options or other causes of pain. Surgical investigations and management may be considered in the woman whose pain is persistent despite medical treatment or if there are intolerable side effects. Neuromodulators such as amitriptyline and gabapentin may also be considered in conjunction with a pain specialist, with frequent patient review. It is important to assess for side effects of these medications and treat or cease medication as appropriate.

For the woman who has refractory CPP, it is likely that her management will require a combination of treatments. The multifactorial nature of chronic pelvic pain, the difficulty in obtaining a 'cure' means that the necessity of promoting management that allows functionality is imperative. A good working relationship with the woman is important and a partnership needs to be established to ensure an optimal management program with regular follow-up. Multidisciplinary review may be required to expand treatment options, create realistic expectations of treatment outcomes, and ensure that there is no diagnosis that is not considered or investigated. This will include the gynaecologist, physiotherapist, general practitioner, and a chronic pain team with pain specialist and pain psychologist. Multiple or scheduled surgeries expose the woman to increased risk without the benefits of significant reduction in her symptoms, and so clearly defined parameters for surgical intervention are necessary. CPP is a common, time intensive, and debilitating medical problem for women and their healthcare providers. Management options need to be tailored to the patient's current situation with a view to her long-term goals and the likelihood of success.

FURTHER READING

Abbott JA, Hawe JA, Clayton R, Garry R. The effects and effectiveness of laparoscopic excision of endometriosis: A prospective study with 2–5 year follow-up. Hum Reprod 2003;18(9):1922–7.

Al-Azemi M, Jones G, Sirkeci F, et al. Immediate and delayed add-back hormonal replacement therapy during ultra long GnRH agonist treatment of chronic cyclical pelvic pain. Br J Obstet Gynaecol 2009;116:1646–56.

Chapron C, Barakat H, Fritel X, et al. Presurgical diagnosis of posterior deep infiltrating endometriosis based on a standardized questionnaire. Hum Reprod 2005;20(2):507–13.

Ferrero S, Abbamonte LH, Giordano M, et al. Uterine myomas, dyspareunia, and sexual function. Fertil Steril 2006;86(5):1504–10.

Garry R, Clayton R, Hawe J. The effect of endometriosis and its radical laparoscopic excision on quality of life indicators. Br J Obstet Gynaecol 2000;107(1):44–54.

Haugstad GK, Haugstad TS, Kirste UM, et al. Posture, movement patterns, and body awareness in women with chronic pelvic pain. J Psychosom Res 2006;61:637–44.

Jiang QY, Wu RJ. Irritable bowel syndrome. Prim Care 2011;38:433–47.

Laparoscopy patient information sheet on laparoscopy. Online. Available from: www.alanahealthcare.com.au/pdfs/Laparoscopy.pdf.

Royal College of Obstetricians and Gynaecologists. The initial management of pelvic pain. Guideline No. 41. April 2005. Online. Available from: www.rcog.org.uk.

Sweet RL. Pelvic inflammatory disease: current concepts of diagnosis and management. Curr Infect Dis Rep 2012. epub. Available from: www.ncbi.nlm.nih.gov/pubmed/22298157. doi: 10.1007/s11908-012-0243-y.

Tokushige N, Markham R, Russell P, Fraser IS. Different types of small nerve fibres in eutopic endometrium and myometrium in women with endometriosis. Fertil Steril 2007;88(4):795–803.

Won HR, Abbott J. Optimal management of chronic cyclical pelvic pain: an evidence-based and pragmatic approach. International Journal of Women's Health 2010;2:263–77. doi: http://dx.doi.org/10.2147/IJWH.S7991.

World Endometriosis Society. Online. www.endometriosis.ca.

MCQS

Select the correct answer.

1   A 33-year-old woman complains of a 6-month history of worsening deep dyspareunia and dysmenorrhoea. Vaginal examination reveals tender nodules on the uterosacral ligaments. Which of the following is the most likely diagnosis?

   A   pelvic inflammatory disease
   B   endometriosis
   C   adenomyosis
   D   pelvic floor myalgia
   E   interstitial cystitis

2   A 19-year-old women presents with a 3-year history of moderated dysmenorrhoea. She has been sexually active for 2 years with the same partner, uses condoms for contraception, and has a normal examination and pelvic ultrasound. What would be your next steps in management?

   A   Recommend OCP, consider danazol, discuss laparoscopy.
   B   Recommend NSAIDS, consider OCP, discuss laparoscopy.
   C   Recommend laparoscopy, consider post-op GnRH analogues.
   D   Recommend laparoscopy, consider Depo Provera, discuss GnRH analogues.
   E   Recommend NSAIDS, consider GnRH analogues, discuss laparoscopy.

3   A 26-year-old women presents with a 3-year history of isolated dyspareunia. She had a laparoscopy 2 years ago that showed no sign of endometriosis, has normal bowel function, and has been using the OCP for the last 2 years. On examination, the vulval skin is normal; she has pain immediately over the puborectalis and extending infero-laterally. The uterus is anteverted and mobile and there is no tenderness in the posterior compartment. What would you recommend as the next line of management?

   A   physiotherapy
   B   repeat laparoscopy
   C   gabapentin
   D   danazol
   E   colonoscopy

OSCE

Jane is a 22-year-old woman with a 7-year history of chronic pelvic pain. She is presenting to you for the first time today.

What are the features on history and examination that you wish to address with Jane? What investigations and management are important?

Chapter 9

The physiological changes of pregnancy

Martha Finn

KEY POINTS

The primary cardiovascular change in pregnancy is peripheral vasodilatation.

The cardiac output increases by 40%: the maximum is achieved at 24–28 weeks' gestation and is preserved until term. A further acute increase occurs immediately postpartum.

It is important to be aware of the supine hypotensive effect of maternal position in late pregnancy.

The pregnant woman is susceptible to pulmonary oedema due to reduced colloid oncotic/pulmonary capillary pressure gradient.

The relatively greater expansion in plasma volume compared to red cell mass results in the 'physiological haemodilution' of pregnancy.

In pregnancy, there is a three-fold increase in iron demand and 10–20-fold increase in the demand for folate.

Glomerular filtrate rate increases due to increased cardiac output and renal flow. Creatinine clearance rises by 50%.

Reduced renal tubular reabsorption of glucose and amino acids lead to glycosuria and aminoacidura in the absence of hyperglycaemia or renal disease.

Pregnancy is a hypercoaguable state. The risk of venous thromboembolism is increased six-fold and is a leading cause of maternal death.

The physiological hyperventilation of pregnancy leads to a fully compensated respiratory alkalosis. It may be experienced as mild breathlessness.

Pregnancy is a state of physiological insulin resistance and relative glucose intolerance.

In the first trimester, elevated serum hCG levels associated with hyperemesis may precipitate hyperthyroidism.

Progesterone-mediated smooth muscle relaxation may lead to urinary stasis and infection, varicose veins, gastric reflux and constipation.

In pregnancy, increased maternal calcium absorption meets the fetal demand for bone mineralisation, while sparing the maternal skeleton.

Enlargement of the pituitary due to lactotroph hyperplasia makes the gland vulnerable to ischaemia following severe peripartum haemorrhage hypotension.

Levels of both free and bound cortisol increase during pregnancy and contribute to glucose intolerance.

The three-fold increase in aldosterone levels maintains sodium balance in a relatively underfilled expanded vascular system.

The functions of the placenta comprise gas exchange, nutrition and waste elimination.

The pregnant woman undergoes profound anatomical and physiological changes in almost every organ system in adaptation to the needs of the growing fetus. Successful implantation associated with rising human chorionic gonadotrophin stimulates continued ovarian production of oestrogen and progesterone, which are responsible for many of these changes. After the first trimester this function is taken over by the placenta.

The respiratory and cardiovascular changes in pregnancy serve to ensure optimal growth and development of the fetus. Oxygen delivery to the placenta and fetus is dependent on the maternal oxygen saturation, haemoglobin concentration and uterine blood flow. This is largely achieved by a sustained increase in cardiac output mediated by peripheral vasodilatation and increased blood volume. Glucose metabolism is altered to direct more of the available glucose and amino acids for the fetus. Increased hepatic synthesis of clotting factors protects the mother from the risks of haemorrhage at delivery. These physiological changes evolve during pregnancy and delivery, after which there is a complete return to the prepregnant state within weeks.

It is important to appreciate the influence of these changes on the pregnant woman. Normal physiological changes may mimic organ pathology in the non-pregnant state. Laboratory normal ranges of organ function differ in the non-pregnant and pregnant woman. Some adaptations may be exaggerated and lead to serious consequences, gestational diabetes and venous thromboembolism being salient examples. Normal physiological changes occurring in a woman with preexisting medical condition such as cardiac or renal compromise may cause serious complications. An understanding of the physiological changes of pregnancy is therefore essential for optimal care of the pregnant woman.

CARDIOVASCULAR CHANGES

The primary cardiovascular event is peripheral vasodilatation, mediated by decreased vascular responsiveness to the pressor effects of angiotensin II and adrenaline, increased endothelial prostacyclin and nitric oxide production, and increased vessel compliance.

Peripheral vasodilatation leads to a fall in systemic vascular resistance, which reduces cardiac afterload. An increased blood volume (see haematological and renal changes) increases cardiac preload, and these two factors combined result in increased cardiac output. The changes commence early in gestation. By 8 weeks' gestation the cardiac output has already increased by 20%. Indeed, the first evidence of pregnancy in women with preexisting cardiac disease may be sudden deterioration, with cardiac failure at 10 weeks' gestation.

Before the increase in cardiac output can adequately compensate for the fall in systemic vascular resistance, blood pressure begins to fall in the second trimester of normal pregnancy until the nadir is reached by about 22–24 weeks' gestation. From then onwards, there is a steady increase to prepregnant levels until term.

The cardiac output increases by 40%, this maximum occurring at about 24–28 weeks' gestation (Figure 9.1). An increase in stroke volume is possible due to the increase in ventricular wall muscle mass and end-diastolic volume (but not end-diastolic pressure) seen in pregnancy. The heart is physiologically dilated and myocardial contractility is increased. Although stroke volume declines towards term, the increase in maternal heart rate (by 10–20 beats per minute) is maintained, thus preserving the increased cardiac output.

There is a profound haemodynamic effect of maternal position in late gestation. In the supine position, the enlarged uterus may compress the vena cava, reducing venous return to the heart and thus resulting in a decrease of cardiac output, maternal blood pressure and uterine perfusion. The maternal compensatory response comprises increased sympathetic tone causing vasoconstriction

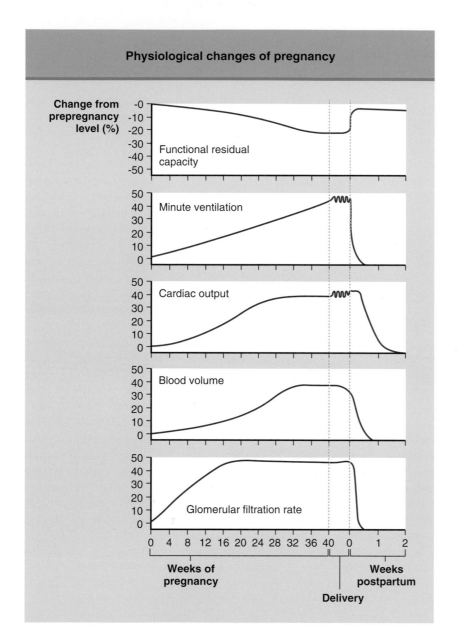

Figure 9.1

Physiological changes of pregnancy. Schematic representaton of some of the physiological changes occurring during pregnancy and the postpartum period.

(Albert: Clinical Critical Care Medicine; 1st ed. 9780323028448. Copyright © 2006 Mosby, An Imprint of Elsevier; Figure 59.2. Chapter 59 – Pregnancy-Related Critical Care. Stephen E. Lapinsky)

and tachycardia, and diversion of blood flow from the lower limbs through the vertebral plexus and azygos veins to the right atrium. In 10% of women this may not be sufficient to maintain blood pressure, resulting in severe hypotension and loss of consciousness. This supine hypotensive syndrome may be relieved by placing the woman in the left lateral position or inserting a wedge under her right hip. This is especially important when the woman is administered anaesthetic agents, which reduce stroke volume, and neuroaxial blockade (spinal or epidural), which causes sympathetic blockade.

Although blood volume and stroke volume increase in pregnancy, pulmonary capillary pressure and central venous pressure do not increase significantly, as pulmonary vascular resistance also decreases approximately 30% in normal pregnancy.[1] As serum colloid osmotic pressure is, however, reduced by about 10–15%, the colloid oncotic pressure / pulmonary capillary pressure gradient is reduced by almost 30%, making pregnant women particularly susceptible to pulmonary oedema. Pulmonary oedema will be precipitated if there is either an increase in cardiac pre-load (such as infusion of fluids), or increased pulmonary capillary pressure (such as in preeclampsia), or both.

Intrapartum and postpartum haemodynamic changes

During labour there is a further increase in cardiac output (15% in the first stage and 50% in the second stage; Figure 9.2). Uterine contractions lead to autotransfusion of 300–500 mL of blood back into the circulation, and the systemic response to pain and anxiety further elevates heart rate and blood pressure.

Following delivery there is an immediate rise in cardiac output due to the relief of inferior vena cava obstruction and contraction of the uterus emptying blood into the systemic venous system. Cardiac output increases by 60–80%, followed by a rapid decline to pre-labour values within about 60 minutes of delivery. Transfer of fluid from the extravascular space increases venous return and stroke volume further. The second stage of labour and immediate postpartum period are thus the most dangerous time for women with cardiovascular compromise. The cardiac output remains elevated at the levels seen in late pregnancy for about 2 days postpartum.

Normal findings on examination of the cardiovascular system in pregnancy

Symptoms of breathlessness, fatigue and reduced exercise tolerance may occur in normal pregnancy and do not necessarily indicate cardiac compromise. Peripheral oedema may occur due to progesterone-mediated smooth muscle dilatation and increasing venous obstruction due to the gravid uterus.

The hyperdynamic circulation of pregnancy due to peripheral vasodilatation and increased cardiac output may be associated with a bounding pulse, higher basal heart rate and louder heart sounds, with splitting of both sounds in late pregnancy and a soft ejection systolic murmur found in almost 90% of women (Figure 9.3). A third heart sound is not uncommon, and occasionally supraventricular ectopic beats may be identified. Diastolic murmurs are uncommon and may reflect increased flow through the mitral or tricuspid valve, but are more likely to represent a pathological condition.

The enlarged heart undergoes anterior and lateral rotation, leading to physiological changes in the ECG: QRS axis leftward shift, ST segment depression and T wave inversion in inferior and lateral leads, and Q wave inversion and inverted T wave in

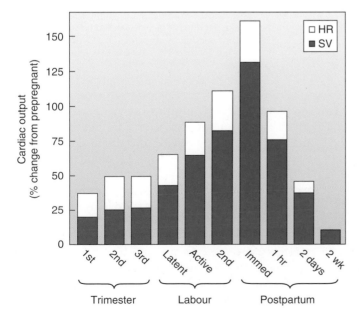

Figure 9.2
Cardiac output during pregnancy, labour, and the puerperium. Values during pregnancy are measured at the end of the first, second, and third trimesters. Values during labour are measured between contractions. For each measurement, the relative contributions of heart rate (HR) and stroke volume (SV) to the change in cardiac output are illustrated.

(The Heart and Circulation. Chestnut: Obstetric Anesthesia, 4th ed. 9780323055413; Figure 2.1. Copyright © 2009 Mosby, Inc. The Heart and Circulation)

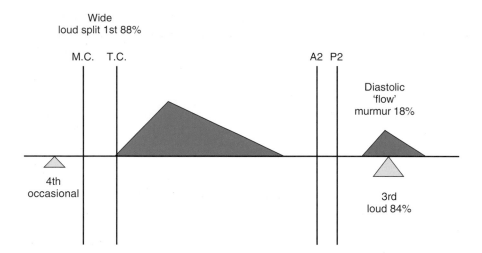

Figure 9.3
The findings on auscultation of the heart in pregnancy. MC, mitral closure; TC, tricuspid closure; A2 and P2, Aortic and pulmonary elements of the second sound.

(Gabbe: Obstetrics: Normal and Problem Pregnancies, 6th ed. 9781437719352; Figure 3.5. Copyright © 2012 Saunders, An Imprint of Elsevier. From Cutforth R, MacDonald C: Heart sounds and murmurs in pregnancy. Am Heart J 1966;71:741, p. 747, with permission.)

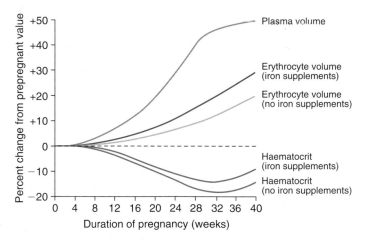

Figure 9.4
Plasma and erythrocyte increase during pregnancy.

(Otto: Valvular Heart Disease, 3rd ed. 9781416058922 Figure 25.1. Copyright © 2009 Saunders, An Imprint of Elsevier. From Pitkin RM. Nutritional support in obstetrics and gynecology. Clin Obstet Gynecol 1976;19:489–513, with permission.)

lead III. In the pregnant woman, these physiological changes should be recognised and not confused with those of cardiac compromise or pulmonary embolism in a non-pregnant woman.

Haematological changes

The plasma volume increases progressively throughout normal pregnancy, from 10–15% in the first trimester to a maximum at 30–34 weeks' gestation (Figure 9.4). The total gain at term averages 1100–1600 mL and results in a plasma volume of 4700–5200 mL, 30–50% above that found in non-pregnant women.[2]

Elevated renal production of erythropoietin (50% increase) induces a rise in red blood cell mass to meet the growing metabolic demand for oxygen in pregnancy. This red blood cell mass begins to increase at 8–10 weeks' gestation and in women taking iron supplements steadily rises by 20–30% above non-pregnant levels by the end of pregnancy. A smaller increase of 15–20% in red cell mass occurs in women not on iron supplements (Figure 9.4).

Because the expansion in plasma volume is greater than the increase in red cell mass, there is a fall in the haemoglobin concentration, haematocrit, and red cell count. This is recognised as the physiological haemodilution of pregnancy.

In pregnancy there is a two- to three-fold increase in the need for iron for both maternal haematological and enzymatic function and fetal development. There is a 10–20 fold increase in folate requirement. Provided adequate supply of iron and folic acid, there is usually no change in the mean corpuscular volume (MVC) or mean corpuscular haemoglobin concentration (MCHC).

The lower limit of normal haemoglobin concentration in pregnancy is 10.5 g/dL. Women who are already anaemic prior to pregnancy may become rapidly symptomatic, with tiredness, dizziness or fainting. Most cases of anaemia present in the third trimester, when the demand for iron is greatest.

The platelet count tends to fall progressively during normal pregnancy but usually remains within normal limits. In a proportion of women (5–10%), the count will reach levels of $100–150 \times 10^6/L$ by term. In practice, therefore, a woman is not considered to be thrombocytopenic in pregnancy until the platelet count is less than $100 \times 10^6/L$.

Leucocytosis is observed in pregnancy, in particular a neutrophilia. The rise in white blood cell (WBC) count starts after 8 weeks of pregnancy, reaching a plateau in the late second trimester, when total WBC counts range from 9000 to $15\,000 \times 10^6/L$. Further increases may occur in labour up to $29\,000 \times 10^6/L$. The levels return to prepregnant levels by 6 days postpartum. Because of the rapid production of WBC, precursors such as myelocytes or metamyelocytes may be seen in the peripheral circulation. In healthy women, the concentration of lymphocytes (T and B lymphocytes) and monocytes remains unchanged in pregnancy. The basophil count may reduce slightly and the eosinophil count may increase slightly.

RENAL CHANGES

Glomerular filtration rate (GFR) increases significantly due to elevations in both cardiac output and renal blood flow (Figure 9.1). The hormonal vasodilator relaxin produced by the ovary and the placenta increases nitric oxide production in the renal circulation, leading to generalised vasodilatation and subsequent increase in renal blood flow, which peaks at approximately 80% above baseline levels by the early second trimester and then declines slowly towards term, but remains above 50%. Creatinine clearance

rises by about 50%, resulting in a fall in serum urea and creatinine levels. Indeed serum urea levels within the non-pregnant range may represent renal compromise in the pregnant woman.

The plasma osmolality falls to a new set point of about 270 mosmol/kg, with a proportional decrease in plasma sodium concentration of 4–5 meq/L. This is one of the main reasons for water retention, with an average increase at term of 3 L. The physiological response to changes in osmolality above or below this threshold (i.e. thirst and release of antidiuretic hormone from the pituitary) is intact. This physiological hyponatraemia of pregnancy resolves within 6–8 weeks after delivery.

Pregnancy is associated with reduction in tubular reabsorption of glucose, amino acids and beta microglobulin, resulting in higher rates of urinary excretion. Glycosuria and aminoaciduria may thus occur in the absence of hyperglycaemia or renal disease. The upper limit of normal protein excretion in pregnancy is 300 mg/24 hours.

Progesterone-mediated ureteral smooth muscle relaxation results in dilatation of the urinary collecting system. This is aggravated by compression of the ureters by the enlarging uterus. Renal calyceal and ureteral dilatation is more pronounced on the right, due to pressure from the dextro-rotated uterus. Urinary stasis may predispose to asymptomatic bacturia, acute cystitis, or acute pyelonephritis. The latter increases the risk of preterm labour.

CLOTTING SYSTEM

Pregnancy is a hypercoagulable state, designed to mimimise bleeding following delivery. It is, however, a double-edged sword, as pregnancy increases the risk of venous thromboembolism (VTE) sixfold and this is a leading cause of maternal mortality. In the period 1997–2005, in Australia, there were 14 maternal deaths attributed to venous thromboembolism.[3]

The concentrations of clotting factors II, VII, VIII, X, XII and XIII are increased by 20–200%. Fibrinogen levels rise by up to 50%. Activity of the fibrinolytic inhibitors PAI-1 and PAI-2 is increased, although fibrinolytic activity may not be impaired. The concentration of endogenous anticoagulants such as Protein S falls slightly. Pregnancy-related changes return to baseline by 6–8 weeks postpartum.

The risk of VTE is present from the first trimester to at least 6 weeks postpartum. Venous stasis in the lower limbs is more marked on the left due to compression of the left iliac vein by the left iliac artery and the ovarian vein. The iliac artery only crosses the vein on the left.

In-vitro tests of clotting, such as the activated partial thromboplastin time (aPTT) and prothrombin time (PT) remain normal in the absence of anticoagulants or a coagulopathy. Bleeding time remains unchanged in pregnancy.

RESPIRATORY CHANGES

The increased metabolic rate in pregnancy leads to 20% increased oxygen consumption. This demand is met by a 40–50% increase in minute ventilation, mostly due to an increase in tidal volume rather than in respiratory rate. The functional residual capacity decreases by approximately 20% during pregnancy, due to the upward displacement of the diaphragm by the growing uterus and decreases in the expiratory reserve volume and residual volume. The inspiratory capacity also gradually decreases as pregnancy progresses because of this splinting of the diaphragm, resulting in a minimal decrease in total lung capacity, from 4.2 L to 4.0 L. Forced expiratory volume (FEV1) is unchanged during pregnancy, indicating stable large airway function.

The maternal hyperventilation causes arterial pO_2 to increase and arterial pCO_2 to decrease, with a compensatory fall in serum bicarbonate to 18–22 mmol/L. A mild fully compensated respiratory alkalosis is therefore normal in pregnancy (arterial pH 7.44). Increased awareness of this physiological hyperventilation may lead to a subjective feeling of breathlessness in up to 75% of women at some stage during pregnancy. Interestingly, similar respiratory function is seen in women with singleton and twin pregnancies.[4]

Anatomical changes in pregnancy include widening of the anteroposterior and transverse chest diameters and widened costal margin to compensate for the elevated position of the diaphragm (Figure 9.5). Diaphragmatic function remains normal.

GLUCOSE METABOLISM

Pregnancy is a state of physiological insulin resistance and relative glucose intolerance caused by opposing action of placental hormones, chorionic somatomammotrophin (human placental lactogen), glucagon and cortisol. There is almost doubling of insulin production from the end of the first trimester to the third trimester.

Fasting levels of glucose are decreased due to increased tissue storage of glycogen, increased peripheral glucose utilisation and the continuous fetal draw, particularly in late pregnancy. Insulin resistance results in higher postprandial glucose levels or higher levels following a glucose load compared to the non-pregnant state facilitating placental glucose transfer.

The maternal adaptation is characterised by a switch from carbohydrate to fat utilisation. Insulin resistance leads to inhibition of amino acid uptake into cells resulting in increased plasma levels of this substrate. Increased lipolysis also occurs, which allows the mother to preferentially use fat for fuel. The net effect is preservation of much of the available glucose and amino acids for the fetus, while providing free fatty acids, triglycerides and ketone bodies as sources of maternal fuel. Gestational diabetes mellitus (GDM) develops in women in whom there is insufficient insulin secretion to compensate for the insulin resistance. In 2005–06, in Australia, the risk of GDM increased with age: from 1% among 15–19-year-old women to 13% among women aged 44–49 years. Women aged 30–34 years accounted for more than one-third of GDM cases in the period 2005–06.[5]

THYROID FUNCTION

Hepatic synthesis of thyroid-binding globulin (TBG) is increased. Total levels of thyroxine (T4) and triiodothyronine (T3) are increased commensurably. The level of free T4 is thus relatively unchanged but does fall slightly in the second and third trimesters. Commensurately, levels of thyroid-stimulating hormone (TSH) increase as pregnancy progresses, and in the third trimester TSH levels have increased to the upper limit of normal compared to those in the non-pregnant woman.

Serum concentration of TSH falls in the first trimester as concentrations of human chorionic gonadotrophin (hCG) rise. The latter is structurally similar and has TSH-like activity. This explains the hyperthyroidism (biochemical and occasionally clinical) associated with elevated hCG and hyperemesis gravidarum.

Pregnancy is a state of relative iodine deficiency. Active transport of iodine to the fetus and two-fold loss of iodine in the urine due to increased glomerular filtration and reduced renal tubular reabsorbtion lead to a fall in plasma iodine concentration. This in turn leads to a three-fold uptake of iodine from

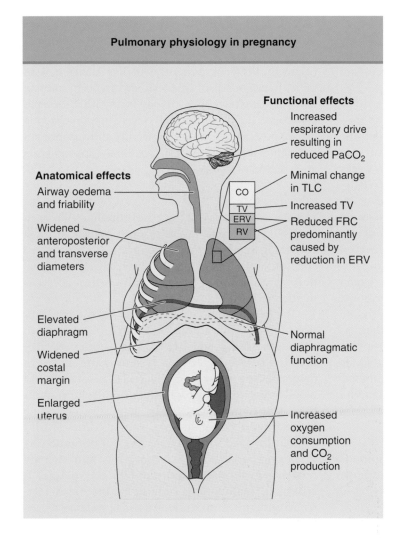

Pulmonary physiology in pregnancy

Functional effects

Increased respiratory drive resulting in reduced PaCO$_2$

Minimal change in TLC

Increased TV

Reduced FRC predominantly caused by reduction in ERV

Normal diaphragmatic function

Increased oxygen consumption and CO$_2$ production

CO
TV
ERV
RV

Anatomical effects

Airway oedema and friability

Widened anteroposterior and transverse diameters

Elevated diaphragm

Widened costal margin

Enlarged uterus

Figure 9.5
Pulmonary physiology in pregnancy. Anatomical and functional effects of pregnancy that influence pulmonary physiology. ERV: expiratory reserve volume; FRC: functional residual capacity; RV: residual volume; TLC: total lung capacity.

(Albert: Clinical Critical Care Medicine, 1st ed. 9780323028448, Figure 59.1. Copyright © 2006 Mosby, An Imprint of Elsevier. Chapter 59 – Pregnancy-Related Critical Care. Stephen E. Lapinsky)

the blood by the thyroid. If a woman already has dietary insufficiency of iodine, the thyroid gland hypertrophies to trap a sufficient amount of iodine, and goitre is observed.

CALCIUM METABOLISM

There is a high fetal demand for calcium to promote fetal bone mineralisation, particularly in the third trimester. The placenta produces an increased amount of 1,25 cholecalciferol, which enters the maternal circulation and acts on the intestine to increase calcium absorption. Calcium is actively transported across the placenta, facilitated by parathyroid hormone-related peptide also produced by the placenta. The fetus is relatively hypercalcaemic compared to the mother. Hypercalcaemia inhibits fetal parathyroid hormone activity and stimulates fetal calcitonin release, which minimises bone

resorption. This environment of high calcium, low PTH and high calcitonin is optimal for bone mineralisation.

In the maternal circulation total calcium concentration falls because of the physiological hypoalbuminaemia (40% of calcium is normally bound to albumen). Free ionised calcium concentration does not change, however, despite increased renal excretion. In pregnancy, increased intestinal calcium absorption satisfies the fetal need, while relatively sparing the calcium of the maternal skeleton.

The calcium needed for breast milk production is, however, met through renal calcium conservation and, to a greater extent, by mobilisation of calcium from the maternal skeleton. Women experience a transient loss of approximately 3–7% of their bone density during lactation, which is rapidly regained after weaning.[6]

PITUITARY CHANGES

The volume of the anterior pituitary progressively increases during pregnancy by up to 35%. Postpartum return to normal size is slower in women who breastfeed.

Anterior pituitary

Prolactin levels increase up to 10-fold under the influence of oestrogen and progesterone, returning to normal in the non-lactating woman by 2 weeks postpartum. Luteinising hormone (LH) and follicle-stimulating hormone (FSH) are suppressed by high circulating oestrogen and progesterone. Basal growth hormone (GH) concentrations are unchanged in pregnancy. The placenta, however, produces a specific growth hormone and somato-mammotrophin (human placental lactogen), which closely resembles pituitary-derived growth hormone. Pituitary levels of adrenocorticotrophic hormone (ACTH) are unchanged in pregnancy but the placenta produces its own ACTH and corticotrophin-releasing hormone (CRH). Thyrotrophin (TSH) secretion is modestly reduced in the first trimester in response to the thyrotrophic effect of rising hCG levels.

Intermediate lobe

Melanocyte-stimulating hormone secretion is increased from the first trimester, contributing to the increased pigmentation of pregnancy.

Posterior pituitary

Levels of antidiuretic hormone (ADH, arginine vasopressin) are unchanged in pregnancy. Oxytocin levels increase throughout gestation, and this hormone is involved in the process of parturition and the 'let down' response during lactation. Its release is promoted by nipple stimulation.

The enlargement of the pituitary in pregnancy is mainly due to hyperplasia of lactotroph cells in the anterior pituitary. Because of this enlargement, the pituitary is vulnerable to ischaemia, particularly in the peripartum period. In 1937 Sheehan attributed the deaths of 11 women to anterior pituitary infarction following severe haemorrhage and hypotension. It is still the most common cause of pan-hypopituitarism in women of childbearing age, particularly in developing countries. The condition may be life-threatening, with hypotensive shock and acute adrenal insufficiency, or more commonly may present with a more gradual onset of failure to lactate, rapid breast involution, amenorrhoea, loss of axillary and pubic hair, depigmentation, fatigue, and weight loss. Growth hormone deficiency may occur in 90% of patients, ACTH deficiency in 66%, hypogonadism in 65%, and hypothyroidism in approximately 40% of patients with Sheehan's syndrome. Less common is severe hyponatraemia due to posterior pituitary ischaemia and vasopressin deficiency. Symptoms and signs may appear years after delivery.

ADRENAL GLAND

Hepatic synthesis of cortisol-binding globulin (CBG) is increased. Levels of both bound and free cortisol increase during pregnancy, with serum free cortisol levels almost trebling by term. The normal diurnal variation in ACTH and cortisol levels is maintained in pregnancy.

The renin–angiotensin system is the primary determinant of adrenal aldosterone secretion, although ACTH and hyperkalaemia also contribute. The renin–angiotensin system is stimulated in pregnancy by the reduced vascular resistance and blood pressure and progressive vascular unresponsiveness to angiotensin. Plasma levels of aldosterone are increased threefold in the first trimester and 10-fold by the third trimester. Aldosterone, by increasing renal sodium absorption and thereby restoring extracellular fluid and blood volume, is critical in maintaining sodium balance in a relatively underfilled expanded vascular system.

The concentration of urinary catecholamines is unchanged in pregnancy.

GASTROINTESTINAL SYSTEM

The absorptive and secretory functions of the gastrointestinal tract (GIT) are relatively unaffected by pregnancy. Progesterone-mediated smooth muscle relaxation leads to reduced tone and motility throughout the GIT. Heartburn, due to gastro-oesophageal reflux, is a common symptom in pregnancy. Reduced cardiac sphincter tone and delayed gastric emptying may be further aggravated by anaesthetic agents and increase the risk of pulmonary aspiration of stomach contents. Increased small- and large-bowel transit times occur, and constipation is common. Haemorrhoids, or varicosities of the anal canal, are exacerbated by the increased intraabdominal pressure and constipation. Reduced gallbladder motility predisposes to stone formation.

Nausea and vomiting in pregnancy affect at least 50% of women, with an exaggerated response of hyperemesis gravidarum ocurring in up to 1% of pregnancies. The severity of this disorder parallels the level of hCG and is more common in twin and molar pregnancies.

Oropharyngeal changes include gingival swelling and inflammation; pregnancy epulis (granuloma gravidarum), a benign lesion of the interdental papilla which may bleed during pregnancy; change in taste sensation; and increased salivation. Increased attention to oral hygiene is advised.

In pregnancy liver function is relatively unchanged. Serum bilirubin and fasting total bile acid concentrations remain within the normal range. Serum alkaline phosphatase concentration, a marker of liver function, is markedly higher (up to 2–4 times normal) in the third trimester, due primarily to placental synthesis. Because of physiological haemodilution, serum albumen is reduced. Serum total cholesterol and triglyceride concentrations increase markedly during pregnancy, in association with increased insulin resistance.

SKIN, HAIR AND NAILS

Increased skin pigmentation occurs in the first trimester and fades postpartum. The pink areola become darker. Specific areas of pigmentation appear, such as the abdominal linea nigra (former linea alba) and the facial melasma (chloasma, mask of pregnancy), which may affect up to 70% of women in the second half of pregnancy. The prominences of the forehead, cheeks and chin are particulary affected.

Oestrogen causes vascular distention and proliferation of blood vessels in pregnancy. Spider naevi occur on the face, chest and arms. The majority regress after pregnancy.

Palmar erythema may be present in up to 70% of women by late pregnancy, resolving within a week of delivery. Saphenous, vulval and haemorrhoidal varicosities all occur more frequently during pregnancy.

Connective tissue changes such as striae gravidarum appear as pink linear skin 'stretch marks'. While they may fade, they never completely disappear. The aetiology is believed to be a hormonal-mediated diminution of elastin fibres in the dermis.

Scalp hair grows denser during gestation due to a longer anagen (growth) phase of the hair growth cycle. Hair loss may occur between 4 and 20 weeks

postpartum, and represents a correspondingly prolonged physiological telegen (resting) phase. The hair loss is thus diffuse, but recovery generally occurs within 6 months.

Generalised pruritus without rash or cholestasis may be a feature in up to 20% of pregnancies. Liver function should be checked to exclude cholestasis.

Nails grow faster during pregnancy but can become dystrophic, becoming soft and brittle with transverse grooves and distal onycholysis (painless separation of the nail from the nail bed). Apocrine activity is reduced in pregnancy but rebounds postpartum. As a result hidradenitis suppurativa improves during pregnancy.

MUSCULOSKELETAL SYSTEM

The musculoskeletal system is affected by maternal weight gain and hormonal influences. There is a marked increase in lumbar lordosis because of the enlarged uterus (Figure 9.6). Forward flexion of the neck and downward movement of the shoulders occur to compensate for the change in centre of

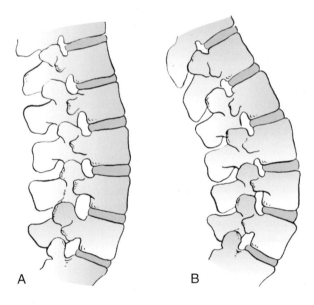

Figure 9.6
Effects of pregnancy on the lumbar spine.
A: Non-pregnant. B: Pregnant. There is a marked increase in lumbar lordosis and a narrowing of the interspinous spaces during pregnancy.

(Chestnut: Obstetric Anesthesia, 4th ed. 9780323055413; Figure 2.9. Copyright © 2009 Mosby, Inc. Modified from Bonica JJ. Principles and Practice of Obstetric Analgesia and Anesthesia, Volume 1. Philadelphia: FA Davis, 1967, p. 35.)

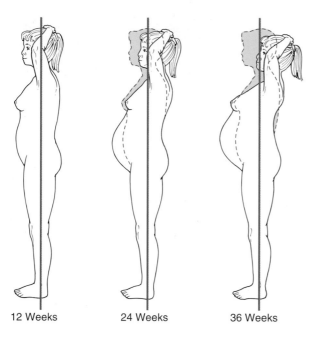

12 Weeks   24 Weeks   36 Weeks

Figure 9.7

Changes in posture during pregnancy. The first figure and the subsequent dotted-line figures represent a woman's posture before growth of the uterus and its contents have affected the centre of gravity. The second and third solid figures show that as the uterus enlarges and the abdomen protrudes, the lumbar lordosis is enhanced and the shoulders slump and move posteriorly.

(Chestnut: Obstetric Anesthesia, 4th ed. 9780323055413; Figure 2.7. Copyright © 2009 Mosby, Inc. Redrawn from Beck AC, Rosenthal AH. Obstetrical Practice. Baltimore, Williams & Wilkins, 1955:146.)

gravity (Figure 9.7). Stretching of the abdominal muscles and laxity of the longitudinal ligaments of the spine further impede neutral posture and place further strain on the paraspinal muscles. The pelvis tilts anteriorly, leading to increased use of the hip extensor and abductor muscles. The woman's stance is widened to maintain trunk movement.

The sacroiliac joints and pubic symphysis widen. The increased mobility of these joints facilitates passage of the fetus through the birth canal. Occasionally marked ligamental softening and widening of the pubic symphysis occur, leading to severe pain and difficulty in walking. Fluid retention may cause compression of nerves in fascial sheaths such as the median nerve in the carpal tunnel and lateral cutaneous nerve of the thigh under the fascia lata, giving rise to paraesthesia and numbness.

REPRODUCTIVE SYSTEM

The uterus develops into the most powerful human muscle at term. Uterine muscle undergoes both hyperplasia and hypertrophy under the influence of oestrogen (Figure 9.8). It increases from 50 g in non-pregnant state to 1000 g at term, with a capacity of 4 mL in non-pregnant state and up to 4000 mL at term.

As the uterus grows it may compress the bladder anteriorly, giving rise to symptoms of urinary frequency. As it further enlarges, it undergoes dextro-rotation, due to presence of the rectosigmoid colon on the left side. This may compress the right ureter and result in renal hydronephrosis, which is usually asymptomatic. From midtrimester, the uterus undergoes irregular painless contractions called Braxton Hicks contractions. They may cause some discomfort late in pregnancy and may account for false labour pain. Uterine blood flow increases progressively and reaches about 500 mL/minute at term. After 12 weeks, the isthmus starts to expand gradually to form the lower uterine segment at term.

In pregnancy the mature breast differentiates into the lactating organ. After the second month the breasts increase in size. The primary areola becomes deeply pigmented. The nipples become larger, deeply pigmented, and more erectile. Montgomery's follicles, which are hypertrophic sebaceous glands, appear as non-pigmented elevations in the primary areola. During the fifth month, a pigmented area called the secondary areola appears around the primary areola.

At the cellular level, the lactogenesis process occurs, whereby the mammary glands develop the ability to produce and secrete milk. As a result of rising levels of oestrogen, progesterone, prolactin, and human somatomammotrophin, the terminal duct lobular units expand and secretory cells begin to differentiate. Prolactin induces the transcription of β-casein and lactalbumin genes. Large numbers of fat droplets accumulate in the alveolar cells. The glandular fluid contains lactose, total protein, and immunoglobulin (Figure 9.9).

After delivery the inhibitory effect of progesterone on prolactin secretion no longer occurs and leads to the production of milk. Maternal insulin, growth hormone, cortisol and parathyroid hormone also play a part in the formation of the colostrum. The continued production and secretion of milk occurs in response to sensory signals from suckling transmitted to the paraventricular and supraoptic

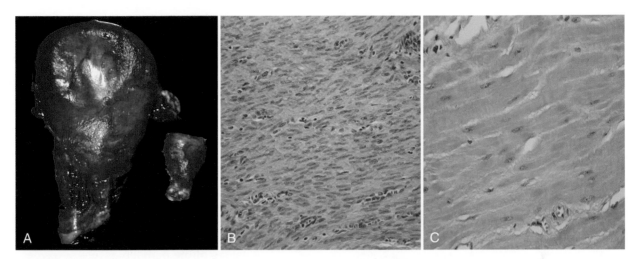

Figure 9.8
Physiological hypertrophy of the uterus during pregnancy. **A**: gross appearance of a normal uterus (right) and a gravid uterus (left) that was removed for postpartum bleeding; **B**: small spindle-shaped uterine smooth muscle cells from a normal uterus. Compare this with **C**: large, plump hypertrophied smooth muscle cells from a gravid uterus (B and C, same magnification).

(Kumar: Robbins and Cotran Pathologic Basis of Disease, Professional Edition, 8th ed. 9781437707922; Figure 1.3. Copyright © 2009 Saunders, An Imprint of Elsevier)

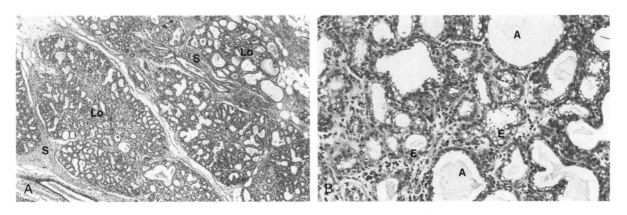

Figure 9.9
Breast during pregnancy. **A**: Haematoxylin and eosin (H & E) stain ×20; **B**: H & E ×100. At low magnification in micrograph A, the breast lobules (Lo) are seen to have enlarged greatly at the expense of the intralobular tissue and interlobar adipose tissue, although septa S of interlobular tissue still remain. At higher magnification in B, the acini (A) are dilated. The lining epithelial cells (E) vary from cuboidal to low columnar and contain cytoplasmic vacuoles. The intralobular stroma is much less prominent and contains an infiltrate of lymphocytes, eosinophils and plasma cells. As pregnancy progresses, the acini begin to secrete a protein-rich fluid called colostrum, the accumulation of which dilates the acinar and duct lumina as seen in micrograph B.

(Young: Wheater's Functional Histology, 5th ed. 9780443068508; Figure 19.39. Copyright © 2006 Elsevier)

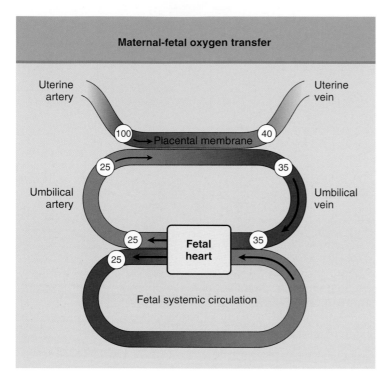

Maternal–fetal oxygen transfer

Uterine artery

Uterine vein

100 → Placental membrane   40

25   35

Umbilical artery

Umbilical vein

25   35

Fetal heart

25

25

Fetal systemic circulation

Figure 9.10

Maternal–fetal oxygen transfer. The circled numbers represent approximate values of the partial pressure of oxygen (mmHg).

(Albert: Clinical Critical Care Medicine, 1st ed. 9780323028448; Figure 59.3. Copyright © 2006 Mosby, An Imprint of Elsevier. Determinants of fetal oxygen. Adapted from Lapinsky SE, Kruczynski K, Slutsky AS. Critical care in the pregnant patient. Am J Respir Crit Care Med 1995;152:427–455.)

nuclei of the hypothalamus. This releases oxytocin from the posterior pituitary and causes myoepithelial cell contraction and milk release.

FETAL PHYSIOLOGY

The functions of the placenta are threefold: gas exchange, nutrition, and waste elimination. The maternal and fetal circulations interact via a concurrent exchange program (Figure 9.10). Oxygen delivery to the placenta and fetus is dependent on the maternal oxygen saturation, haemoglobin concentration and uterine blood flow. Uterine blood flow at term is about 10% of cardiac output (600–700 mL/min) compared with 50 mL/min in the non-pregnant state. The placental membrane allows transfer of oxygen and nutrients. The fetal umbilical vein transports oxygenated blood to the fetal circulation, and the fetal umbilical artery carries deoxygenated blood back to the placenta.

The fetus has several adaptive processes to ensure optimal oxygen extraction from the circulation. The fetus has a higher haemoglobin concentration (15 g/dL) and the fetal haemoglobin is 80–90% saturated at a pO_2 of 30–35 mmHg. This is in contrast to adult haemoglobin, which is only 30% saturated at this pO_2. The fetus achieves this by a leftward shift of the fetal oxygen saturation curve.

The fetus has about 42 mL of oxygen reserves and its oxygen consumption is 20 mL/min.[7] In the face of complete hypoxia in the fetus, only 2 minutes of oxygen reserve would be expected; however the fetus may survive 10 minutes by shunting blood flow to vital organs and decreasing oxygen consumption.

A fetus is considered viable when the gestational age reaches 24 weeks, at which stage the average weight is 750 g. In many Australian tertiary centres, the limit of viability at this gestational age may be as low as 450 g. Gestational age and maturity of the fetal organs, in particular the respiratory system, plays a more important role than birth weight in determining survival without handicap.

REFERENCES

1   Clark SL, Cotton DB, Lee W, Bishop C, et al. Central hemodynamic assessment of normal term pregnancy. Am J Obstet Gynecol 1989;161:1441.

2   Larsson A, Palm M, Hansson L-O, Axelsson O. Reference values for clinical chemistry tests during normal pregnancy. BJOG 2008;115:874.

3   Sullivan EA, Hall B, King JF. Maternal deaths in Australia 2003–2005. Maternal deaths series no. 3. Cat. no. PER 42. Sydney: AIHW National Perinatal Statistics Unit; 2007.

4   McAuliffe F, Kametas N, Costello J, et al. Respiratory function in singleton and twin pregnancy. BJOG 2002;109:765.

5   Templeton M, Pieris-Caldwell I. Gestational diabetes mellitus in Australia, 2005–2006. Cat. no. CVD 44. Canberra: AIHW; 2008.

6   Kalkwarf HJ, Specker BL. Bone mineral changes during pregnancy and lactation. Endocrine 2002;17(1):49.

7   Chesnutt AN, Matthay MA, DiFederico EM. Critical illness in pregnancy. Clin Pulm Med 1998;5(4):240.

MCQS

Select the correct answer.

1   Concerning changes in the cardiovascular system in pregnancy:

    A   the primary cardiovascular change is peripheral vasodilatation.
    B   cardiac output increases by a maximum of 20%.
    C   systemic blood pressure rises in midtrimester.
    D   following delivery there is an immediate fall in cardiac output.
    E   pregnancy reduces the risk of pulmonary oedema.

2   The major physiological change to the haematological system in pregnancy is that:

    A   plasma volume expansion lags behind an increase in red cell mass.
    B   iron supplementation does not affect the haematocrit.
    C   blood viscosity is decreased.
    D   factor VII, X and fibrinogen levels decrease.
    E   the risk of thrombosis is only present in the third trimester.

3   The respiratory system is affected by pregnancy so that:

    A   demand is met by a 20% increase in minute ventilation.
    B   a mild physiological respiratory acidosis is common.
    C   there is a 20% increase in oxygen consumption.
    D   FEV1 is reduced, indicating reduced large airway function.
    E   diaphragmatic function is restricted.

4   The impact of pregnancy on the endocrine system means that:

    A   pregnancy is characterised by increased insulin sensitivity.
    B   in pregnancy fetal demand for calcium occurs at the expense of the maternal skeleton.
    C   prolactin levels are doubled by the third trimester.
    D   hyperthyroidism may occur in the first trimester.
    E   renin–angiotensin activity is reduced.

5   Effects of pregnancy on the gastrointestinal system mean that:

    A   pregnancy predisposes to pulmonary aspiration of gastric contents.
    B   intestinal motility is increased 50% throughout pregnancy.
    C   hyperemesis gravidarum occurs in at least 10% of women.
    D   attention to oral hygiene is irrelevant.
    E   pregnancy is characterised by impaired liver function.

6   Dermatological and musculoskeletal effects of pregnancy include:

    A   diffuse hair loss may occur in late pregnancy.
    B   pruritus without cholestasis may occur in 80% of women.
    C   marked lumbar kyphosis leads to a change in the centre of gravity.
    D   skin hypopigmentation is a common occurrence.
    E   fluid retention may cause nerve compresson in the carpal tunnel.

7   An effect of pregnancy on the reproductive system is that:

   A   uterine blood flow at term reaches 500 mL/min.
   B   relaxin induces uterine muscle hyperplasia and hypertrophy.
   C   uterine laevo-rotation is associated with left renal hydronephrosis.
   D   prolactin secretion is inhibited after delivery.
   E   suckling stimulates oxytocin release from the anterior pituitary.

8   The following is a feature of fetal physiology:

   A   The fetal umbilical vein carries deoxygenated blood to the placenta.
   B   A primary placental function is gas exchange.
   C   Fetal and maternal haemoglobin concentrations are similar.
   D   Fetal oxygen saturation is 30% at a pO_2 of 30–35 mmHg.
   E   Hypoxic selective vasodilatation reduces oxygen consumption.

Chapter 10

Problems in early pregnancy

Thomas G Tait

KEY POINTS

Bleeding per vaginam (PV) in early pregnancy is a common and distressing symptom.

Miscarriage (loss of a pregnancy at less than 20 weeks' gestation) is common.

History, examination, pregnancy test and ultrasound imaging are important for diagnosis of problems in early pregnancy.

Ectopic pregnancy (extrauterine) has the potential to be life-threatening.

Diagnosis of ectopic pregnancy may be challenging. Quantitative serum hCG and ultrasound imaging are the most important diagnostic tools.

Management options for miscarriage and ectopic pregnancy include conservative (observational), medical and surgical.

Emotional support is important for women and families suffering early pregnancy loss.

The most common problem in early pregnancy is bleeding per vaginam. It is emotionally distressing to the woman and family, and warrants careful evaluation. The causes include implantation bleeding, spontaneous miscarriage, ectopic pregnancy, lesions involving the lower genital tract, perineal infections and, rarely, gestational trophoblast disease. This chapter deals with spontaneous miscarriage and ectopic pregnancy.

MISCARRIAGE
Definition and epidemiology

In Australia, a miscarriage is defined as the spontaneous loss of an intrauterine pregnancy before 20 weeks' gestation. This definition may vary in different countries. Miscarriage is now the preferred terminology, rather than abortion, which is reserved for the legal system.

Spontaneous miscarriage occurs in 10–20% of all clinical pregnancies, and perhaps as many as 60% of conceptions are lost. This equates to only a 25% chance of successful pregnancy per ovulation in fertile couples. The incidence of miscarriage for women aged 35–40 years is 21%, and for women over 40 years it is 41%. Eighty per cent of miscarriages are diagnosed between 8 and 12 weeks' gestation. The risk of miscarrying decreases with advancing gestational age (Figure 10.1).

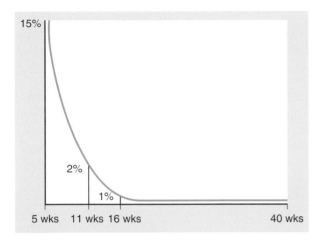

Figure 10.1
Risk of spontaneous miscarriage.

(James High Risk Pregnancy. 4th ed. 2010.)

Missed or delayed miscarriage is the failure to expel the products of conception after death of the embryo.

Recurrent miscarriage refers to three or more consecutive pregnancy losses before 20 weeks of gestation. This affects 1% of couples trying to conceive.[1]

Aetiology and pathophysiology

Most spontaneous miscarriages result from the death of the embryo or the failure of the embryo or placenta to develop normally. This is followed by haemorrhage into the decidua basalis, which causes necrotic changes at the site of placentation. At the same time, there is a fall in oestrogen and progesterone concentrations, causing decidual sloughing. All these changes result in vaginal bleeding and uterine irritability, leading to uterine contractions and expulsion of the products of conception.

As many as 50–60% of embryos miscarried in the first trimester will have a chromosomal abnormality. Autosomal trisomies are the most common, involving chromosomes 13, 16, 18, 21 and 22 in 50–60% of cases, and with karyotype 45XO present in 7% of cases.

Other causes of miscarriage include factors such as age (paternal age greater than 40 years as well as maternal age over 35 years), uterine abnormalities such as bicornuate or subseptate uterus, and an incompetent cervix. Less commonly, thrombophilias, antiphospholipid syndrome, immunological conditions (e.g. systemic lupus erythematosus) and other diseases (e.g. diabetes mellitus and coeliac disease) are associated with miscarriage. Infections (e.g. toxoplasmosis, ureaplasma urealyticum, *Chlamydia*, cytomegalovirus, herpes simplex) and environmental toxins, such as cigarette smoking, high-dose radiation and cytotoxic drugs, have also been implicated.

Diagnosis

The classic clinical presentation is with per vaginam (PV) bleeding and lower abdominal pain.

With *threatened miscarriage*, the typical history is one of vaginal spotting or light bleeding with minimal pelvic or lower back pain. On vaginal examination, the cervix is closed. An ultrasound scan reveals a live intrauterine fetus.

Inevitable miscarriage is characterised by lower abdominal pain and vaginal bleeding. On vaginal examination, the lower uterus appears to be ballooning, while the internal os is closed. The products of conception have not yet been passed.

Incomplete miscarriage presents with a history of increasing bleeding, cramping lower abdominal pain and passage of some products of conception. On vaginal examination, the internal os of the cervix is open and often products of conception are present in the canal.

Septic miscarriage presents with fever, bleeding, and significant tenderness in the lower abdomen and uterus.

In *complete miscarriage*, products of conception are passed and on pelvic examination the cervix is closed. An ultrasound scan reveals an empty uterine cavity.

Missed or delayed miscarriage is often diagnosed when a first-trimester ultrasound scan reveals an absence of embryonic (6–9 weeks) or fetal (>9 weeks) heartbeat (Figure 10.2a; compare the live 7-week embryo shown in Figure 10.2b). Another common finding on ultrasound imaging is an empty sac (formerly known as anembryonic pregnancy or blighted ovum), where the sac size is such that an embryo should be visible (at least 25 mm average diameter; Figure 10.2c). Clinically, the woman loses the symptoms of pregnancy. On examination, the uterus is smaller than expected for length of amenorrhoea and the cervix is closed.

For most women, the diagnosis will be clear following history, examination, urine pregnancy test and transvaginal ultrasound scan. For some, it will be difficult to distinguish between ectopic

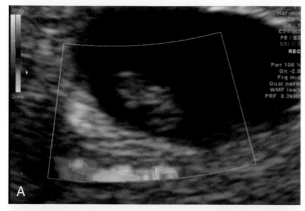

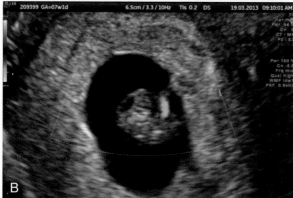

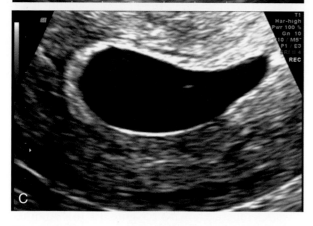

Figure 10.2

A: Transvaginal image of small-for-dates embryo at 8 weeks gestation. Colour Doppler illustrates vascularity only in the myometrium, confirming no embryonic cardiac activity. B: Live 7 week embryo for comparison. C: Large empty gestation sac of >25 mm diameter indicative of missed miscarriage.

(Images courtesy of D Sutton and W Brown.)

pregnancy and early miscarriage, so quantitative estimation of serum β hCG is required in cases occurring early in the first trimester.

Management

Early pregnancy assessment units provide care by a supportive, multidisciplinary team and have been found to improve the quality of outpatient care.[2] Not all women in Australia have access to such units, but care is given along similar guidelines by other health services, particularly in rural and remote areas.

If a live embryo is seen on ultrasound scan and the cervix is closed, the woman is reassured and follow-up is organised. Patients with complete miscarriage may need serum β hCG follow-up.

Surgical evacuation of the uterus with suction curettage was standard treatment until recently. This option may be preferred for patients who have heavy bleeding or who wish to avoid the inconvenience of not knowing when a miscarriage will take place. It is a necessity if haemodynamically unstable or if signs of sepsis are present. Serious complications of surgical evacuation include perforation, cervical tears, intraabdominal trauma, haemorrhage, and intrauterine adhesions (Ashermann's syndrome). All at-risk women undergoing surgical uterine evacuation should be screened for *Chlamydia trachomatis*. Tissue obtained at the time of miscarriage should be examined histologically to confirm products of conception and to exclude ectopic pregnancy and gestational trophoblastic disease.

Expectant management may be a solution for women in the first trimester. In a randomised controlled trial, up to 80% of patients were managed expectantly, but they needed regular follow-up, and some still needed surgical evacuation. This management option is more successful with incomplete miscarriage (94%) than with a missed miscarriage (28%).[2]

Medical evacuation is an accepted alternative using misoprostol (prostaglandin analogue) and/or mifepristone (antiprogesterone).[2] Incomplete miscarriage is usually managed with misoprostol alone. In missed miscarriage, higher doses and longer duration of use may be needed, or priming with antiprogesterone. Success rates are high (85%) but bleeding may continue for 14–21 days after treatment. Patient acceptance of this option has been reported as higher than with the surgical option.

Non-sensitised Rhesus-negative women require 250 IU of anti-D IgG within 72 hours of miscarriage if the gestation period is 12 weeks or less, and 625 IU if bleeding occurs after 12 weeks. There is insufficient evidence to recommend administration of anti-D in threatened miscarriage (ongoing pregnancy) under 12 weeks.[3]

Women with recurrent miscarriages should be referred to specialised services with expertise in dealing with recurrent pregnancy loss. It is reasonable to refer and start investigation after at least two miscarriages under 12 weeks and after one second-trimester loss. After one miscarriage, the risk of another is the same as for the general population. After two miscarriages, the risk is 25% and after three it is 40%. Investigations are undertaken to look for modifiable factors such as thrombophilia, medical disorders, and structural abnormalities.

Cytogenetic analysis should be performed on products of conception of the third and subsequent consecutive miscarriages. Parental karyotyping may identify abnormal chromosome status, and if this is found genetic counselling should be offered to discuss risk to future pregnancies.

Low-dose aspirin, heparin and supportive care are the cornerstones of management. Women with unexplained recurrent miscarriages have an excellent prognosis for future pregnancy outcome without pharmacological intervention if offered supportive care alone in the setting of a dedicated early pregnancy assessment unit.[1]

Cervical incompetence can cause miscarriage of a fetus in the second trimester. Often spontaneous rupture of the membranes occurs, leading to fetal loss. Trauma to the cervix is the most significant risk factor. Diagnosis can be made if an ultrasound shows a characteristic appearance of 'funnelling' of the membranes and shortening of cervical length.

Treatment usually consists of the insertion of a cervical suture, with bed rest and close observation for signs of infection. Transabdominal cervico-isthmic cerclage is sometimes indicated in the management of previous recurrent second-trimester loss and preterm delivery. Occasionally, a woman may be managed conservatively with strict bed rest.

Early pregnancy loss will evoke a range of emotions in different women and can significantly affect women and their families. Women need to be informed of the available support and follow-up. Often the time of presentation is not the appropriate time to counsel, but the woman must be managed with empathy and reassured as far as possible.

ECTOPIC PREGNANCY

An ectopic pregnancy results from implantation of the fertilised ovum (blastocyst) in tissue other than the endometrium of the uterine cavity.

Epidemiology

Ectopic pregnancy remains a major health concern for women of reproductive age, and is a cause of pregnancy-related deaths. It is still the principal cause of maternal death in the first trimester. In developed countries, the incidence of ectopic pregnancy has increased six-fold over the last 20 years, although in recent years there is some evidence of reduction. The incidence of ectopic pregnancy in the general population is 1 in 200; in a high-risk population it can be as high as 1 in 30. With IVF, there is a risk of ectopic and heterotopic pregnancy (coexisting intrauterine and ectopic pregnancies) in 1.4% of pregnant cycles (6.6% of early pregnancy losses in clinical pregnancies).[4]

Sites

The fallopian tube is the most common site for ectopic pregnancy (97%): 70% ampulla, 12% in the isthmus, 11% fimbrial end, 2% interstitial segment (cornual) (Figure 10.3). Other sites include the ovary, cervix, broad ligament, caesarean section scar, and peritoneal cavity.

Pathophysiology of tubal damage

Ectopic pregnancy is believed to be due to endothelial tubal damage secondary to salpingitis, disturbed

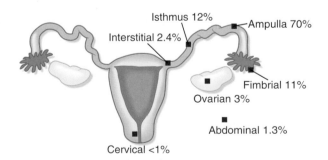

Isthmus 12%
Interstitial 2.4%
Ampulla 70%
Fimbrial 11%
Ovarian 3%
Abdominal 1.3%
Cervical <1%

Figure 10.3
Sites and rate of occurrence at each site of ectopic implantation.

(Adams: Emergency Medicine. 2nd ed. 2012 Saunders; 9781437735482; Figure 119.2)

tubal oocyte transport or proliferation of refluxed endometrial tissue arrested within the fallopian tube. History of salpingitis often cannot be obtained, but histological evidence of previous salpingitis such as deciliation is frequently found.

Risk factors for ectopic pregnancy include sexually transmitted infections, prior ectopic pregnancy, prior tubal surgery including tubal ligation, hormonal factors such as diethylstilbestrol exposure and progestogens, contraceptive failures (e.g. intra-uterine devices), increasing age, and cigarette smoking. Proliferation of refluxed endometrial tissue arrested within a tube could provide the epithelial characteristics of a uterine environment, and this is the pathophysiological explanation involving endometriosis.[5] There is also an increased risk with assisted reproduction techniques (IVF).

Diagnosis

Ectopic pregnancy is frequently misdiagnosed at the initial visit. At present, we rarely see patients who present in shock because of ruptured ectopic pregnancy. The main symptoms are pelvic pain, delayed period or abnormal bleeding. Pain is initially unilateral but it may become more generalised.

On examination, the patient should be assessed for signs of shock, such as pallor, tachycardia and hypotension. On abdominal examination, there might be unilateral or generalised guarding and peritonism. On vaginal examination, there may be bleeding, a closed cervix, a small uterus for gestational age, an adnexal mass (with or without tenderness) and localised tenderness.

Currently, transvaginal ultrasound scan (TVS) and serial β hCG determinations remain the two most important diagnostic tools. The absence of an intrauterine gestation sac on TVS when β hCG is above 1000–1500 IU/mL is strongly associated with ectopic pregnancy. In units with experienced gynaecological ultrasound specialists most ectopic pregnancies will also be visualised.[6] Figure 10.4 shows the characteristic 'doughnut' shape of the ectopic gestation in the fallopian tube.

Clinical findings are associated with a higher probability of ectopic pregnancy, even when β hCG and TVS are below algorithm threshold. In these situations, findings of free fluid in the pouch of Douglas (POD) and adnexal mass on TVS are useful. A β hCG rise of at least 60% over 48 hours and progesterone values over 25 nmol/mL are

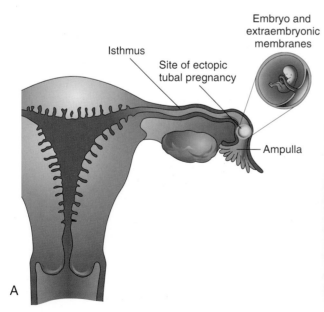
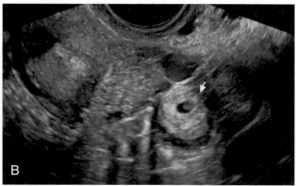

Figure 10.4
A: Coronal section of the uterus and the uterine tube illustrating an ectopic pregnancy in the ampulla of the tube. B: Ectopic tubal pregnancy (6 weeks). The sonogram of the uterine tube (left) shows a small gestational sac (arrow).

(Ultrasound image courtesy of I Peters of Monash Ultrasound for Women.)

predictors of live pregnancy, but do not determine the site of pregnancy. A suboptimal rise of less than 60% in β hCG increases the suspicion of an ectopic pregnancy.

Emergency treatment

When a patient has haemorrhagic shock, she must be operated on as soon as possible by the most expedient method. Open laparotomy may be preferable to laparoscopy, after securing intravenous access and blood for blood group, crossmatch, FBC and β hCG, even before blood and fluid have been replaced.

Management and implications

As diagnosis becomes possible at increasingly earlier gestation, it is possible to observe the ectopic pregnancy when indicated and await natural resolution. The success rate of expectant management is up to 70% in selected cases with low β hCG, no haemoperitoneum and a tubal mass less than 2 cm diameter. Rupture of ectopic pregnancy can still happen, and expectant management has a poor efficiency. Follow-up requires measurement of β hCG until it disappears, which might take up to 50 days. Operation is indicated as soon as there is deterioration in clinical symptoms/signs, or administration of methotrexate if the only change is increasing β hCG.[6]

The most common surgical approach is by laparoscopy (Figure 10.5). Laparoscopy is associated with less blood loss, shorter hospital stay, lower analgesic requirements and quicker postoperative recovery compared with laparotomy. Laparoscopic salpingectomy or salpingostomy can be performed. There is no difference in the intrauterine pregnancy (IUP) rate following these two procedures if the contralateral tube is healthy. Failure to completely remove trophoblast and continuing development of trophoblastic tissue with potential for further intraabdominal bleeding/tubal rupture is possible after conservative surgery. It is therefore important to follow β hCG levels to <5 IU/mL if conservative surgery (e.g. salpingostomy) has been performed. It is reported that recurrent ectopic pregnancy is higher after salpingostomy.[7]

In selected cases — e.g. the asymptomatic patient with no free fluid in POD, small tubal ectopic pregnancy on TVS, absence of fetal heart beat and low serum β hCG (<3500 IU) — it is possible to give methotrexate, an antimetabolite that prevents the

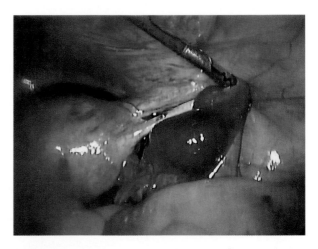

Figure 10.5
Ectopic pregnancy in the right fallopian tube, seen at laparoscopy.

(Lentz: Comprehensive gynecology 6e 2012 Mosby; 9780323069861; Figure 10-13 Ectopic pregnancy in the right fallopian tube. Courtesy of B Beller MD, Eugene, OR.)

growth of rapidly dividing cells by interfering with DNA synthesis. The most widely used medical treatment at present is intramuscular methotrexate given as single dose. Serum β hCG levels are checked on days 4 and 7 and further dose given if β hCG levels fail to fall by >15% between these days. It has been reported that about 14% of patients will require more than one dose and 90% will avoid surgical intervention.[7] These patients require serum β hCG follow-up until it is less than 5 IU. A management algorithm for diagnosis and management of suspected tubal ectopic pregnancy is illustrated in Figure 10.6.

Non-tubal ectopic pregnancies (cervical, ovarian or in the caesarean scar) are rare, and standardisation in diagnosis and management is complex. With the aid of methotrexate, a more conservative approach has recently evolved. Other forms of therapy for cervical pregnancy include embolisation, Foley catheter tamponade and suction curettage.[8]

All non-sensitised Rhesus-negative women should receive 250 IU of anti-D IgG.

Fertility outcomes

If infertility has not been a problem, the rate of IUP following an ectopic pregnancy is 85%, with 7.5% recurrence and 7.5% infertility. Future fertility is unrelated to size of ectopic pregnancy,

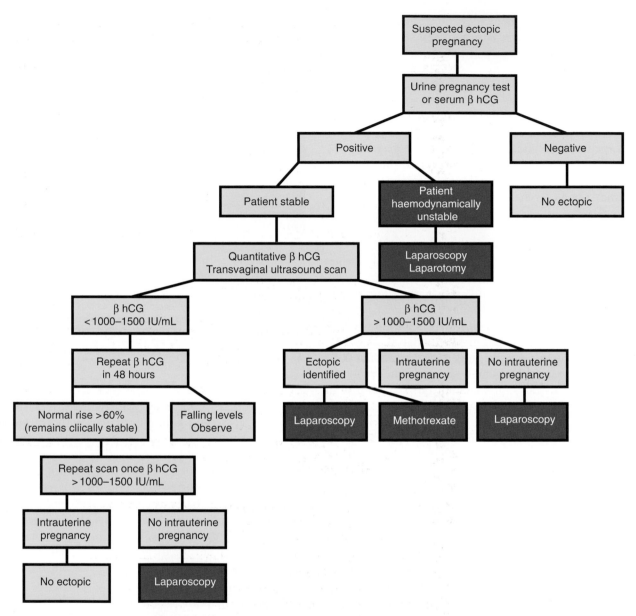

Figure 10.6
Management of suspected ectopic pregnancy.

haemoperitoneum or tubal rupture. It is significantly affected by the presence of periadnexal adhesions. Patients should be advised to have early assessment by transvaginal ultrasound at 5–6 weeks gestation in subsequent pregnancies, to ensure early identification of intrauterine pregnancy.

The patient should be involved in the selection of the most appropriate treatment. She should be reviewed in a follow-up clinic and have appropriate counselling regarding future fertility. Support for the grieving process related to pregnancy loss should be provided if necessary.

REFERENCES

1   Royal College of Obstetricians and Gynaecologists. The investigation and treatment of couples with recurrent first-trimester and second-trimester miscarriage. Guideline No 17, April 2011.

2   Royal College of Obstetricians and Gynaecologists. The management of early pregnancy loss. Guideline No 26, October 2006.

3   National Blood Authority Approved by NHMRC 06 June 2003 Guidelines on the prophylactic use of Rh D immunoglobulin (anti-D) in obstetrics. Online. Available from: www.nba.gov.au/pubs/pdf/glines-anti-d.pdf.

4   Wang YA, Macaldowie A, Hayward I. Assisted Reproductive Technology in Australia and New Zealand. Assisted Reproductive Series No 15, Cat no. PER 51. Canberra: Australian Institute of Women's Health and Welfare; 2009.

5   Hunter RH. Tubal Ectopic Pregnancy: A patho-physiological explanation involving endometriosis. Human Reprod 2002;17(7):1685–91.

6   Condous G. Ectopic pregnancy: challenging accepted management strategies. Aust N Z J Obstet Gynaecol 2009;49(4):346–51.

7   Royal College of Obstetricians and Gynaecologists. The management of tubal pregnancy. Guideline No 21, May 2004, reviewed 2010.

8   Tulandi T, Sammour A. Evidence based management of ectopic pregnancy: Review. Curr Opin Obstet Gynecol 2000;12(4):289–92.

MCQS

Select the correct answer.

1   Which of the following statements is correct?

    A   The risk of miscarriage rises with advancing gestation beyond 10 weeks.
    B   The risk of miscarriage is increased in non-smokers.
    C   The risk of miscarriage is not increased if the fetus has trisomy 21.
    D   The risk of miscarriage rises with increasing maternal and paternal age.
    E   Spontaneous miscarriage occurs in up to 35% of clinical pregnancies.

2   Suction curettage is the indicated/necessary treatment for:

    A   incomplete miscarriage with light bleeding.
    B   heavy bleeding in association with miscarriage.
    C   missed miscarriage with empty gestation sac.
    D   tubal ectopic pregnancy.
    E   threatened miscarriage.

3   The finding of no intrauterine gestation sac on TVS in a woman with positive pregnancy test, light vaginal bleeding and mild lower abdominal pain:

    A   is strongly associated with diagnosis of ectopic pregnancy if β hCG>1500 IU/L.
    B   is strongly associated with diagnosis of ectopic pregnancy if β hCG<1000 IU/L.
    C   is diagnostic of ectopic pregnancy.
    D   confirms complete miscarriage.
    E   excludes an early intrauterine pregnancy.

4   Which of the following statements about ectopic pregnancy is true?

    A   In a subsequent pregnancy diagnostic laparoscopy should be performed early in the pregnancy to exclude another ectopic.
    B   Anti D gamma globulin administration to non-sensitised Rhesus-negative women is not necessary after surgical management.
    D   A normally rising serum β hCG level excludes ectopic pregnancy.
    D   Visualisation of an intrauterine gestation sac excludes an ectopic gestation.
    E   Follow-up β hCG levels are necessary after surgical management by salpingostomy.

OSCE

Joanne, a 23-year-old woman, presents with lower abdominal pain and some per vaginam spotting of dark blood. Her vital signs are normal with pulse rate 85 beats/min, BP 118/70 and temperature 36.8°C. She performed a home urine pregnancy test, which was positive.

What are the important features to be elicited from the history and examination? What further investigations and possible management will be required?

Chapter 11

Antenatal care

Lucy Bowyer and Andrew Bisits

KEY POINTS

Midwives, obstetricians and GPs may provide antenatal care.

Women should be advised to take folic acid periconceptually.

Smoking cessation programs should be encouraged in order to stop smoking in preparation for and during pregnancy.

The average length of pregnancy is 280 days.

Average weight gain in pregnancy is 10–14 kg.

Summary of evidence for antenatal care:

- Women who receive antenatal care have lower perinatal and maternal mortality rates.
- Ultrasound is more effective at providing accurate gestational dating than the last menstrual period.
- Screening for syphilis is cost-effective.
- Folic acid supplementation reduces the incidence of neural tube defects.
- First trimester screening is sensitive for the detection of Down syndrome.
- Antenatal ultrasound detects some fetal anomalies and placental location.

Routine antenatal testing should include:

- full blood count
- blood group and antibodies
- syphilis, hepatitis B, hepatitis C and HIV serology
- rubella immunity
- midstream urine culture.

Ultrasound investigations in pregnancy include:

- first trimester screening at around 12 weeks' gestation
- fetal morphology and placental ultrasound at 18–20 weeks gestation.

Antenatal assessment includes:

- blood pressure measurement
- urine analysis
- fundal height measurement
- fetal lie and presentation
- auscultation of the fetal heart.

The majority of women in Australia and New Zealand entering pregnancy will have antenatal care. A healthy mother and baby is the aim that all who care for pregnant women aspire to, and a large body of evidence has accumulated that shows the environment the fetus grows in is crucial to the future health of the child. It is also true that pregnancy is 'a stress test' for life, and so is an excellent opportunity to improve the health of the woman and unearth potential physical or mental health problems that may occur in the future.

WHO PROVIDES CARE FOR PREGNANT WOMEN?

Around the world, many different models exist for the care of pregnant women during pregnancy, delivery and postpartum. Women in Australia and New Zealand are able to choose from: standard public hospital care; shared care with a general practitioner at a public or private hospital; midwifery group practice; birth centre attached to a hospital; private obstetric consultant care; and home birth. For most women a midwife ('with woman') will look after the woman at some stage during her pregnancy or birth.

The health of the pregnant woman and the nature of her pregnancy play a large part in dictating who cares for the pregnant woman. For example, an older woman with a multiple pregnancy and diabetes is very likely to have a greater involvement with obstetricians than a young healthy woman with a singleton pregnancy.

PRE-CONCEPTION COUNSELLING: HEALTH EDUCATION FOR OPTIMAL PREGNANCY

Pre-conception counselling and antenatal care provide excellent opportunities for improving the health outcomes of women before and during pregnancy. For example, controlled trials have demonstrated that the following interventions lower adverse outcomes for babies and/or improve maternal wellbeing:

- behavioural strategies to stop smoking during pregnancy[1]
- pre- and periconceptual vitamins, particularly folic acid, to prevent neural tube defects[2]
- dietary and insulin management of gestational diabetes.[3]

Such interventions can have a flow-on effect in improving the health of women and their families. For women with chronic medical conditions such as diabetes, epilepsy, hypertension and haematological disorders, pre-conception counselling is always advisable, since optimising the maternal health, and sometimes changing medication prior to pregnancy,

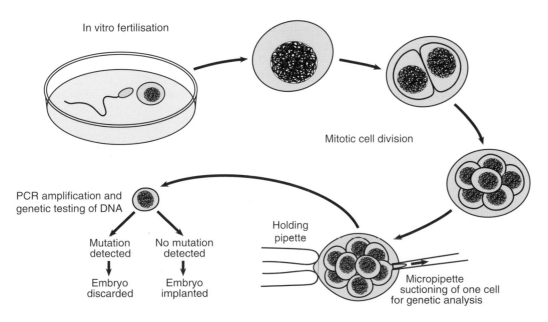

Figure 11.1
Pre-implantation genetic diagnosis.

(Lentz: Comprehensive Gynecology, 6th ed. 9789323069861; Figure 1.8. Courtesy of Edith Cheng MD)

reduces the chances of teratogenesis and poor outcomes for the mother.[4]

Certain genetic conditions require investigation pre-conceptually. For example, if a family carries the mutation for haemophilia, genetic counselling would enable them to decide if they wished to undertake pre-implantation genetic diagnosis (see Figure 11.1). This would mean the couple needs to consider in-vitro fertilisation as part of the process of conceiving.

BOOKING VISIT: THE FIRST ANTENATAL CONSULTATION

It is important that women be given appropriate advice at the beginning of pregnancy about a suitable model of care for their individual needs. Hence the priority of taking an accurate medical and obstetric history (Box 11.1).

The history taken at the booking visit (the woman's first consultation in her pregnancy) will elucidate factors that cannot be altered; such as age, genetic background, ethnicity, social class and previous medical and obstetric history, and those that can; such as body mass index (BMI), smoking and behavioural patterns that are relevant to pregnancy. The history should be followed by an examination (Box 11.2); for most women this will occur in the first trimester of pregnancy. For women who book later in pregnancy the examination will need to include a fetal examination.

The majority of women will have a low-risk pregnancy and are able to choose different models of care for their pregnancy and birth. Women with high-risk medical or obstetric histories should be triaged to hospital care with a consultant obstetrician, and may need to be seen in consultation with other specialists.

Australia and New Zealand are complex, multifaceted societies with many recent migrants. There are groups of women within our society who, for a variety of reasons, will require special consideration when they present for antenatal care. They may be Indigenous or from a non-English-speaking background. They may be very young, depressed, victims of domestic violence, or socially disadvantaged. The history taken at the first antenatal visit should identify any factors that need consideration when providing care for the individual woman so as to enhance her care and her experience of pregnancy.

Dating the pregnancy

The average length of gestation is 280 days, but this varies according to ethnic group, with Caucasian

---

Box 11.1 Taking a medical and obstetric history

The medical and obstetric history includes:

- Date of the first day of the last menstrual period
- Characteristics of the woman's normal menstrual cycle: how many days from one cycle to the next
- Calculation of the expected date of delivery
- Prior contraception
- Date of last Pap smear
- Parity (number of pregnancies proceeding beyond 20 weeks)
- Gravidity (number of any pregnancies)
- History of previous pregnancies including miscarriages, ectopic pregnancies, stillbirths and live births, mode of delivery, gestation, complications, postnatal course
- Breastfeeding history
- Past medical history, including surgical history and response to anaesthesia
- Medications being taken, including vitamins and supplements
- Allergies
- Family history: inherited conditions, parental health, history of the woman's own birth
- Social history: whether with a partner or single, social support situation, employment, smoking, alcohol, recreational drugs.

> **Box 11.2 Examination at booking visit**
>
> - Weight and height, and hence BMI
> - Blood pressure
> - Cardiovascular examination
> - Thyroid examination
> - Breast examination
> - Abdominal examination and if possible auscultation of the fetal heart (usually after the first trimester).

women having longer gestations than Indian or Afro-Caribbean women.[5] Historically the gestational age was always calculated from the first day of the last menstrual period, since most women knew when that occurred, but the actual date of conception was uncertain for many. Nowadays, some women know when they ovulate and so can be more certain of the day of conception. Diagnosis of pregnancy is possible with highly reliable pregnancy test kits, which use a monoclonal antibody to detect the presence (or absence) of the beta subunit of human chorionic gonadotrophin (hCG) and may be positive a few days after the first missed menstrual period. A formal serum assay of hCG levels can confirm ongoing gestation if necessary.

Naegele's rule is still used to calculate the due date: add 280 days to the last menstrual period date. Ultrasound may be used to alter the estimated date of delivery where necessary: the size of embryos (<10 weeks' gestation) is more accurate than the size of fetuses (>10 weeks' gestation), since embryos are more uniform in size than fetuses. Genetic and environmental factors affect the growth of all pregnancies, so altering an expected date of delivery on ultrasound should only occur if the date is more than 5 days different at less than 12 weeks' gestation or greater than 10 days different at between 12 and 20 weeks' gestation.[6]

Minor symptoms and complications

Virtually all women experience some minor complications of pregnancy, and for some women these symptoms can be most distressing. The most common symptoms are urinary frequency, fatigue, nausea, pelvic pressure, insomnia, and lower backache. The most distressing symptoms of the first trimester are usually nausea and vomiting, which may be related to increased hCG and progesterone. These are more severe in multiple pregnancy. Relief measures include frequent small meals, foods low in fat, eating dry carbohydrates before rising, and oral vitamin B1. When nausea and vomiting are severe, the condition is known as hyperemesis gravidarum (see chapter 14) and can lead to significant dehydration if not treated appropriately with rehydration and antiemetic drugs such as metoclopramide and ondansetron.

The principles of management for all minor complications of pregnancy are to exclude more serious underlying pathology, reassure the woman, and provide supportive therapy.

Diet and weight during pregnancy

A small increase in energy requirements occurs during pregnancy (300–500 kJ per day). With the current epidemic of obesity, it is most important to get away from the old-fashioned notion of 'eating for two': in the second trimester the extra energy requirements equate to 200 mL of low-fat yogurt and a couple of plain sweet biscuits. In Australia and New Zealand half of all pregnant women will commence pregnancy overweight. It is not in the maternal or the fetal interest to gain excessive weight, since overweight is clearly linked to poorer pregnancy outcomes such as hypertension and diabetes.[7,8]

The average weight gain in pregnancy is 10–14 kg. Low prepregnancy weight (BMI <18.5) increases the risk of intrauterine growth restriction (IUGR), while excess weight gain during pregnancy is associated with larger infants. During famine, the mean birth weight may fall by 550 g, and similarly women who gain excessive weight are more likely to have macrosomic babies.

Protein requirements increase in the final 12 weeks of pregnancy, with 12 g nitrogen being required for the growth of maternal and fetal tissue. Additional folate, riboflavin and polyunsaturated fatty acids promote fetal wellbeing. A balanced diet rich in fruit and vegetables and containing three serves of dairy products each day is ideal. The fetus accrues calcium into its skeleton from 20 weeks of gestation onwards, so a good calcium intake is important. Vitamin D is required to absorb and metabolise calcium: 90% of vitamin D is absorbed via the action of ultraviolet light on the skin (i.e.

sunshine) and 10% through the diet and so vitamin D deficiency is usually easily corrected by increasing sunlight exposure and oral supplementation.

Teratogenesis, alcohol, smoking and recreational drugs

During the first trimester the embryo/fetus is at its most vulnerable to environmental influences (Figure 11.2). Whether the mother ingests teratogenic substances, has a viral infection or has unmanaged diabetes, the fetus at this stage can potentially sustain critical damage to its development and long-term outcome.

Alcohol is teratogenic, and ingestion of large amounts of alcohol can cause fetal alcohol syndrome. This is characterised by pre- and postnatal growth restriction, dysmorphic facial features, and mental retardation. While there is no known safe level of alcohol intake in pregnancy, ingestion of small amounts of alcohol (e.g. two drinks per week) has not been associated with fetal alcohol syndrome.

An increased frequency of low birth weight infants, prematurity and spontaneous miscarriage are well-documented, dose-related complications of maternal smoking. Other associations include placental abruption, fetal death in utero (FDIU), premature rupture of membranes, and sudden infant death syndrome (SIDS). However, the incidence of congenital anomalies is not increased with maternal smoking.

Since marijuana is frequently used in combination with tobacco, it is difficult to study it independently. Its use in pregnancy may be associated with IUGR, an increased risk of prematurity, and delayed mental development in the newborn.[9]

The most dangerous recreational drugs to use in pregnancy are cocaine and amphetamines. Cocaine and amphetamine use has been linked to maternal medical complications including stroke, seizures, acute myocardial infarction, and arrhythmias. Amphetamines have also been implicated with fetal anomalies created by focal vasospasm, for example cerebral haemorrhage and IUGR, prematurity, spontaneous miscarriage and placental abruption. Furthermore, prenatal exposure to cocaine is associated with necrotising enterocolitis and abnormal behavioural development in the newborn.

Maternal opiate use has been associated with spontaneous abortion, hypoxia, passage of meconium, FDIU and hyperactivity of the newborn.

Babies born to mothers who are opiate users need to be observed after birth for detoxification.

Dental care

There is some evidence that periodontal disease in pregnancy may be a risk factor for preterm delivery and low birth weight.[10] These complications can often be prevented by non-surgical procedures such as professional teeth cleaning to remove plaque and local irritants. Precautions should be taken to avoid invasive dental procedures and reduce any risks associated with the administration of medications or diagnostic radiation. Maintenance of oral health in pregnancy is helped by a diet high in protein, calcium, phosphorus and vitamins A, D and C.

Routine blood and other investigations

Blood tests that are routinely ordered include full blood count (FBC), blood group (ABO and Rhesus), red blood cell antibody screen, and serology for syphilis, hepatitis B, hepatitis C, human immuno-deficiency virus (HIV) and rubella.[11] If these tests identify a problem, they enable treatment to be given to improve outcome. For example, if red blood cell antibodies are detected in the mother's blood during pregnancy, further investigation and appropriate treatment can reduce the effects of Rhesus isoimmunisation (see chapter 12).

A sterile mid-stream urine (MSU) sample is also collected and sent for culture and sensitivity, as asymptomatic urinary tract infection is more common in pregnancy and may lead to pyelonephritis if untreated.

First trimester ultrasound

Fetal imaging with ultrasound in the first trimester is performed to establish gestational age, to investigate vaginal bleeding, or to screen for Down syndrome. High-resolution ultrasound, particularly with a high-frequency transvaginal imaging probe, is able to date the pregnancy accurately (±5 days) and identify the presence of a fetal heartbeat from 6–7 weeks amenorrhoea. This demonstrates a live fetus, whether the pregnancy is intrauterine or ectopic, and shows whether the pregnancy is singleton or multiple (Figure 11.3).

Ultrasound can also be used routinely as a screening test for chromosomal abnormality such as Down syndrome (trisomy 21) by measuring fetal nuchal translucency (see Figure 11.4), together with first-trimester biochemical assay of two hormones:

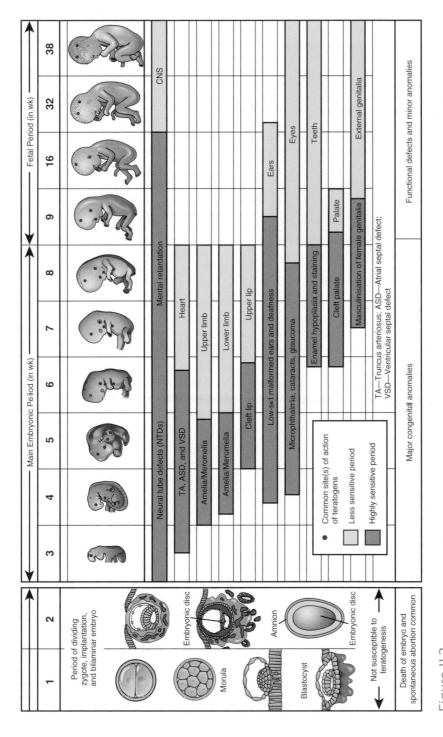

Figure 11.2

Critical periods in human prenatal development.

(Kliegman: Nelson Textbook of Pediatrics, 19th ed. 2011 Saunders; 9781437707557; Figure 6.7. From Moore KL, Persaud TVN: Before we are born: essentials of embryology and birth defects, ed 7, Philadelphia, 2008, Saunders/Elsevier. 9781437720013)

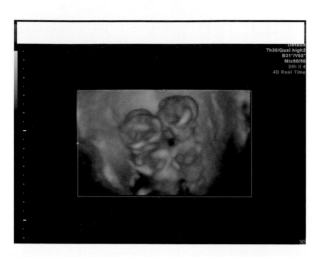

Figure 11.3
3D monochorionic twin pregnancy at 12 weeks' gestation.

(Courtesy of Dr L Bowyer.)

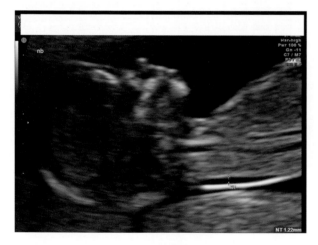

Figure 11.4
Image of nuchal translucency measurement in first trimester.

(Courtesy of Dr L Bowyer.)

free β hCG and pregnancy-associated plasma protein A (PAPP-A). Such a test has an 85–90% detection rate for trisomy 21 (and also for some of the other major chromosomal disorders) and can be used as a population-screening test for women who have been counselled and choose to have this test.[12] Since women are born with all the oocytes they possess to reproduce with, the older the woman the greater the chance of trisomy: aging oocytes are more likely to cause non-disjunction at the time of conception.

Diagnostic tests for karyotype

Chorionic villus sampling at 10–13 weeks involves taking a transvaginal or transabdominal sample, under ultrasound guidance, of chorionic villi for genetic testing to identify chromosomal abnormalities and some hereditary conditions. Amniocentesis is the removal of a sample of amniotic fluid under ultrasound guidance. It is usually performed between 15 and 18 weeks' gestation. It is offered to any woman at increased risk of chromosomal abnormality, for example women over 35 years of age. This procedure carries a 0.5–1% risk of miscarriage.

SECOND TRIMESTER

The second trimester of pregnancy is often a time when the woman is feeling well. Morning sickness has passed and she starts to feel the baby move and to experience the growth of the uterus, but without the later physical limitations of the heavy gravid uterus. She is usually starting to explore what it will be like to be a new mother. She may relate stories she has been told by family and friends about birth and parenting. This can be a frightening as well as joyous time. Each woman's experience will be unique. Her background, culture and social supports strongly influence how she perceives her parenting role.

Antenatal care in the second trimester is based on monitoring maternal health and fetal wellbeing, and providing education and support to the woman and her partner. Care also aims to prevent, identify and manage any obstetric and/or medical problems that arise, including socioeconomic and psychological issues.

Most women will be offered an ultrasound at around 18 weeks' gestation to check the anatomy of the fetus (see Figure 11.5, demonstrating a cleft lip) and the number of fetuses (Figure 11.6), and to confirm the gestational age of the fetus, although after 20 weeks ultrasound is unreliable in confirming gestational age of the pregnancy. Ultrasound is also used to assess fetal wellbeing, for example to check if there is any evidence of delayed fetal growth or other indicators of maternal/fetal compromise (see chapter 12).

In the second trimester, up until 28 weeks' gestation, a woman is recommended to have regular monthly antenatal check-ups with her pregnancy carer (Box 11.3). Randomised controlled trials in developed countries have shown that, in the *low risk* pregnancy, a decrease in antenatal visit frequency is not associated with any negative perinatal outcomes. However, some women feel less satisfied and their expectations of care are not fulfilled.[13]

A comprehensive history taken at the first visit will alert the carer to any problems. At each subsequent visit, the woman is asked about her general wellbeing and fetal activity. Blood pressure is checked — normal blood pressure in pregnancy is accepted as <140/90 mmHg using the phase V Korotkoff sounds (disappearance of sounds).[14] The woman is asked if the baby is moving regularly and often. She is asked to report sudden changes in the fetal activity. In the third trimester, she will feel the baby roll over and kick several times a day.

Symphysis–fundal height (SFH) is measured (see Figure 11.7; generally, fundal height in cm ±3=weeks of gestation). Fetal size, lie (see Figure 11.8), presentation and descent of the presenting part are assessed. Fetal growth is evaluated by comparison with previous SFH measurements. The fetal heart rate is checked with a Pinard stethoscope or Doppler ultrasound.

Urine is tested for proteinuria to screen for infection and preeclampsia. Information about pregnancy and motherhood is provided, and the woman's ability to cope with the transition and her need for social support is assessed. Box 11.4 lists some of the common problems that may arise in the second trimester.

In the mid-second trimester, since 2006, all women in Australia are screened for gestational diabetes using an oral 50 g glucose load (GCT) with measurement of the blood glucose concentration at 1 hour. Women with abnormal glucose tolerance then undergo a full 2-hour formal glucose tolerance assessment. Gestational diabetes has become more common as the populations of Australia and New

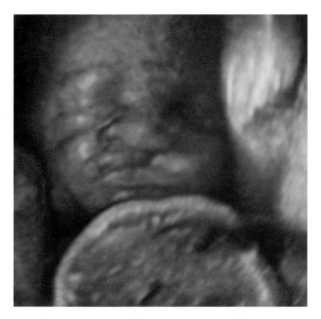

Figure 11.5
Surface-rendered three-dimensional ultrasound image of a 24-week fetus with isolated unilateral left cleft lip.

(In Flint: Cummings Otolaryngology: Head & Neck Surgery, 5th ed. 9780323052832; Figure 186.14. Courtesy of Roya Sohaey MD, Portland, Oregon.)

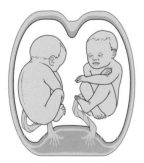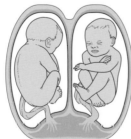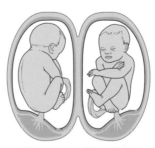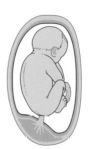

| Monoamniotic Monochorionic | Monochorionic Diamniotic | Dichorionic diamniotic [fused placenta] | Dichorionic diamniotic [separate placenta] |

Figure 11.6
Different types of twinning.

(In Adam: Grainger & Allison's Diagnostic Radiology, 5th ed. 2008 Churchill Livingstone; 9780443101632 Figure 53.8. From Twining P, McHugo J M, Pilling D W (eds.) 2006 Textbook of Fetal Abnormalities, 2nd edition, Churchill Livingstone.)

Box 11.3 Routine antenatal examination

Inspection

- abdominal contour
- operation scars, striae
- pigmentation
- fetal movements

Palpation

- Fundal height: the uterus is first palpable at around 12 weeks' gestation, reaching the umbilicus at 20 weeks. Thereafter SFH rises by 3–4 cm in each 4-week period.
- Fetal lie: using both hands to gently compress the abdomen longitudinally, determine the lie of the long axis of the fetus in the uterus.
- Presentation: using both hands, determine the presenting fetal part and assess descent into the pelvis. The one-hand Pawlic's grip is more uncomfortable for the woman.
- Auscultation: listen to the fetal heart over the area of the fetal shoulder. This area is determined by identifying the position of the fetal back and limbs. The back is felt as a smooth, firm elevation. Fetal limbs are felt by gliding the hands over the surface of the abdomen, seeking the mobile irregularities. The fetal heart is heard directly using a Pinard stethoscope or indirectly using Doppler ultrasound. The normal fetal heart rate is 110–150 bpm.

Box 11.4 Common complications of the second trimester of pregnancy

- Nausea and vomiting (usually resolving by early in the second trimester, but may continue).
- Constipation due to increased progesterone (smooth muscle relaxes in gastrointestinal tract). Relief measures include increasing fluid and fibre intake, exercise, mild laxatives or stool softeners.
- Varicosities due to progesterone-mediated smooth muscle relaxation of the veins, increased blood volume, stasis, and increased pelvic pressure. Relief measures include frequent position changes, elevation of legs, exercise, avoiding lengthy periods of standing, and support stockings.
- Headaches, often worse in those women who have a prepregnancy history of migraine. Consider anaemia, hypoglycaemia. Relief measures include rest, hydration, simple analgesia and cold packs.

Zealand have become more overweight and more indolent. Women who are diagnosed with gestational diabetes are advised to monitor their blood sugar levels through fingerprick testing. They will also receive advice around diet and exercise to achieve normo-glycaemia through the pregnancy. This is an investment in both the woman's and her baby's health. Well-controlled diabetes lessens the incidence of complications at delivery, such as macrosomia, and improves the infant's long-term health, lessening the incidence of diabetes, obesity and hypertension to the child in the future.

At the same time as the glucose challenge, a full blood count should be checked for anaemia. In Rh-negative women, an antibody screen should be performed prior to 28 weeks gestation, and these women should receive 650 IU of anti-D IgG at 28 and 34 weeks if no anti-D has been detected.

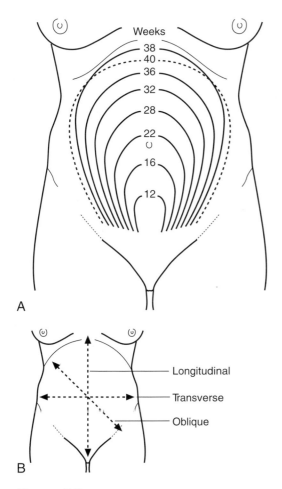

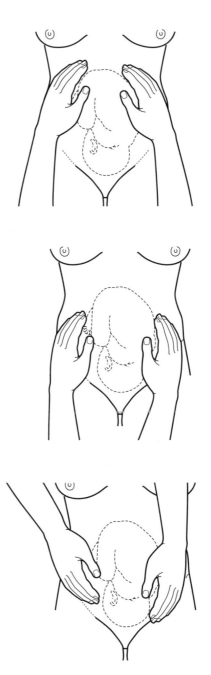

Figure 11.7

A: Progressive increase of fundal height. B: The lie of the baby. This refers to the relationship of the long axis of the fetus to the uterus: longitudinal is normal.

(Based on Hanretty 2003, pp 59, 75)

THIRD TRIMESTER

The third trimester of pregnancy is a time of increasing anticipation about the birth of the baby. It is important that those caring for pregnant women allow adequate space and time for the woman and her partner to voice all their questions in preparation for birth.

The principles of management remain to:

- monitor the progress of pregnancy
- provide advice, reassurance and education about pregnancy, labour and planning for a parenting role, including factors influencing the overall health and wellbeing of women and their families

Figure 11.8

Abdominal palpation.

(Based on Hanretty 2003, p 76)

- identify women at risk of maternal and fetal complications during pregnancy
- manage any obstetric and/or medical problems arising during pregnancy, including socioeconomic and psychological factors.

In the third trimester, antenatal visits will be fortnightly from 28 to 36 weeks, and then weekly to 41 weeks. At each visit, the woman will have the systematic assessment as outlined in the second trimester. The significance of the physical examination becomes more important in the third trimester as delivery approaches (Box 11.5). In particular the lie of the fetus must be assessed (see Figure 11.9).

Blood pressure is of greater significance in the third trimester, because this is when preeclampsia is most likely to occur. The focus of education moves to preparation for labour. One area receiving increasing attention is the prevention and management of major perineal trauma. Pelvic floor exercises antenatally are believed to reduce longer term problems with anal incontinence, stress incontinence and genital prolapse. There is also greater emphasis on assessment of antenatal depression and postnatal depression.

Investigations

Many health centres will perform an FBC at 28 weeks' gestation and an antibody screen at 36 weeks if the woman is Rh-negative. There is no good evidence to support the use of a routine third-trimester

---

Box 11.5 Minor complications of pregnancy in the third trimester

The enlarging uterus can produce the following symptoms:

- gastro-oesophageal reflux due to relaxation of the sphincter. The woman should be advised to eat frequent, small meals, to avoid caffeine and spicy food, and to take antacids if severe.
- increasing difficulty with breathing due to enlargement of the uterus. This can be especially evident at night. Sleeping in a supported lateral position can help.
- oedema and potential median nerve compression, leading to carpal tunnel syndrome. Lower limb oedema is related to peripheral vasodilation, increased blood volume and prolonged standing. Relief measures include wearing support hose and regular exercise. Median nerve compression in the carpal tunnel by oedema may require wrist splints or corticosteroid injection.
- supine hypotension due to aortocaval compression
- postural hypotension due to obstructed venous return from the lower limbs
- urinary frequency due to pressure on the bladder
- loin pain secondary to varying degrees of ureteric obstruction
- back and pelvic pain from the descent of the fetal head and the relaxation of pelvic ligaments. Relief measures include sleeping in the lateral position, massage, heat packs, and pelvic rock exercise.

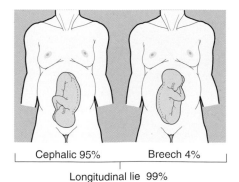

Cephalic 95%   Breech 4%

Longitudinal lie 99%

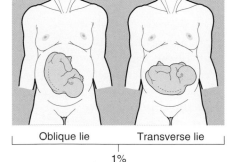

Oblique lie   Transverse lie

1%

Figure 11.9
Fetal lie at term.

(In Ferri: Ferri's Clinical Advisor 2013, 1st ed. 2012 Mosby; 9780323083737; Figure 1.89. Drife J, Magowan B: Clinical obstetrics and gynecology, Philadelphia, 2004, Saunders)

ultrasound scan; this should be done only if fetal growth problems are suspected from the history or examination.

Physiology

Further breast enlargement occurs during the third trimester and colostrum production commences. The uterus contracts irregularly throughout pregnancy, but in the third trimester it contracts more frequently in preparation for the labour. Contractions commence as painless tightenings but become more painful closer to the onset of labour. The cervix undergoes a process of ripening. This involves breakdown of collagen so that with the pressure of the amniotic sac and the presenting part, the cervix assumes a more anterior position in the vagina, becomes shorter (effaces), and dilates. As a result of this, women will notice an increasing amount of discharge or the loss of a discrete mucous plug.

The precise trigger for the onset of labour is not known but the following are important events leading up to it:

- Oestrogen promotes the development of gap junctions between myometrial cells, thus facilitating coordinated contractions in labour
- Oestrogen also promotes the production of prostaglandins from the membranes.
- Another placental hormone, corticotrophin-releasing hormone (CRH), is produced in increasing amounts.
- The action of progesterone is removed, possibly through a change in receptor subtypes.
- Fetal maturation also seems to contribute to the onset of labour.[15]

MULTIPLE PREGNANCY

Twin and higher order multiple (HOM) (triplets, quadruplets and so on) pregnancies have become more common since the advent of routine fertility treatments over the last 20 years. Indeed, as many as one in four pregnancies from IVF result in a multiple birth.[16] While the natural occurrence of twin pregnancy used to be 1 in 80, the incidence seen in a modern Australian population is much greater.

The antenatal care of twins and HOM pregnancies should always include consultation with an obstetrician, and women carrying these pregnancies should be advised to book into a hospital with appropriate neonatal care. Multiple pregnancy per se is a clear risk factor for preterm birth, meaning that women and their families need to be counselled with regard to their individual risk factors and where birth would be most appropriate for them.

Twin pregnancies should be classified by chorionicity

All women with multiple pregnancies will require increased antenatal care. In addition to the increased risks of prematurity, obstetric complications of multiple pregnancy are much more common, including gestational diabetes, gestational hypertension, preeclampsia, placenta praevia, and postpartum haemorrhage.

Antenatal ultrasound surveillance of fetal growth with be required. For uncomplicated dichorionic diamniotic twins, 4-weekly ultrasound surveillance of growth is recommended. For monochorionic diamniotic twins, there is approximately a 15% risk of twin–twin transfusion syndrome and a 30% risk of growth discordance, and therefore fortnightly ultrasound surveillance is recommended. Monoamniotic twins and higher order multiple pregnancies should have care linked in routinely with a maternal fetal medicine department. Figure 11.6 depicts the different categories of chorionicity.

PREPARATION FOR BIRTH

All women will have many questions about the signs of labour, the length of labour, what contractions feel like, pain management options, who will care for them, or other concerns about labour based on their own past experiences or those of others. Every woman should be encouraged and supported to explore the changes occurring in her body and her life during pregnancy, and to prepare for birth and parenthood.

A woman should be advised to stay at home until the contractions are regular and becoming more frequent, for example once every 5 minutes. She should contact her health service when the membranes rupture, or if she is bleeding, experiencing reduced fetal movements, or is feeling distressed.

SOCIAL CONSIDERATIONS DURING THE ANTENATAL PERIOD
Seatbelts

It is a legal requirement that all motor vehicle drivers and passengers, including pregnant women, wear seatbelts. During pregnancy, the lap belt should be worn low under the enlarging abdomen and over both anterior and superior iliac spines and the symphysis pubis. If a shoulder harness is used, the straps should be placed so that they pass diagonally across the body between the breasts. It is important to avoid placing the lap belt over the anterior abdominal wall and the underlying uterus as, should an accident occur, the forward momentum of the uterus against the seatbelt at the time of impact may result in trauma to the uterus. In particular, placental abruption and fetal death may occur.

Air travel

Provided the woman has an uncomplicated pregnancy, there is no reason for restricting air travel prior to 32 weeks gestation for international flights and 36 weeks' gestation for domestic flights. Pregnant women should consult the airline before making arrangements to fly.

Exercise

In the absence of medical or obstetric complications, 30 minutes of moderate exercise a day is recommended for pregnant women. Exercise reduces the incidence of diabetes by producing insulin from the muscle pump. After the first trimester, exercise in the supine position should be avoided to prevent supine hypotension secondary to inferior vena caval occlusion. Contact sports and recreational activity with an increased risk of falling should be avoided.

Occupational work

Evidence suggests that physically demanding work and prolonged standing are associated with preterm birth and reduced birth weight.[17] Shift and night work may also be associated with preterm birth and higher incidences of hypertensive complications of pregnancy. However, long working hours and preterm birth are not associated. Exposure to toxic chemicals and radiation in the work environment is best avoided during pregnancy.

Sexual activity

Variable changes in sexual feelings are normal in pregnancy, ranging from a significant increase to a decrease in desire. Sexual intercourse is not usually contraindicated at any time during normal pregnancy, but it is best avoided when the membranes have ruptured prematurely or when antepartum haemorrhage has occurred, particularly if there is a placenta praevia. In women with threatened miscarriage, it may be wise to advise against sexual intercourse for several days after symptoms and signs have disappeared.

REFERENCES

1 Lumley J, Oliver S, Waters E. Interventions for promoting smoking cessation during pregnancy. Cochrane Database Syst Rev 2001;2.

2 Lumley J, Watson L, Watson M, et al. Periconceptional supplementation with folate and/or multivitamins for preventing neural tube defects. Cochrane Database Syst Rev 2002;1.

3 Crowther CA, Hiller JE, Moss JR, et al. The effect of gestational diabetes mellitus on pregnancy outcomes. N Engl J Med 2005;352:2477–86.

4 NICE Guideline. Antenatal care: routine care for the healthy pregnant woman. London, UK: RCOG Press; 2008.

5 Patel RR, Steer P, Doyle P, et al. Does gestation vary by ethnic group? Int J Epidemiol 2003;33:107–13.

6 Mongelli M, Wilcox MD, Gardosi MD. Estimating the date of confinement: Ultrasonographic biometry versus certain menstrual dates. Am J Obstet and Gynecol 1996;174(1):278–81.

7 Hedderson, MM, Gunderson EP, Ferrara A. Gestational weight gain and risk of gestational diabetes mellitus. Obstet Gynecol 2010;115:597–604.

8 Gardner B, Wardle J, Poston L, et al. Changing diet and physical activity to reduce gestational weight gain: a meta-analysis. Obes Rev 2011;12:e602–e20.

9 Faden VB, Graubard BI. Maternal substance use during pregnancy and developmental outcome at age three. J Subst Abuse 2000;12:329–40.

10 Offenbacher S, Katz V, Fertik G, et al. Periodontal infection as a possible risk factor for preterm low birth weight. J Periodontol 1996;67:1103–13.

11 Connor N, Roberts J, Nicoll A. Strategic options for antenatal screening for syphilis in the United Kingdom: a cost effectiveness analysis. J Med Screen 2000;7:7–13.

12 Spencer K, Spencer CE, Power M, et al. Screening for chromosomal abnormalities in the first trimester using ultrasound and maternal serum biochemistry in a one-stop clinic: a review of three years prospective experience. BJOG 2003;110(3):281–6.

13 Villar J, Carroli G, Khan-Neelofur D, et al. Patterns of routine antenatal care for low-risk pregnancy. 2003. In: Cochrane Database Syst Rev. Online. Available: http://www.update-software.com/cochrane.

14 Brown MA, Hague WM, Higgins J, et al. The detection, investigation and management of hypertension in pregnancy: full consensus statement (Australasian Society for the Study of Hypertension in Pregnancy). Aust N Z J Obstet Gynaecol 2000;40(2):139–55.

15 Challis JRG. Characteristics of parturition. In: Creasy and Resnick, Maternal fetal medicine — principles and practice. Philadelphia: WB Saunders; 2001. p. 691–724.

16 Human Fertilisation & Embryology Authority. Latest UK IVF figures — 2008. London: HFEA; 2011.

17 Berkowitz GS, Papiernik E. Epidemiology of preterm birth. Epidemiologic Reviews 1993;15:414–43.

MCQS

Select the correct answer.

1 Which of the following statements is correct?

   A Behavioural strategies to stop smoking during pregnancy are unsuccessful.
   B Social support during pregnancy prevents preterm labour.
   C Air travel during pregnancy is contraindicated after 28 weeks' gestation.
   D Folic acid supplementation reduces the risk of neural tube defect.
   E Treatment of periodontal disease should be delayed until after parturition.

2 Which of the following blood tests is **not** routinely performed at the first antenatal visit for all women?

   A vitamin C status
   B hepatitis B serology
   C HIV serology
   D full blood count
   E rubella serology

3 Which of the following statements is true?

   A All fetuses with Down syndrome look abnormal on a scan at 18 weeks' gestation.
   B All cases of spina bifida will have an elevated maternal serum alphafetoprotein (MSAFP) blood test result.
   C Most cases of Down syndrome are detectable by first-trimester screening with nuchal translucency ultrasound.
   D A scan at 18 weeks should be done only on women who are at high risk of fetal malformations.
   E Amniocentesis can detect the vast majority of fetal malformations.

4 With respect to screening tests in the second trimester, which of the following statements is correct?

   A Measurement of the symphysis–fundal height is not a screening test.
   B Screening for gestational diabetes is not carried out in the second trimester.
   C An Rh-negative woman in whom no anti-D was detected in the first trimester does not need to be tested for anti-D antibodies at 28 weeks.
   D Umbilical artery Doppler evaluation is a useful screening tool for intrauterine growth restriction.
   E The 18–20 week ultrasound is aimed to detect fetal morphological abnormalities.

OSCE

You are a general practitioner. Anne is 30 years old and is trying to get pregnant. She has regular menstrual cycles. She has type 1 diabetes and comes to you for advice. What factors do you want to know about her and how will you advise her?

Chapter 12

Fetal growth and development

Alec Welsh

KEY POINTS

Pregnancy should be accurately dated by a combination of dating from the menstrual cycle and by ultrasound.

Small for gestational age describes a fetus that is suspected of having a fetal weight below the 10th centile for gestational age.

Large for gestational age is a fetus who is suspected of having a fetal weight above the 90th centile for gestation.

Clinical examination and ultrasound are the main tools used to monitor fetal growth.

Rhesus isoimmunisation can occur where a woman with a Rhesus(D)-negative blood group carries a fetus with a Rhesus-positive blood group.

THE PLACENTA AND ITS EMBRYOLOGY

Far from being a simple passive barrier, the placenta is a highly active organ. It is responsible for:

- transport of nutrients to and elimination of waste products from the fetus by a variety of methods
- supply of oxygen and removal of carbon dioxide as the respiratory organ for the fetus
- production of a number of key hormones that regulate the mother's response to the pregnancy and the environment for the fetus.

The importance of the placenta is highlighted by the fact that, embryologically, at the morula stage, one-third of cells form the inner cell mass from which the embryo arises, and two-thirds form the trophoectoderm from which the placenta develops. A normal pregnancy relies upon optimal placental development and compensatory responses of the placenta to any exogenous insults. The quality of placental implantation is the major determinant of fetal growth and wellbeing, and depends on multiple genetic and epigenetic, maternal, fetal, and environmental factors.

The human placenta is described as haemochorial, meaning that maternal blood bathes the placental trophoblast cells. By day 18–20 fetal capillaries grow into developing placental villi at the same time as maternal spiral arteries penetrate the basal plate to open into intervillous spaces. Between these two circulations is the outer lining of the placenta, which is made up of syncytiotrophoblast cells that form a single barrier or syncytium. As the placenta implants into the endometrium it does so in two waves, with placental cells invading and lining maternal spiral artery walls so that they lose their muscular lining and convert the spiral arterial tree into channels with a low resistance to flow, thereby facilitating a high-volume smooth blood supply from the mother. Failure to implant normally may result in the later development of intrauterine growth restriction in the fetus or preeclampsia in the mother.

EVALUATION OF FETAL GROWTH AND WELLBEING

Each fetus has its own normal anticipated pattern of growth, dependent upon a number of

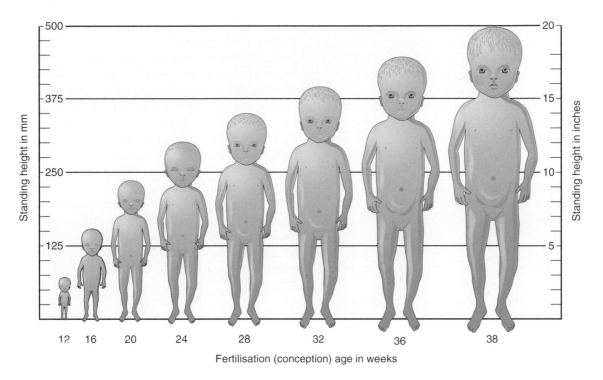

Figure 12.1
Evaluation of fetal growth and wellbeing.

constitutional, ethnic and genetic factors. The majority of fetuses will achieve their potential and will be healthy and well-grown (Figure 12.1).

Reduced fetal growth for any reason may mean an increase in perinatal mortality and morbidity as well as cardiovascular, developmental and endocrine consequences for the child. Increased fetal growth is associated with an increase in the risk of stillbirth and also in labour dystocia. The in-utero environment plays a major role in the health of that individual into their adult life. This role was initially described over 20 years ago as the Barker hypothesis after one of its main proponents, then later as 'fetal programming', and now as the 'developmental origins of health and disease' (DOHAD). Each fetus is intended to experience a certain level of nutrition throughout its development in-utero and in the early neonatal period (particularly for those born prematurely). Those that are undernourished in-utero are prone to cardiovascular disease and a number of associated features that together have been described as the 'syndrome X' features.

Methods for establishing gestational age and their accuracy

Without accurate knowledge of the true gestational age it is impossible to comment on whether a fetus is growing appropriately. It would be most accurate to know the precise timing of intercourse and conception, though in many cases this is unknown. An exception to this is pregnancies resulting from IVF where date of implantation and age of embryo are known exactly.

The estimated date of delivery (EDD) is determined as 280 days from the first day of the last period (LMP). The typical menstrual cycle lasts 28 days with ovulation around day 14, though this may not be precisely the case even with a regular cycle. Conception may occur within a 4–5 day window around ovulation. Naegele's rule states that the EDD may be calculated by adding 7 days to the first day of the LMP and subtracting 3 months. Ovulation tracking by ultrasound, basal body temperature measurement or luteinising hormone levels may help to pinpoint ovulation, though it has been shown that more than 50% of pregnancies are unintended so by default the LMP is often used as the dating method.

Inaccuracies may exist in LMP dating due to cycle irregularity, inaccurate recall by the woman, bleeding that simulates light menstruation, breastfeeding, and recent use of oral contraceptives.

While a regular 28-day cycle with known ovulation on day 14 may provide a clearly accurate EDD, it has been shown that *first trimester* ultrasound examination of the fetus is most accurate for dating the pregnancy. As pregnancy progresses the range of fetal size diverges, reducing the accuracy of ultrasound dating. In early pregnancy the crown–rump length is most commonly used to date pregnancy. It has an accuracy of ±5 days. If the LMP is relatively certain, and the ultrasound dates are within this range, then the LMP is kept to calculate the EDD. If outside of this range then the dates are calculated based upon the ultrasound. In early pregnancy transvaginal sonography is more accurate as the probe is directly adjacent to the cervix and uterus.

The toolkit for assessment of fetal wellbeing

Methods for evaluation of fetal wellbeing include:
- fetal movements
- maternal symphysio-fundal height (SFH)
- ultrasonography: growth; amniotic fluid; blood flows; structures; movements
- infection screen, chromosomal evaluation
- cardiotocography.

Fetal movement

A healthy well fetus will move well every day, whether general body movements, isolated limb movements, breathing or hiccupping. The maternal perception of movements is one of the simplest, clinically useful but frequently overlooked methods of fetal surveillance. Generally a woman perceives fetal movements from around 20 weeks' gestation in a first pregnancy, and earlier in a second or subsequent pregnancy. Up to 50% of women who experience a stillbirth have a reduction in fetal movements in the days before intrauterine death. An unhealthy fetus will rest to conserve energy.

Reduction in fetal movements is a frequent cause for presentation to delivery suites (up to 15% of pregnancies). Such presentations should be encouraged, in order to detect the rare cases of fetuses truly at risk. Perception of fetal activity, as well as being individual, decreases near full-term from 17% to 7% of the time. Differing fetal behavioural states mean that movement is intermittent and periods of quiescence are normal, though these do not generally exceed 2 hours. A presentation with reduced fetal movement requires further history-taking, examination and investigation, including cardiotocography and ultrasound.

Assessment of maternal symphysio-fundal height

Between 20 weeks when the uterine fundus is at the level of the umbilicus and 38 weeks when the uterine fundus is at the xiphisternum, the SFH is generally equal in centimetres to the number of weeks of gestation ±3 cm. A measurement outside this range is taken to be abnormal, requiring ultrasound investigation. The sensitivity of routine SFH assessment for restricted growth is only approximately 40%, with a high false-positive rate. Suspicion of a small or large fetus is more likely *not* to be confirmed, so the overall tone of counselling should be one of reassurance. Measurement of the SFH is charted on the maternity record and may be compared between visits.

Ultrasound

Ultrasound may be used to measure with some accuracy the size of the fetal structures, the amount of fluid around the fetus, the blood flows within, to and from the fetus, the fetal anatomy, and fetal body and breathing movements. Fetal biometry refers to measurement of fetal size using anatomically defined planes. The most commonly used measurements are the femur length (FL), biparietal diameter (BPD), head circumference (HC), and abdominal circumference (HC).

To estimate growth, one of many formulae is applied to these measurements to generate an estimated fetal weight (EFW). These formulae assume certain proportions and density and have been shown to have an accuracy of ±10–15%, though less so for very small or very big babies.

Individual measurements may be plotted against population. Most fetuses have relative symmetry and so the centiles such as AC and HC should be approximately equal. If they are not then the growth is described as asymmetrical, most notably when there is asymmetrical growth restriction (described later this chapter).

The main aim of plotting fetal centiles for measurement is to detect the truly small or large fetus. Each fetus has its own projected normal growth pattern, however, so universal application of a single growth chart may result in a significant false positive screening rate (and consequent maternal anxiety). In order to overcome this, customised ultrasound centile charts have been proposed. These take into account factors such as sex, maternal weight, height, ethnicity, and parity.

It is important to evaluate the fetus carefully for any signs suggestive of infection, chromosomal or genetic syndromic abnormality, as these will influence fetal growth and may be useful for a diagnosis. Examples include calcifications, microcephaly or cataracts seen with in-utero cytomegalovirus infection, or atrioventricular cardiac septal defects seen in Down syndrome.

Amniotic fluid volume

Up to 16 weeks gestation, much of the amniotic fluid comes from placental exudate. After this stage, most of the amniotic fluid is fetal urine. In later pregnancy, the healthy fetus passes urine continually, breathes fluid in and out (with a net outflow of lung fluid), and swallows the fluid. A reduction in amniotic fluid volume (oligohydramnios) is the result of ruptured membranes or reduced fetal urine output. An increase in amniotic fluid volume (polyhydramnios) is a result of a fetal inability to swallow or an excess in production, for example polyuria from diabetes.

Blood flows

Doppler ultrasound uses the alteration in frequency that occurs when an ultrasound wave hits a moving particle, much the same as the change in pitch from an ambulance siren as it approaches and then goes away. The change in frequency detects movement, which is primarily blood flow. When pulsatile vessels such as arteries are scanned it is possible to show the fluctuation of flow with the cardiac cycle. This fluctuation allows measurement of ratios of flow between systole and diastole. A number of blood vessels in the uteroplacental environment can be used in the comprehensive evaluation of fetal wellbeing (Figure 12.2).

UMBILICAL ARTERIES

The umbilical arteries (UmAs) take blood from the fetus to the placenta. Their waveform shows the balance between the strength of cardiac activity and the placental resistance. Normally the placental resistance is low and the cardiac activity is strong, so there is good flow in diastole. If the placenta is suboptimal or there is cardiac impairment, the resistance increases, eventually leading to either absent or even reversed blood flow in diastole.

MIDDLE CEREBRAL ARTERY

The middle cerebral artery (MCA) supplies blood to the fetal brain from the Circle of Willis. It usually has a high resistance to flow. In the presence of fetal hypoxia this vessel dilates to supply more blood to the fetal brain, so it reduces its resistance.

DUCTUS VENOSUS

The ductus venosus (DV) arises from the intrahepatic vein after it returns from the umbilical artery. It directs blood away from the fetal liver to the inferior vena cava and channels this highly oxygenated blood towards the fetal heart and brain. It has a characteristic double pulsation in its waveform. In the presence of fetal hypoxia this vessel can dilate dramatically to bypass the liver and send highly oxygenated blood via the inferior vena cava into the right atrium and then through the foramen ovale to the left side of the heart and the fetal brain.

UTERINE ARTERIES

The uterine arteries (UtAs) represent the maternal perfusion of the uterus and respond to placental implantation. In early pregnancy the uteroplacental circulation (spiral arteries and arterioles) have a muscular lining giving a high resistance to flow and a muscular recoil or 'notch' to blood flow. Normal placental implantation results in removal of the muscular lining by syncytiotrophoblast cells so the resistance reduces and the 'notch' disappears. Evaluation of these vessels after 23 weeks can therefore give a good indication of normality of placental implantation and may act as a screen for later uteroplacental insufficiency (manifesting as IUGR or preeclampsia).

Karyotype, infection and results of screening tests

As well as considering the relevant presentation, history and examination before interpreting any ultrasound, it is important to consider any relevant investigations that may have been performed, most importantly chromosomal assessment (karyotyping) or estimation of risk for chromosomal abnormality (aneuploidy) such as first-trimester screening with nuchal translucency and placental protein evaluation. An abnormal karyotype may be the reason for the abnormality in growth. For example fetuses with trisomy 21 (Down syndrome) are usually smaller than average.

Various bacterial or viral infections can affect fetal growth and development. These include rubella, cytomegalovirus, herpes, varicella, toxoplasmosis, syphilis and listeria, and are covered in

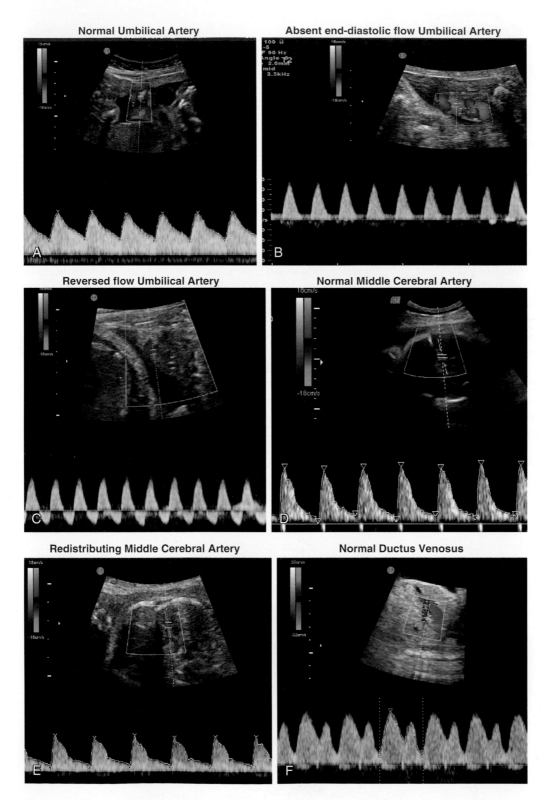

Figure 12.2
Blood flow waveforms.

(Images courtesy of GE Healthcare and acquired with Voluson™)

chapter 13. When investigating abnormal fetal growth, the presence of infection in the pregnancy must be considered.

THE SMALL FETUS

Measurement of the fundal height as 4 cm or more less than anticipated labels a fetus as 'clinically small-for-dates'. In fact most of these babies are of normal size but ultrasound confirmation is warranted. The fetus is labelled small when the estimation of the fetal weight on ultrasound is below the 5th or 10th percentile for gestation. Choice of centile for definition influences sensitivity and specificity for babies that are truly small and at risk of perinatal compromise. Four potential reasons why a fetus may be small are outlined below. If the fetus is small and there is evidence that it is failing to reach its true growth potential, then it is showing signs of *intrauterine growth restriction* (IUGR).

Causes of small babies may be extrinsic to the fetus (e.g. maternal disease or hypertension, smoking, drug use or abuse, or fetal infection), or intrinsic to the fetus (e.g. fetal abnormality including genetic or chromosomal).

Normal small

This fetus is following along its own centile, which is where it is genetically or ethnically meant to be. Clues may be that the parents are slight or from a smaller ethnic group, have had previously small healthy babies, or may have small feet. Ultrasound should show a structurally normal symmetrically small fetus, amniotic fluid and Dopplers. There is no cause for concern.

Incorrectly diagnosed small

This fetus has mistakenly been labelled as small as the dates are wrong. In fact the fetus is simply earlier in gestation than anticipated. Clues may be that the LMP is uncertain (such as conception following oral contraceptive use, or after breastfeeding), and there may not have been an ultrasound to confirm dates early in pregnancy. Once the mistake in dating is certain, a new EDD should be generated. As with the normal small fetus, ultrasound will show a symmetrically small biophysically well fetus that grows along its centile.

Abnormal small

This fetus is small because unfortunately it has a problem such as a chromosomal or structural abnormality or genetic syndrome, or more rarely has been damaged by an infection or external agent such as a drug exposure. Clues may be an abnormal karyotype result or high risk for aneuploidy on previous screening. Ultrasound will show the fetus to be symmetrically small or asymmetrically small. Amniotic fluid volume may be normal, reduced or increased. Dopplers are most likely to be normal. There may be structural abnormalities detected on ultrasound. Management needs to be tailored to the underlying cause for the abnormality.

Starved small

This is the fetus that has intrauterine growth restriction (IUGR) (see Figure 12.3). This fetus has not realised its true growth (centile) potential and may need to be delivered early. Note the terminology is *restriction* and not *retardation*, a term previously used but which is highly stigmatising to parents. In the vast majority of cases IUGR is not associated with neurodevelopmental delay.

Commonly IUGR results from uteroplacental insufficiency, with the placenta being poorly implanted. There may be underlying maternal conditions that are responsible for this, including diabetes, hypertension, vascular disease or a number of coagulopathies. In most cases, however, there are no

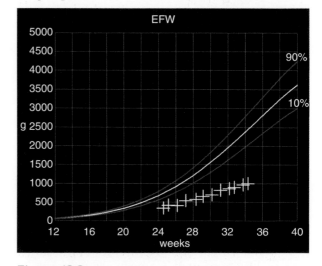

Figure 12.3
Profound IUGR presenting at 24½ weeks' gestation. Chromosomally and structurally normal fetus. Serial growth scans are shown. Eventual decision for delivery at 34 weeks' gestation with an estimated fetal weight of 1000 g. Delivery of a live healthy male infant who has had no significant compromise in early childhood life.

(Images courtesy of GE Healthcare and acquired with Voluson™)

clear causes. A first pregnancy is most commonly affected.

Less commonly, if the IUGR commenced in early gestation then the growth is likely to be symmetrical. If the onset was in later gestation, the growth is likely to be asymmetrical (i.e. HC>AC). This reflects the fact that the fetus conserves as much nutrition as it can to preserve the brain, at the expense of peripheral organs and storage in the liver (the source of the AC).

There is a relatively well known pattern of Doppler changes in the uteroplacental IUGR fetus. The UmA often shows increased resistance from the placenta as an early change. The MCA may show reduced resistance as the baby diverts blood with nutrients and oxygen to the brain. The DV may show signs of dilatation as it diverts blood away from the liver. Careful monitoring of these vessels along with other signs of fetal wellbeing allows timing of delivery to be optimised.

These cases must be closely monitored with careful timing of delivery to avoid stillbirth.

Management

Management for the growth-restricted fetus may be conservative or active. Administration of maternal corticosteroids has been shown to significantly reduce the risk of neonatal death, intraventricular haemorrhage and necrotising enterocolitis.

Decision for delivery needs to be based upon both the maternal and fetal condition. For example, in the case of preeclampsia delivery may be indicated to preserve the maternal health regardless of gestation. In the majority of cases, the main factor influencing outcome for the small fetus is that of gestational age at birth, followed by the birth weight, sex (female fetuses fare better than male), and other factors such as structural anomalies, infections, perinatal trauma, and neonatal complications.

Neonatal facilities are stratified between different hospitals, with specialised care for the extreme preterm baby available only in major tertiary institutions. Diagnosis of IUGR may allow transfer to one of these units for ongoing management and delivery, as neonatal outcomes are significantly better with in-utero transfer than with ex-utero 'retrieval'.

Many fetuses near full term with IUGR can be successfully delivered vaginally. They require continuous electronic fetal monitoring (CTG) in labour as contractions of the uterus may cause fetal hypoxia and acidaemia. At very early gestations caesarean delivery is recommended as the very small, very early fetus will almost certainly not tolerate the impact of labour.

Unfortunately there is no treatment for uteroplacental insufficiency. There is no evidence to support strategies such as prolonged bed rest or high-protein diets. The placenta is a relatively defined active barrier, and maternal nutrition and hydration do not significantly influence fetal nutrition or hydration.

LARGE-FOR-DATES FETUS

The vast majority of large babies are healthy normal large babies. Like the small-for-dates fetus, the large fetus may not in fact be truly large (wrong dates), may be constitutionally large, or pathologically large. The constitutionally large fetus may be suspected by being symmetrically large, structurally normal, and in some cases of the parents having a previous history of large babies being born or with the parental weights being large at birth.

There are fewer cases of pathologically large babies than pathologically small, so the approach to counselling is more reassuring. One of the few intrinsic pathological causes is Beckwith–Wiedemann, which is associated with an increased liver size, large tongue, and mid-face hypoplasia. The prognosis for this condition is good. The most common extrinisic pathological cause for the large fetus is diabetes, whether preexisting or gestational (Figure 12.4). Screening should be performed by glucose challenge or tolerance testing.

As with the clinically small-for-dates fetus, ultrasound is used to clarify whether the fetus is genuinely large. If so (>90th or >95th percentile), then it is again useful to evaluate the symmetry of the fetus. If there has been excessive deposition of glycogen, then the abdomen will be relatively large secondary to a large liver, and the AC centile will be much greater than the HC. A constitutionally large fetus will be symmetrically large.

The influence of diabetes on the fetus has been summarised by the Pederson hypothesis: maternal hyperglycaemia is reflected by fetal hyperglycaemia and consequent hyperinsulinaemia as the fetus has intact pancreatic islet cell function (Figure 12.5). The hyperosmolar state in the fetus creates polyuria and increased amniotic fluid. This is often the presenting feature that causes the uterus to measure large-for-dates. Insulin acts as a growth hormone in the fetus causing overall growth, as well as the deposition of a large amount of glycogen in the liver that causes a disproportionately large AC. After birth neonatal

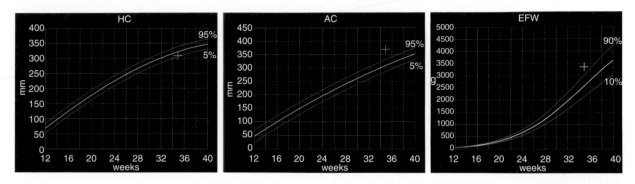

Figure 12.4
Ultrasound of the clinically large-for-dates fetus with diabetes showing an appropriate sized head circumference (HC) but a disproportionately enlarged abdominal circumference (AC) that contributes to an overall increased estimated fetal weight (EFW).

(Images courtesy of GE Healthcare and acquired with Voluson™)

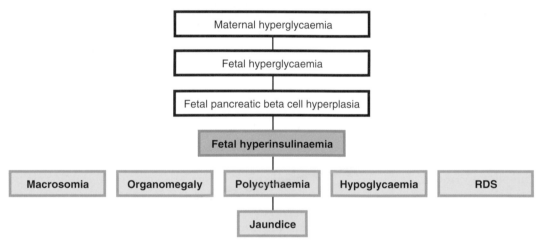

Figure 12.5
The Pederson hypothesis.

(Image courtesy of author)

hypoglycaemia and respiratory distress syndrome are common in infants of diabetic mothers.

There is no current evidence to support a routine policy of induction of labour for the large fetus, as the increase in fetal circumferences with advancing gestation is balanced against cervical favourability and accommodation of the perineum and pelvic floor. In extreme cases where the fetus is >97%, is asymmetrically large and there is maternal diabetes, consideration may be given to delivery by caesarean section due to the risk of shoulder dystocia.

FETAL WELLBEING IN LATE PREGNANCY AND LABOUR

Fortunately stillbirth remains rare, with an incidence of 4–60 per 1000 worldwide and 3.5 per 1000 in recent Australian statistics. However it still occurs, and it frequently happens in the absence of any identifiable risk factors. Conditions known to be associated with fetal compromise include maternal infection, medical conditions such as hypertension, diabetes and autoimmune disease, and therapeutic or illicit drug administration.

In labour the fetus may be considered as being subject to an additional 'stress'. It is generally felt that this stress is beneficial, with a positive influence on the hypothalamic–pituitary–adrenal axis, as well as benefits on absorption of lung fluid with a reduction in respiratory distress and transient tachypnoea of the newborn. However the 'stress' of labour, in some cases, may result in true fetal compromise or 'distress', and this stress may reduce oxygen supply to the fetus and create fetal hypoxia.

During both pregnancy and labour the fetus aims always to conserve oxygen and glucose for the brain. When the oxygen supply is reduced the fetus will preferentially stream oxygenation to the brain, sometimes known as redistribution. If the fetus becomes truly hypoxic, it streams blood preferentially to the brain, heart, placenta and adrenals but not to its peripheries. As a result there is an increase in peripheral anaerobic metabolism. Instead of generating carbon dioxide this generates lactic acid. The fetus then becomes progressively acidaemic, and it is a combination of hypoxaemia and acidaemia that can cause fetal damage. Control of acid–base balance in the fetus is summarised, as in the adult, in the Henderson–Hasselbalch equation, with the newly generated acid being buffered to maintain a normal pH. While carbon dioxide can be blown off after birth, lactic acid crosses the placenta only slowly, and so, after a period of buffering, the pH will drop.

Monitoring fetal wellbeing

Principal methods of evaluating fetal wellbeing in late pregnancy and labour are:
- fetal heart monitoring including cardiotocography
- fetal movement evaluation
- ultrasound
- fetal blood sampling in labour.

Fetal heart monitoring and fetal scalp sampling

Along with routine examination of the mother and abdominal palpation, it is mandatory to monitor the fetal heart rate at each antenatal visit and for it to be monitored in labour.

In the low-risk situation, it is sufficient to intermittently auscultate the fetal heart in labour. There is evidence that over-reliance on the CTG results in an increase in intervention with no appreciable improvement in outcome. A perfectly normal fetal heart rate at full term should be in the range of 110–160 bpm with variability of 5–25 bpm, some accelerations of 15 bpm for 15 seconds (usually in response to movement), and no decelerations (Box 12.1). Other patterns need to be carefully evaluated in context, including presence or absence of labour, associated risk factors, and gestation and clinical history.

The CTG was introduced as a tool to monitor the fetal heart rate in labour, with the assumption that this would reduce the incidence of cerebral palsy, which was believed to be mostly attributable

Table 12.1 Normal ranges for scalp and cord blood sampling

Parameter	Range
Fetal scalp pH	7.25–7.35 normal 7.21–7.25 pre-acidaemia <7.21 acidaemia
Cord pH	7.25–7.45 arterial 7.18–7.38 venous
Base excess	<–8 mmol/L
Scalp lactate	<4.2 mmol/L normal 4.2–4.8 mmol/L pre-acidaemia >4.8 mmol/L acidaemia

to intrapartum asphyxia. Unlike modern diagnostic tools, CTG was introduced after demonstration of changes in the heart rate in animal models, but no randomised controlled trials were ever used to demonstrate its validity. Nearly 40 years later, the CTG is almost ubiquitous, the rate of cerebral palsy remains constant, and obstetric intervention in labour has increased. At the same time, there is a strong medicolegal reliance upon the CTG as a predictive or diagnostic tool, such that it will be impossible to abandon its use until a proven tool emerges. Many minor alterations in the CTG are of no functional significance, but there are clear features that do indicate likely fetal hypoxia and if these are overlooked there may be significant harm to the fetus.

Reassurance of fetal wellbeing or confirmation of the fetus at risk can be performed by looking at a capillary sample taken from the fetal scalp. Use of fetal scalp sampling reduces the need for caesarean delivery (increasing the true positive rate for screening). See Table 12.1.

HYPOXIC–ISCHAEMIC ENCEPHALOPATHY

When labour does not go well, the fetal brain may be damaged by hypoxia (reduced oxygen supply) or ischaemia (reduced blood supply), causing hypoxic–ischaemic encephalopathy (HIE). This affects approximately 1–4 per 1000 births. Severe asphyxia may cause acute encephalopathy in a previously normal brain. It is important to remember that severe asphyxia will affect the whole fetus and not just the brain, so other organs such as the gut and

---

Box 12.1 CTG descriptive features and normal ranges

Baseline

Mean fetal heart rate (FHR) when stable, determined over 5–10 minutes. Higher in the preterm fetus. Normal range 110–160 beats per minute (bpm). Bradycardia ≤110. Tachycardia ≥160.

Baseline variability

Minor fluctuations in baseline FHR, the bpm between highest peak and lowest trough in 1-minute segments. Normal 5–25 bpm; reduced 3–5 bpm; absent <3; increased >25 bpm.

Accelerations

Transient increases in FHR of ≥15 bpm above the baseline for ≥15 seconds.

Decelerations

Transient decreases in FHR of ≥15 bpm below the baseline for ≥15 seconds.

EARLY

Uniform, repetitive, slow onset early in contraction, returning to baseline by end of the contraction.

VARIABLE

Repetitive or intermittent. Rapid onset and recovery, variable relationship with the contraction, most commonly simultaneously with contractions.

COMPLICATED VARIABLE

Has features that may increase the likelihood of hypoxia: rising baseline or tachycardia; reducing baseline variable; slow return to baseline; large amplitude (by 60 bpm or to 60 bpm) and/or long (60 seconds); loss of brief increases in FHR before or after (shouldering); temporary increase in baseline afterwards.

PROLONGED

≥15 bpm for longer than 90 seconds but less than 5 minutes.

LATE

Uniform, repetitive, usually slow onset at middle to end of contraction, lowest point >20 seconds after peak and ending after the contraction.

Adapted from RANZCOG Guidelines on Intrapartum Fetal Surveillance 2nd ed. 2006.

cardiac function will also be impaired. The damage caused to the brain by HIE and consequent neuronal cell death occurs in two phases. The first phase is primary cell death, followed by secondary or delayed cell death between 8 and 72 hours of age. Major neurological and developmental deficits in the infant and young child can result from hypoxic–ischaemic injury to the brain.

A diagnosis of HIE requires knowledge that there has been true hypoxia or acidaemia. Neonatally, HIE is graded from mild to severe to allow an estimation of prognosis (Box 12.2). Fortunately the prognosis for mild and moderate HIE is good, most commonly with no long-term sequelae. Severe HIE with EEG changes and seizures has a poorer neuro-developmental prognosis.

There is now strong evidence that cerebral hypothermia has a protective effect for the baby at risk or showing signs of HIE, so current treatment in the neonatal nursery includes either head or whole body cooling as well as respiratory and cardiovascular support. Other treatment strategies have included use of glutamate, which is felt to be neuroprotective, though this remains experimental.

> ## Box 12.2 Grading of hypoxic-ischaemic encephalopathy
>
> ### Mild
>
> Increased muscle tone, brisk reflexes. Transiently abnormal behaviour such as poor feeding, irritability or excessive crying. Normal by 3–4 days.
>
> ### Moderate
>
> Lethargy and hypotonia, diminished reflexes. Possible apnoeic periods and seizures in the first 24 hours of life. Full recovery in 1–2 weeks may occur and is associated with better long-term outcome.
>
> ### Severe
>
> Stupor or coma. Irregular breathing, hypotonia, absent neonatal reflexes. Disturbed ocular motion, pupils may be dilated, fixed or poorly reactive. Early seizures that may not respond well to conventional treatment. Multi-organ dysfunction may occur (cardiac, respiratory, renal, hepatic, haematological, neurological).

CEREBRAL PALSY

Cerebral palsy (CP) is a term used to cover a broad range of non-progressive brain lesions involving motor or postural abnormalities that are noted during early development. Its incidence is approximately 2 per 1000 live births. It may be further classified by the type of motor disorder (spastic, athetotic, dyskinetic, ataxic or mixed), distribution (hemiplegia, diplegia or quadriplegia), or the severity. Spasticity may be gradual in onset and abnormal movements may not appear until up to 18 months of age. In the majority of cases, higher cerebral function is well-maintained despite a variety of handicapping elements.

Up to 80–90% of cases of CP are now known to be associated with intrauterine events prior to the onset of labour. These causes include:
- infections in pregnancy
- thyroid abnormalities
- complications of multiple pregnancy
- antepartum haemorrhage
- prematurity
- growth restriction
- chromosomal, syndromic or metabolic abnormalities in the fetus
- coagulation disorders.

Less than 10% of cases are likely to be caused by true intrapartum hypoxia, and an equal number are likely to be related to events postpartum.

PERINATAL MORTALITY

Perinatal mortality is a composite of stillbirths and neonatal deaths. As care is perinatal (i.e. decisions are frequently made by obstetricians and neonatologists regarding timing of birth), it is a useful overall statistic for outcome of pregnancy. Common causes include prematurity and fetal anomaly.

Stillbirth is defined in Australia as 'the complete expulsion or extraction from its mother of a product of conception of at least 20 weeks gestation or 400 grams birth weight who did not, at any time after birth, breathe, or show any evidence of life such as a heartbeat'.

Neonatal death is defined in Australia as 'the death of a liveborn infant within 28 days of birth'.

Australia is fortunate to have one of the lowest international perinatal mortality rates, between 8 and 9 per 1000. Of these approximately 70% are stillbirths and 30% are neonatal deaths. Rates are significantly higher among the Indigenous population (up to 12–18 per 1000). Internationally, in 2000 the WHO reported perinatal mortality rates of approximately 60 per 1000 in Africa and 50 per 1000 in Asia. The most common recorded cause for perinatal death is congenital abnormality (20–25%). Other common reported causes include perinatal infection, hypertension, antepartum haemorrhage, maternal disease, specific perinatal conditions, hypoxia, IUGR, and prematurity.

RHESUS ISOIMMUNISATION

Approximately 17% of Caucasians are negative for the Rh(D) antigen and are termed Rhesus-negative (Rh(D)-negative). This blood type is rare in people of Asian or Australian Aboriginal origin. Rh(D) positive individuals may be heterozygous or homozygous for the D antigen. A heterozygous father has a 50% chance of passing on the D antigen. If a woman is Rh(D)-negative and her partner is heterozygous, each fetus has a 50% chance of being Rh(D) positive or Rh(D) negative.

More than 40 different red cell antigens have been reported to cause haemolytic disease of the fetus/newborn (HDN). However, only anti-Rh(D), anti-Rh(c) and anti-Kell cause serious fetal problems. Other antibodies (Rh E, C, e), Duffy (Fya), Kidd (Jka) and Lutheran (Lua) are common but usually cause only mild to moderate HDN.

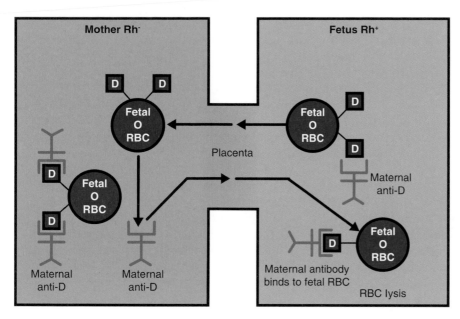

Figure 12.6
Mechanism of Rhesus isoimmunisation secondary to fetal red cells entering into maternal circulation.

(From Gilbert Barness: Potters Pathology of the Fetus, Infant and Child. 2nd Ed. 9780323034036; Figure 291.5)

Pathophysiology

During pregnancy, fetal cells may cross the placenta and enter the maternal circulation, exposing the mother to 'foreign' red cell antigens that the fetus has inherited from the father. This fetomaternal haemorrhage (FMH) is most likely to occur at delivery (60% of pregnancies), but may also occur spontaneously during pregnancy and in association with threatened or complete miscarriage, after trauma and after invasive procedures such as amniocentesis, chorionic villus sampling (CVS), external cephalic version (ECV) or abruptio placentae.

Exposure to foreign fetal red-cell antigens may result in the development of maternal antibody (Figure 12.6). Development of isoimmunisation depends on a number of factors, including the antigenicity of the antigen, the dose of antigen to which the mother is exposed and the responsiveness of her immune system, and ABO compatibility between the mother and the fetus. Rh(D) is the most immunogenic of the red-cell antigens. A single pregnancy with an Rh(D)-positive, ABO-compatible fetus initiates immunisation in about 1 in 6 Rh(D)-negative women.

Antibodies of the immunoglobulin G (IgG) class are actively transferred from mother to fetus. The amount of antibody transferred is small in the first 12 weeks of pregnancy, increases slowly between 12 and 24 weeks, and thereafter increases exponentially until term. HDN occurs when the life span of the infant's red cells is shortened by the action of a specific antibody derived from the mother by placental transfer. Antibody-coated red cells are removed from the circulation by the fetal liver and spleen, leading to anaemia.

In mild cases of HDN, the fetus may be born without major clinical problems, and simple postnatal observation of the infant may be all that is required. In other cases, phototherapy or an exchange transfusion may be required for severe hyperbilirubinaemia. Early onset of severe disease may result in fetal anaemia in utero, which leads to increased extramedullary erythropoeisis (enlarged liver and spleen), cardiac decompensation and hydrops fetalis (so-called immune hydrops) with ascites, pleural and pericardial effusions, and polyhydramnios. Untreated, this usually results in fetal death. The effect on the fetus of isoimmunisation usually increases in severity with subsequent pregnancies.

Investigations

The presence of red cell antibodies in maternal blood is detected by an indirect antiglobulin test (IAT). Antibody levels are monitored by either titration or quantitation. Once the titre exceeds 1 in 16, investigations are instituted to determine if the fetus is affected.

Pre-formed antibodies detected at the booking visit may have developed during another pregnancy (a miscarriage, termination of pregnancy or ectopic pregnancy). They may also have occurred as a result of a blood transfusion (rare in Australia) or after sharing needles (in injecting drug users). As red-cell antigens do not form until approximately 6 weeks' gestation, it is unlikely that a maternal immune response would be evoked this early in a first pregnancy. Where antibodies are detected very early in the pregnancy, antibody titres should be repeated after 20 weeks' gestation.

Fetal haemoglobin concentration may be measured by cordocentesis: fetal blood sampling from the umbilical cord. However, since this invasive procedure is associated with a significant risk to the fetus (1–2% chance of fetal loss), a variety of indirect measurements of severity are also used. In particular the peak systolic flow in the middle cerebral artery reflects anaemia: the faster the flow, the more anaemic the fetus. Liver length, spleen perimeter and flow velocity changes in other fetal vessels have also been used to detect fetal anaemia. If cordocentesis confirms anaemia, then an intrauterine transfusion can be performed. Intrauterine transfusions are usually stopped around 34 weeks' gestation and the fetus delivered at 36–37 weeks. In less severe disease, where the maternal blood titres do not rise above 1 in 16, delivery is usually planned after 37 weeks' gestation.

Prevention of Rhesus isoimmunisation

Since the mid-1960s, there has been considerable success in preventing Rh(D) immunisation in Rh(D)-negative women. The principle of prevention is that of passive immunisation. Rh(D)-negative women are given an injection of anti-D antibody at a time when it is likely that fetal cells may have entered the maternal circulation. The injected anti-D antibody binds to any Rh(D)-positive fetal cells present in the maternal circulation, allowing these cells to be rapidly cleared by the maternal liver and spleen before an immune response can take place.

Anti-D is given to Rh(D)-negative women who have no pre-formed antibody in the following circumstances during pregnancy:

- threatened or spontaneous miscarriage, invasive procedures, trauma, placental abruption (increased risk of FMH)
- routinely at 28 and 34 weeks' gestation
- routinely at delivery if the baby is Rh(D)-positive.

The dose of anti-D given must be sufficient to remove all fetal cells from the maternal circulation. The Kleihauer–Betke test, which identifies fetal cells in maternal blood, is used to determine the volume of FMH and thus the dose of anti-D that should be administered after sensitising events in the second and third trimester and after delivery. Anti-D immunoglobulin should be given as close to the sensitising event as possible, and within 72 hours. Administration of Rh(D) immunoglobulin to all Rh(D)-negative women who have not developed anti-D antibodies at 28 and 34 weeks' gestation and after each sensitising event reduces the development of sensitisation to less than 0.2% (NHMRC 1999).

REFERENCES AND FURTHER READING

1   Wiberg-Itzel E, Lipponer C, Norman M, et al. Determination of pH or lactate in fetal scalp blood in management of intrapartum fetal distress: randomised controlled multicentre trial. BMJ 2008;336(7656):1284–7.

2   Fenlady V, MacPhail J, Gardener G, et al. Detection and management of decreased fetal movements in Australia and New Zealand: A survey of obstetric practice. Aust N Z J Obstetr Gynaecol 2009;49:358–63.

3   Neonatal and Perinatal Mortality 2004. Country, Regional and Global Estimates. World Health Organization. Accessed February 2012: http://www.who.int/reproductivehealth/publications/monitoring/9789241596145/en/index.html.

4   Burton GJ, Fowden AL. Review: The placenta and developmental programming: Balancing fetal nutrient demands with maternal resource allocation. Placenta 2012;33(Suppl):S23–7. doi: 10.1016/j.placenta.2011.11.013.

5   Himmelman K, Ahlin K, Jacobsson B, et al. Risk factors for cerebral palsy in children born at term. Acta Obstet Gynecol Scand 2011;90:1070–81.

6   Mahendru AA, Lees CC. Is intrapartum fetal blood sampling a gold standard diagnostic tool for fetal distress? Eur J Obstet Gynecol Reprod Biol 2011;156:137–9.

7   Nyberg DA, Abuhamad A, Ville Y. Ultrasound assessment of abnormal fetal growth. Seminars in Perinatology 2004;28(1):3–22.

8   Intrapartum Fetal Surveillance. Clinical Guidelines – Second Edition. Royal Australian and New Zealand College of Obstetricians and Gynaecologists. Accessible through www.ranzcog.org.au.

9   NHMRC. Guidelines on the prophylactic use of Rh D immunoglobulin (Anti-D) in obstetrics. Main Report. Canberra: National Health and Medical Research Council; 1999.

MCQS

Select the correct answer.

1   A 42-year-old woman presents at 34 weeks' gestation in her first pregnancy. Her pregnancy appears clinically small for dates. Which of the following is correct?

    A   She is at risk of preeclampsia.
    B   Diabetes is a likely cause.
    C   She should be advised that the fetus should be delivered as there is a risk of death from intrauterine growth retardation.
    D   She will have to have a caesarean section.
    E   Ultrasound is inaccurate in detecting fetal growth.

2   A 35-year-old woman with diabetes mellitus is at **significant** risk of having:

    A   a growth-restricted fetus.
    B   a traumatic delivery associated with shoulder dystocia.
    C   a fetus that succumbs to intrauterine asphyxia.
    D   a macrosomic fetus.
    E   Rhesus disease.

3   Which of the following is correct in the assessment of fetal wellbeing?

    A   Isolated abnormal fetal umbilical artery Doppler resistance reliably predicts a hypoxaemic fetus.
    B   Amniotic fluid volume reflects uterine perfusion and the processes of fetal swallowing, fetal breathing and renal function.
    C   A fetus with a normal cardiotocograph is likely to be acidotic.
    D   The use of fetal scalp sampling for acid-base status in labour has been associated with an increase in caesarean section rates.
    E   All of the above.

OSCE

Ping Yin, aged 27, comes for a 30-week antenatal visit. She is highly anxious since all her friends and family have told her she looks small and must have a small baby. How do you approach the consultation and what examination would you perform?

Chapter 13

Infections in pregnancy

Amanda Henry

KEY POINTS

Infections in pregnancy may have severe consequences to the mother, baby or both.

Infections causing teratogenesis include:

- rubella
- cytomegalovirus
- varicella
- parvovirus B19
- toxoplasmosis
- syphilis.

Infections causing maternal illness, miscarriage or serious damage to the neonate include:

- listeria
- group B streptococcus
- herpes simplex
- hepatitis B
- hepatitis C
- HIV
- any infection leading to chorioamnionitis.

Infections in pregnancy may have their major effects on the mother, the fetus, or both. In general, any maternal infection leading to sepsis or grave maternal illness can harm the fetus, and influenza

and urinary tract infections are discussed as examples. There are also a number of infections that usually have a mild maternal clinical presentation, but may have severe effects on fetal development, growth and wellbeing, for example rubella or cytomegalovirus (CMV) (Table 13.1). Lastly, maternal infections such as HIV, where perinatal transmission and chronic health consequences may occur, are discussed.

SERIOUS MATERNAL INFECTION WITH FETAL CONSEQUENCES

Influenza

Epidemiology and pathophysiology

Approximately 10% of pregnant women have serological evidence of exposure to seasonal influenza.[1] Influenza is an RNA virus, where mutation and reassortment of genes leads to both seasonal changes and, on occasion, epidemics. Pregnant women are more likely to be severely affected by influenza than the general population, probably secondary to physiological changes in pregnancy such as increased oxygen consumption and decreased lung capacity.

Clinical presentation

Similar to the non-pregnant population, including fever, cough, rhinorrhoea, sore throat, headache, shortness of breath, and myalgia.

Diagnosis

Initially clinical to allow prompt use of antiviral treatment. Confirmatory laboratory tests are

Table 13.1 Fetal susceptibility to damage during development

Time period	Susceptibility	Events
0–2 weeks	High rate of lethality Usually not sensitive to damage ('all or nothing' effect)	From fertilisation to complete implantation of blastocyst in endometrial stroma Uteroplacental circulation established
3–8 weeks	Organogenesis Time of greatest susceptibility Each organ has susceptibility window	Embryonic development in a cephalocaudal fashion. Susceptibility starts with eyes and brain, then moves towards lower limbs Agents causing serious defects include viral infections, alcohol, maternal diabetes, medications
9–40 weeks	Functional maturation Susceptibility decreases	Fetal development can be affected by agents such as alcohol or cigarette products Effects depend on dose and duration of exposure

available, but take 24–48 hours, and rapid tests are not yet sufficiently reliable.[2]

Management and outcomes

Pregnant women are more likely to be hospitalised with influenza-like illness during influenza season, and are more likely to die during influenza epidemics, than those in the general population.[1,3] Early antiviral therapy with neuraminidase inhibitors after symptom onset lowers this risk, and should be standard management along with supportive care including antipyretics.

Influenza virus is probably not directly teratogenic, but untreated associated fever may, however, increase the risk of birth defects such as neural tube defects. There is some association with an increased risk of miscarriage, preterm delivery, low birth weight, and birth of a small-for-gestational age infant.

Influenza vaccination is **safe** for use during pregnancy and it is recommended for all pregnant women. In addition to protective maternal effects during pregnancy, the risk of influenza in the first six months of life is decreased by approximately two-thirds in infants whose mothers were vaccinated during pregnancy.[4]

Urinary tract infection

Epidemiology and pathophysiology

Five per cent of pregnant women have asymptomatic bacteriuria, similar to the rate in non-pregnant women. If untreated, up to 30% will develop pyelonephritis, a much higher incidence than outside of pregnancy.[5] Untreated urinary tract infection (UTI) is associated with miscarriage, premature labour, low birth weight, and perinatal mortality.[5]

Urinary tract infections are more common in women than in men, with the shorter female urethral length increasing the rate of bacterial contamination of the bladder with sexual activity. In pregnancy, high levels of progesterone and relaxin, plus ureteric compression by the uterus, lead to decreased ureteric muscle tone and peristalsis, altered bladder tone and increased bladder capacity, increasing the risk of ascending infection. Eighty per cent of UTIs are due to *Escherichia coli*; other pathogens include group B streptococcus (GBS) and gram-negative bacteria.[5]

Clinical presentation

As in the non-pregnant population, UTI symptoms include frequency, dysuria, urgency and nocturia. Pyelonephritis features include fever, nausea/vomiting, and costovertebral angle and suprapubic tenderness. Premature labour may occur.

Diagnosis

The definition of a urinary tract infection is a pure growth of bacteria (at least 10^5 bacterial colonies per mL) in a midstream or catheter specimen of urine. Positive leucocytes and nitrites on urinalysis are suspicious but **not** diagnostic of UTI. However if clinical features of pyelonephritis are present, antibiotics should be commenced while awaiting culture results. Large numbers of epithelial cells on microscopy indicates a contaminated specimen, and the test should be repeated.

Management and outcomes

First-trimester urine culture is recommended in all pregnant women. Antibiotic treatment of asymptomatic bacteriuria in pregnancy has been found to reduce bacteriuria rates, pyelonephritis, and low birth weight.[5] Treatment for 5 days with cephalexin, nitrofurantoin or amoxicillin clavulanate is recommended.[6]

The optimal duration of antibiotic therapy for symptomatic UTI in pregnancy is unknown, and antibiotic guidelines should be followed.[6] Pregnant women presenting with a severe febrile illness and possible septicaemia should be treated with intravenous cephalosporin.[6] Oral therapy should not replace intravenous until the woman has been afebrile for at least 24 hours, and the total antibiotic course should continue for 10–14 days. Urine should be re-cultured 1 week after the initial antibiotic course is finished.

Screening and treatment of asymptomatic bacteriuria decreases but does not eliminate the risk of bacteriuria or pyelonephritis, so urine culture should be repeated every trimester for those with bacteriuria and monthly for those with symptomatic UTI or pyelonephritis. Recurrent infections make prophylaxis appropriate, with nightly nitrofurantoin or cephalexin for the remainder of the pregnancy.

MATERNAL INFECTION WITH DIRECT FETAL CONSEQUENCES (MALFORMATION AND/OR NEONATAL ILLNESS)

A number of viral infections have a (usually) mild clinical picture in the mother, but may lead to malformation syndromes and/or severe neonatal illness.

Serologic testing usually involves paired samples, that is samples taken at exposure/clinical suspicion and 2–3 weeks later, looking for seroconversion. If booking serology from early pregnancy is available (Australian laboratories keep antenatal serology for 12 months when adequate serum is collected), this can be used as a baseline comparator.

Other infections discussed in this section (HSV, GBS, chorioamnionitis) do not cause malformation but may lead to severe neonatal illness.

Pathways for transmission of perinatal infection are shown in Figure 13.1.

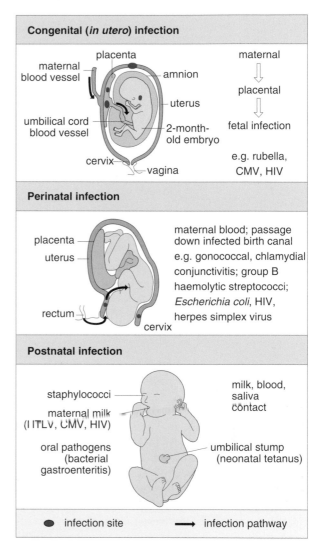

Figure 13.1
Pathways for transmission of perinatal infection.

(Goering: Mims' Medical Microbiology, 5th ed. 2012 Saunders; 9780723436010; Figure 23.4)

Rubella
Epidemiology and pathophysiology

Rubella is a ribonucleic acid (RNA) virus. It is highly teratogenic if maternal viraemia occurs in the first trimester of pregnancy, when there is a greater than 80% risk of transplacental fetal infection leading to miscarriage or congenital rubella syndrome (CRS). The spectrum of CRS defects is shown in Figure 13.2 and includes vision loss, hearing loss, cardiac defects, intellectual disability and behavioural abnormalities. In weeks 13–15

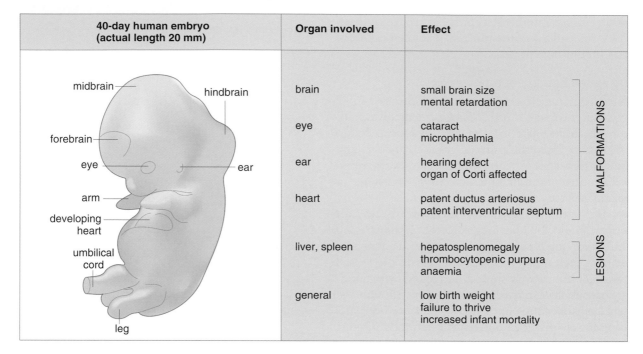

40-day human embryo (actual length 20 mm)	Organ involved	Effect	
	brain	small brain size mental retardation	MALFORMATIONS
	eye	cataract microphthalmia	
	ear	hearing defect organ of Corti affected	
	heart	patent ductus arteriosus patent interventricular septum	
	liver, spleen	hepatosplenomegaly thrombocytopenic purpura anaemia	LESIONS
	general	low birth weight failure to thrive increased infant mortality	

Figure 13.2
Congenital rubella syndrome.

(Goering: Mims' Medical Microbiology, 5th ed. 2012 Saunders; 9780723436010; Figure 23.1)

approximately half of infants will be *infected*, and one-third of these will be *affected*, usually with deafness alone.[7] Infection from 16 weeks may result in growth restriction but does *not* cause CRS.

As rubella is vaccine-preventable, congenital rubella syndrome is now very rare in countries with comprehensive vaccine programs (universal childhood vaccination with booster in adulthood).

Clinical presentation

Mild febrile maternal illness with a fleeting rash 14–21 days after exposure, however 25–50% of cases are asymptomatic. Serious maternal complications such as encephalitis are rare. If serological diagnosis of infection in early pregnancy is not made on first-trimester screening, the first clinical manifestation may be an infant born with CRS.

Management and outcomes

Pre-existing immunity is checked at booking antenatal serology. Any non-immune woman with clinical symptoms or history of exposure to rubella virus in pregnancy should have paired rubella IgM and IgG testing 14–21 days apart (IgM rises 7–10 days after primary infection). Interpretation of serology

results is shown in Figure 13.3. There is no effective post-exposure prophylaxis.

If maternal rubella infection is confirmed in the first 12 weeks of pregnancy, termination of pregnancy should be offered due to the high likelihood of fetal infection and the severe consequences of CRS. Confirmed infection at 13–15 weeks has a 15–20% chance of an affected fetus. If maternal infection is documented as occurring from 16 weeks, surveillance of fetal growth should occur.

Women who are non-immune on prepregnancy screening should be offered vaccination and advised to wait one month before getting pregnant, as the vaccine is live attenuated virus. However, there have been *no* cases of CRS after inadvertent rubella vaccination in the first trimester of pregnancy, and any woman in this situation should be reassured. Women non-immune to rubella on antenatal screening should be offered postpartum immunisation, which is safe. (Breastfeeding is not a contraindication.)

Cytomegalovirus
Epidemiology and pathophysiology

Cytomegalovirus (CMV) is the most common cause of intrauterine infection in developed countries,[8]

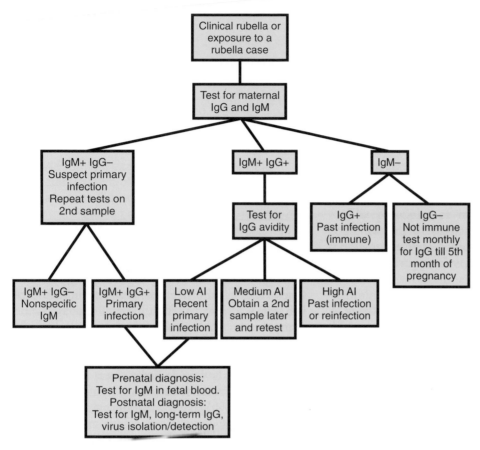

Figure 13.3
Rubella serology after maternal exposure.

(Remington: Infectious Diseases of the Fetus and Newborn, 7th ed. 2010 Saunders; 9781416064008; Figure 28.9. Adapted from Mendelson E, et al. Laboratory assessment and diagnosis of congenital viral infections: rubella, cytomegalovirus [CMV], varicella-zoster virus [VZV], herpes simplex virus [HSV], parvovirus B19 and human immunodeficiency virus [HIV]. Reprod Toxicol 21:350-382, 2006.)

affecting approximately 2–3% of pregnancies and with a birth prevalence of 0.5%. Forty to eighty per cent of women are susceptible to CMV infection during pregnancy.[8] Childcare workers, mothers of a CMV-positive young child, and women of low socioeconomic status are at particular risk if seronegative.

CMV is a member of the herpes virus group. Infectious CMV may be found in urine, saliva, blood, tears, semen and breast milk, and viral shedding may be intermittent and asymptomatic. Infection may be primary or non-primary (reactivation), with primary infection in pregnancy much more likely to lead to congenital sequelae (Figure 13.4).

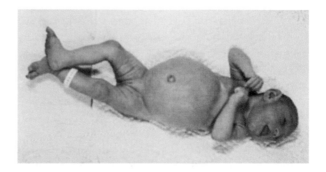

Figure 13.4
CMV-affected neonate.

(Goering: Mims' Medical Microbiology, 5th ed. 2012 Saunders; 9780723436010; Figure 23.3. Courtesy of WE Farrar.)

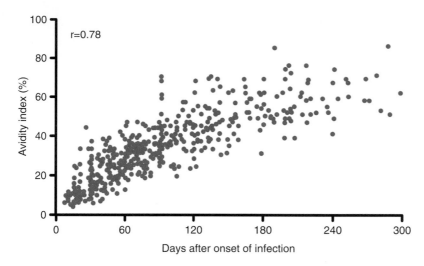

Figure 13.5
CMV avidity index.

(Remington: Infectious Diseases of the Fetus and Newborn, 7th ed. 2010 Saunders; 9781416064008; Figure 23.8. From Revello MG, Gerna G. Diagnosis and management of human cytomegalovirus infection in the mother, fetus, and newborn infant. Clin Microbiol Rev 15:680-715, 2002.)

Clinical presentation

Usually asymptomatic, or mild non-specific illness, unless mother is immunocompromised.

Diagnosis

As CMV status is not currently part of routine antenatal screening, diagnosis is often after the birth of an affected neonate or when ultrasound abnormalities are noted. Diagnosis of maternal infection, infected fetuses, and affected fetuses are all problematic *and care must be taken when interpreting results and discussing their implications with patients.* Recent maternal infection may be diagnosed using paired serology with new appearance of CMV IgG diagnostic of acute infection (IgM is less reliable). Timing of infection is often uncertain, in which case CMV IgG avidity (Figure 13.5) may be helpful, with low avidity suggesting recent infection.

In probable or definite maternal infection, amniocentesis and serial ultrasound may be used to diagnose infected and affected fetuses. Neither of these tests is 100% accurate. Patients in this situation should be referred to specialists with expertise in fetal medicine.

Management and outcomes

As illustrated in Figure 13.6, pregnant women with primary CMV infection have an approximately 30% risk of transmission to the fetus. In 10% of primary infections there is generalised infection in the infant, with symptoms at birth including microcephaly, rash, and hepatosplenomegaly (Figure 13.4). These infants have a 5–10% risk of mortality

and an 80% risk of complications within the first few years of life, including hearing loss, vision impairment, and varying degrees of intellectual disability. In the 90% of infants with no symptoms at birth, up to 15% subsequently develop hearing and neurodevelopmental problems. Non-primary/reactivation CMV infection during pregnancy carries little risk of CMV-related complications.

No therapy is yet proven to reduce the risk of having a baby with congenital CMV. Decision-making is difficult for parents due to the uncertainty of diagnosis and the severity of sequelae in the small percentage of infants who are affected. Some parents where primary CMV infection is proven will elect to have a termination of pregnancy.

Varicella zoster virus

Epidemiology and pathophysiology

Maternal varicella (chickenpox) infection rates are low (1–5 per 10 000 pregnancies), as more than 95% of adults are seropositive secondary to infection in childhood (vaccinated children are just beginning to enter childbearing years). Congenital varicella syndrome (CVS) is rare, less than 1 in 100 000 pregnancies in Australia.[9]

Varicella zoster virus (VZV) is a herpesvirus that causes chickenpox and herpes zoster (shingles). It is spread by droplets or direct contact, and infects more than 90% of susceptible contacts. The incubation period is 10–21 days, with infectivity lasting from 1 to 2 days before the rash appears until all lesions are crusted. Maternal infection may cause serious maternal morbidity and mortality. CVS affects 0.5% of fetuses if maternal infection occurs

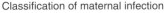

NATURAL HISTORY OF CONGENITAL HCMV
INFECTIONS: 1975–1998

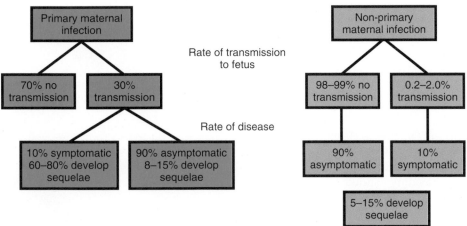

Classification of maternal infection

Primary maternal infection

Rate of transmission to fetus

70% no transmission

30% transmission

Rate of disease

10% symptomatic 60–80% develop sequelae

90% asymptomatic 8–15% develop sequelae

Non-primary maternal infection

98–99% no transmission

0.2–2.0% transmission

90% asymptomatic

10% symptomatic

5–15% develop sequelae

* The transmission rate varies depending on the population. Women of lower socioeconomic status have rates reported as high as 2.0%, whereas women from middle and upper middle class socioeconomic groups have rates less than 0.2%.

Figure 13.6
CMV natural history.

(Remington: Infectious Diseases of the Fetus and Newborn, 7th ed. 2010 Saunders; 9781416064008; Figure 23.6)

at less than 12 weeks, 2% from 12–20 weeks, and rarely thereafter. Neonates are susceptible to varicella infection (not CVS) if maternal infection occurs in the last month of pregnancy, which may be severe. Zoster reactivation is **not** a proven cause of CVS.

Clinical presentation

After a 1–4 day prodrome of fever, malaise, and myalgia, a characteristic vesicular rash appears (Figure 13.7). Complicated varicella in pregnancy is most often varicella pneumonia, appearing several days after the rash, and characterised by cough, dyspnoea, fever and tachypnoea, which may progress to hypoxic respiratory failure.

CVS presents by ultrasound or neonatally with cicatricial skin lesions, limb hypoplasia, microcephaly, and ophthalmic lesions.

Diagnosis

History of prior chickenpox is 98% predictive of IgG positivity, and more than 80% of women with no history are also IgG positive due to unrecognised childhood exposure.[10] If there is history of clinical exposure in a woman of uncertain immunity,

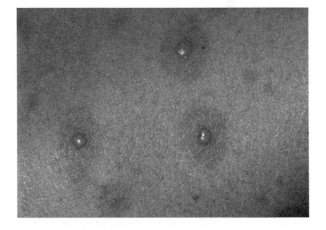

Figure 13.7
Varicella.

(James: Andrews' Diseases of the Skin: Clinical Dermatology, 11th ed. 2011 Saunders; 9781437703146; Figure 19.13)

serology (VZV IgG and IgM) should be performed. If rash is already present, the diagnosis is clinical.

There is no specific antenatal test for CVS, although limb abnormality seen on ultrasound after maternal varicella infection would be suggestive.

Management and outcomes

Varicella pneumonia occurs in 10–20% of VZV during pregnancy, and maternal mortality is 3–14% of cases when varicella pneumonia occurs. A varicella-seronegative pregnant woman with exposure to VZV infection should be offered zoster immune globulin (ZIG) within 96 hours of exposure to decrease her risk of varicella. Prophylactic oral acyclovir is considered for those who miss this window.[11]

Pregnant women who develop varicella pneumonia or other complications of VZV (e.g. haemorrhagic rash, neurological signs) should receive intravenous acyclovir. Babies born to women with VZV infections in the peripartum period should be given ZIG, and breastfeeding should be encouraged.[11]

Pregnant women with no history of VZV who are found to be seronegative should be offered postpartum vaccination.

Parvovirus B19
Epidemiology and pathophysiology

Parvovirus B19 causes a common childhood febrile illness known as fifth disease, erythema infectiosum or 'slapped cheek syndrome'. Thirty-five to fifty per cent of pregnant women have preexisting immunity to parvovirus. Approximately 3–4% of pregnant cohorts have primary parvovirus infection in pregnancy;[12] this is 3–4 times higher in risk groups such as schoolteachers and daycare workers.

Parvovirus causes a small percentage of non-immune fetal hydrops cases and intrauterine fetal death, secondary to fetal anaemia. Fifty per cent of these cases occur 2–5 weeks after maternal infection and more than 90% by 8 weeks after maternal infection. Severe maternal complications are rare.

Clinical presentation

Up to one-third of adults with this infection are asymptomatic. Classically, the illness lasts 1–3 weeks, with a characteristic red rash on the cheeks (Figure 13.8) and a lace-like rash on the trunk and limbs that may fade and reappear.

Diagnosis

Paired parvovirus B19 IgG and IgM serology (IgM appears within 10 days after infection). Direct diagnosis of fetal infection involves invasive testing and a small risk of miscarriage, so the usual method is for close ultrasound surveillance for development of fetal anaemia.

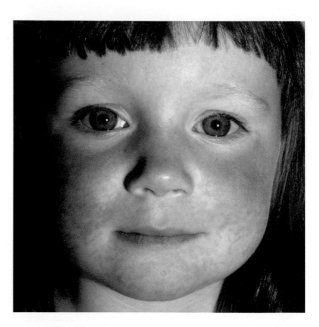

Figure 13.8
Parvovirus rash.

(Habif: Clinical Dermatology, 5th ed. 2009 Mosby; 9780723435419; Figure 14.17)

Management and outcomes

The chance of fetal anaemia developing after maternal parvovirus infection is 3–5% for infection diagnosed before 32 weeks, and less than 1% thereafter. Overall, the fetal loss rate for maternal infection diagnosed at less than 20 weeks is 11%, and at more than 20 weeks it is 0.6%.[12]

No maternal treatment or vaccine is available. Weekly fetal ultrasound surveillance for signs of anaemia is recommended for 8–12 weeks after infection. In several small series, intrauterine transfusion if ultrasound signs of severe anaemia develop appears to decrease the chance of fetal death. This is performed in specialised fetal medicine centres.

Toxoplasmosis
Epidemiology and pathophysiology

Approximately 30% of pregnant women in Australia have had toxoplasmosis prior to pregnancy. Congenital toxoplasmosis usually results from primary infection during pregnancy rather than reactivation. The incidence varies between populations, but is likely to be less than 1 in 1000 in Australia. Fetal infection (without sequelae) is more likely if

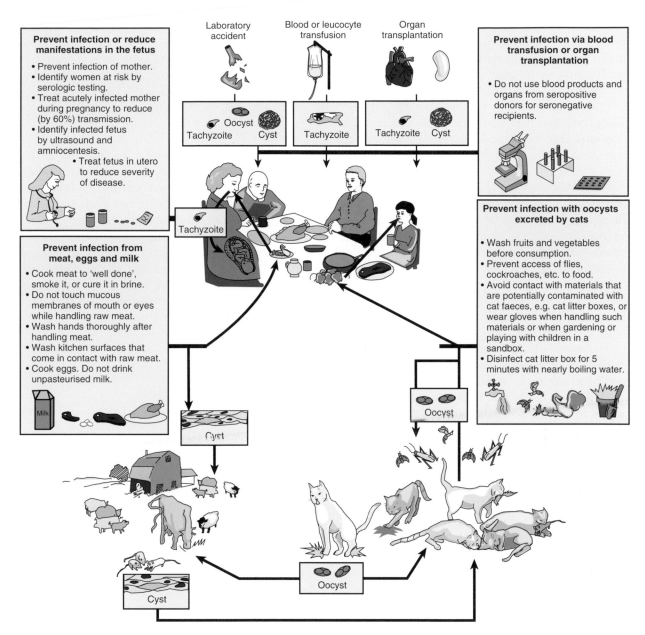

Figure 13.9
Toxoplasmosis life cycle.

(Kliegman: Nelson Textbook of Pediatrics, 19th ed. 2011 Saunders; 9781437707557; Figure 282.1)

maternal infection occurs late in pregnancy, but sequelae are more common for those babies who are infected early in pregnancy.

Pathophysiology

The definitive host of the parasite *Toxoplasma gondii* is the cat, but humans, domestic animals (e.g. cows) and wild animals (e.g. marsupials) may all act as intermediate hosts (Figure 13.9). Ingested cysts transform into tachyzoites, which cause tissue destruction and may be transmitted to the fetus in the maternal bloodstream. The fetal neural and ocular tissues are particularly susceptible. Ingestion of uncooked/undercooked meats, and contact with soil contaminated by *Toxoplasma* oocysts (e.g. cat faeces, vegetables not properly washed), are the major sources of infection. Casual contact with cats is very unlikely to cause infection.

Clinical presentation

Most pregnant women with acute infection are asymptomatic. Non-specific symptoms of low-grade fever, malaise, and lymphadenopathy may occur.

Diagnosis

Serology is tested for specific IgG and IgM. Interpretation is complex as a positive IgM does not necessarily indicate acute infection, and expert advice should be sought. Testing of amniotic fluid for toxoplasma PCR may be performed.

Management and outcomes

Intrauterine infection leads to a fetal syndrome with chorioretinitis, intracranial calcification and hydrocephaly in approximately 10% of cases. Some initially asymptomatic infants may later have visual and/or neurodevelopmental sequelae.

Although their benefit is uncertain, antibiotic regimens are available to attempt to decrease risk of vertical transmission and/or ameliorate severity of congenital disease, and may be used after appropriate specialist consultation.[11]

Pregnant women should be advised to eat only well-cooked meat, and to wash hands and kitchen surfaces/utensils after contact with raw meat. Fruit and vegetables should be washed prior to consumption, and handling cat litter or gardening avoided if possible (see Figure 13.9).

Syphilis

Although very uncommon in the general population, syphilis rates are increasing and a recent survey of Indigenous pregnant women found a prevalence of 2.5%.[13] Routine antenatal screening means pregnancy-associated syphilis is most commonly diagnosed in the latent phase. Perinatal transmission occurs in:

- 50% with primary or secondary syphilis
- 40% with early latent syphilis (within 4 years of infection)
- 10% with late latent syphilis or tertiary disease.

It results in congenital infection and anomalies (most commonly hepatomegaly, rash, generalised lymphadenopathy, and skeletal and dental anomalies),

intrauterine growth restriction, preterm birth, and perinatal death. Penicillin is the gold standard for treatment.[6] With adequate treatment at least one month before the birth, transmission rates drop to less than 2%.

See also chapter 5.

Listeria monocytogenes

This anaerobic gram-positive bacillus is a rare (<1:5000) but important cause of maternal sepsis, chorioamnionitis with intact membranes, and miscarriage (40–50% fetal death rate with second or third trimester infection). As it is principally a food-borne illness it is amenable to prevention, hence dietary recommendations to pregnant women to use safe food-handling practices and avoid high-risk foods such as unpasteurised milk, soft cheeses, pre-prepared salads, uncooked seafood, and processed meat.[11]

MATERNAL INFECTION WITH CONSEQUENCES TO THE NEONATE

Group B streptococcus

Epidemiology and pathophysiology

Group B streptococcus or GBS (*Streptococcus agalactiae*) is a gram-positive diplococcus that colonises the gastrointestinal and genital tracts. Between 15 and 40% of women are asymptomatically colonised with GBS, and approximately 50% of colonised pregnant women will transmit it to their baby at birth. Only 1–2% of babies of colonised mothers develop invasive GBS disease, meaning 1–2 in 1000 untreated neonates develop GBS sepsis. The risk is higher in mothers with a history of an infected infant or GBS bacteriuria, in premature infants, and where there has been premature or prolonged rupture of membranes or history of maternal fever.

GBS is also a cause of maternal UTI, chorioamnionitis, and endometritis.

Clinical features

Usually maternally asymptomatic, GBS may present with UTI symptoms or with maternal endometritis (fever, abdominal pain, offensive vaginal discharge) or rarely with sepsis. In the neonate, invasive GBS usually manifests as sepsis, pneumonia or meningitis in the first 24 hours of life. In a minority of cases invasive GBS is late-onset, up to 6 weeks after birth.

Diagnosis

Maternal colonisation status is best diagnosed by taking a rectovaginal swab at 35–37 weeks gestation,[14] as it is colonisation close to the time of delivery that is most relevant to risk of invasive neonatal GBS. Women with GBS bacteriuria at any time during pregnancy are also considered colonised.

Management and outcomes

Treatment of colonisation does not eradicate maternal GBS. However, the incidence of neonatal disease is significantly reduced by intrapartum intravenous antibiotics, with the first dose at least 4 hours before delivery. Neonatal observations should occur for at least 24 hours post-delivery (+/− neonatal antibiotics if there is clinical suspicion of GBS or significant risk factors).

Universal maternal screening at 35–37 weeks, with intrapartum IV antibiotics for GBS-positive mothers, is the preferred screening and treatment strategy, as there is less risk of failing to identify and treat maternal carriers than if risk factors alone are used to determine treatment.[14] Universal screening and treatment reduces the risk of early-onset disease from approximately 1.5 per 1000 births to 0.3 per 1000; late-onset disease is not reduced.

Mortality of invasive GBS ranges from 2–3% for otherwise healthy term infants to 20% in preterm infants. As maternal GBS is not eliminated by intrapartum chemoprophylaxis, women with clinical illness need appropriate ongoing antibiotic management.

Herpes simplex virus

Epidemiology and pathophysiology

Approximately 75% and 15% of Australian adults have prior exposure to the herpes simplex viruses HSV-1 and HSV-2 respectively. (See also chapter 5.) Both HSV subtypes can result in genital herpes, and pregnant women may have episodes of painful genital ulceration (Figure 13.10) and/or asymptomatic shedding. Active shedding of virus at the time of vaginal delivery may result in neonatal infection, encephalitis and death. This risk is greatest if primary infection occurs in the third trimester of pregnancy (up to 50%), and is rare with recurrent infection.

Diagnosis and management

Diagnosis is on the basis of clinical suspicion, confirmed with genital swabs. For *primary* infection late in pregnancy, antiviral treatment (valaciclovir or acyclovir) is recommended to reduce maternal symptom duration, and caesarean delivery to reduce neonatal risk. For primary infections in early pregnancy and women with recurrent HSV, suppressive therapy from 36 weeks is recommended, with vaginal birth unless there are active lesions present at labour onset or known viral shedding. Caesarean

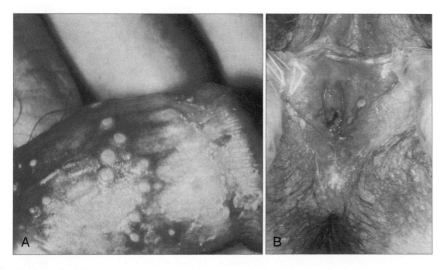

Figure 13.10
Genital herpes.

(Goering: Mims' Medical Microbiology, 5th ed. 2012 Saunders; 9780723436010; Figure 21.15B. Courtesy of JS Bingham.)

delivery substantially reduces the risk of neonatal HSV in women with recent primary infection or active viral shedding at delivery.[15]

Chorioamnionitis

Epidemiology and pathophysiology

Chorioamnionitis is infection of the amniotic fluid, placenta, membranes, and/or decidua. It is primarily due to ascending infection, and usually polymicrobial (Table 13.2). Chorioamnionitis is strongly associated with preterm birth and premature rupture of membranes, occurring in approximately 40% of births at less than 28 weeks compared to 2% of term births. Prolonged labour, multiple intrapartum vaginal examinations, internal fetal heart rate monitoring, and presence of genital tract infections (e.g. STIs, GBS) are other risk factors.

Clinical features and diagnosis

Maternal fever is the most sensitive and specific feature. Maternal or fetal tachycardia, raised white cell count, uterine pain and tenderness, preterm labour, and malodorous or purulent amniotic fluid may all be present.

White cell count is usually raised but this may occur in normal pregnancy, and raised C-reactive protein is insufficiently sensitive and specific. Blood cultures should be analysed.

Management and outcomes

Chorioamnionitis increases the risks of respiratory distress, pneumonia, cerebral haemorrhage, sepsis and death in babies, and preterm labour and bacteraemia/septicaemia in the mother. Cerebral palsy risk increases several fold in both term and preterm babies.[16] Abnormal labour and caesarean deliveries are increased, as is postpartum endometritis.

Aggressive broad-spectrum antibiotic therapy is used to treat chorioamnionitis as soon as the infection is diagnosed, and should be continued after delivery in both mother and baby. Delivery is the treatment for established chorioamnionitis, preferably vaginally if there are no contraindications and the fetal status remains reassuring. Placental swabs and histology should be obtained.

Hepatitis B virus

Epidemiology and pathophysiology

Between 0.5 and 0.8% of the Australian population is estimated to be chronically infected with hepatitis B (HBV).[17] Most pregnant chronic carriers of HBV were born overseas, in high HBV prevalence areas such as the Asia–Pacific, however Indigenous Australians, partners of HBV carriers, and injecting drug users also have an increased HBV prevalence.

Hepatitis B virus is a DNA virus transmitted in blood, semen and saliva, so may be transmitted perinatally (rarely in-utero). The liver damage associated with acute or chronic hepatitis B occurs as a result of attempts by the host's immune response to remove the virus from infected liver cells.

Diagnosis

Three antigens (and their antibodies) are measurable in association with the hepatitis B virus: the e antigen (HBeAg), the core antigen (HBcoreAg), and the surface antigen (HBsAg) (Figure 13.11). In addition, viral load of HBV DNA can be measured directly.

Positive HBsAg denotes past or present contact with the virus, and the anti-HBs antibody is found in immune and immunised individuals. The anti-HB core antibody is usually the first to appear in an infection. HBeAg usually denotes a highly infectious patient with chronic hepatitis. Vertical transmission is less likely when the anti-HBe antibody is found.

Table 13.2 Pathogens responsible for chorioamnionitis

Pathogen	Approximate frequency of culture in chorioamnionitis (%)
Ureaplasma urealyticum	50
Gram-negative anaerobes	40
Bacteroides species	35
Mycoplasma hominis	30
Gardnerella vaginalis	25
Group B streptococcus	15
Others	35

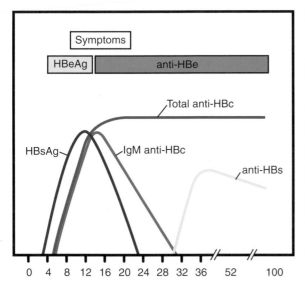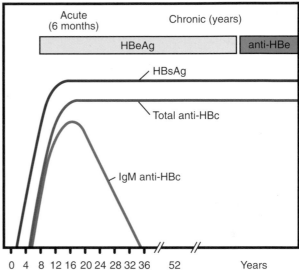

Figure 13.11

Hepatitis B serology time course.

(Mandell: Mandell, Douglas and Bennett's Principles and Practice of Infectious Diseases, 7th ed. 2009 Churchill Livingstone; 9780443068393; Figure 146.8A and B)

HBV DNA is detectable within 2–3 weeks of exposure. It persists, in varying titre, in chronic infection. High HBV DNA levels indicate both increased risk of liver disease progression and increased risk of perinatal transmission.[18] Transaminases (ALT and AST) are also used to monitor disease activity.

Impact and outcomes

Acute adult infection (rare in pregnancy) varies from a severe systemic icteric illness to asymptomatic infection, with 90% acquiring long-term immunity and 10% becoming carriers at risk of progressive liver damage. Acute infection does not appear to be teratogenic, but fetal loss can occur, as with any other febrile illness in pregnancy. Pregnancy in chronic maternal carriage may increase the likelihood of flare or progression of liver disease.[18]

The likelihood of chronic infection is closely tied to age at acquisition. If perinatal infection occurs acute symptoms are rare, but 90% of infants develop chronic infection (versus 10% of acutely infected adults). The lifetime risk of advanced liver disease for infected infants is 20–30%.

Management

Newborns at risk of vertical transmission of hepatitis B should be given hepatitis B immune globulin (HBIG) within 12 hours of birth, and a subsequent course of active hepatitis B vaccination should be commenced within 12 hours of birth. Transmission risk in HBeAg-negative carriers with low viral load ($<10^7$ copies/mL) is approximately 1% with this regimen. Women with high viral load ($>10^8$ copies/mL) or who are HBeAg-positive have a 5–10% perinatal transmission risk *despite* this regimen, and the utility of antenatal antiviral therapy for these women is under study.[18] Vertical transmission occurs in up to 80% of high-risk carriers whose infants do not receive immunoprophylaxis.

Breastfeeding is not contraindicated. Mother and baby should have specialist review for appropriate follow-up and consideration of antiviral therapy. At a community level, HBV is prevented by universal vaccination as per the Australian Immunisation Schedule.

Hepatitis C virus

Epidemiology and pathophysiology

Approximately 1.5% of the Australian population (including pregnant women) is chronically infected with hepatitis C virus (HCV). Injecting drug use (past or present), history of blood transfusion (pre-1990 Australia, anytime overseas), and immigration from high-prevalence regions such as Asia, Africa, and the Middle East are major risk factors. Acute hepatitis C results in chronic infection in at least 70% of cases. Like chronic HBV, HCV can result in end-stage liver disease including cirrhosis, liver cancer, and death.

Diagnosis and management

Initially testing is for anti-HCV. If anti-HCV is detected, viral load (HCV RNA) is performed as this reflects chronic infection. Risk of perinatal transmission is 5% (higher if HIV co-infection) but no specific measures have been shown to decrease this. Accordingly some centres screen for HCV only if risk factors are present. Measures that breach fetal skin intrapartum, for example scalp pH, should be avoided. Breastfeeding is not contraindicated, although if nipples are bleeding expressing milk should be considered.[19] Mother and baby need postpartum follow-up to determine infant antibody status and for consideration of maternal antiviral treatment (these are not safe in pregnancy).

Human immunodeficiency virus

Prevalence of human immunodeficiency virus (HIV) in pregnancy in Australia is low (0.04%), particularly in comparison with developing countries where prevalence is up to 30%. (Refer also to chapter 5.) Universal antenatal screening is recommended to allow appropriate maternal treatment and to minimise the risk of perinatal transmission, which occurs in approximately 30% if no treatment is instituted. Unless maternal progression to AIDS has already occurred, women with HIV generally have uncomplicated pregnancies. Management of these women should be shared with an infectious diseases physician, with regular checking of CD4 count and viral load. The main strategies to decrease perinatal transmission are:

1 Combination antiretroviral therapy (cART) — Most women with known HIV will already be on a cART regimen; if not it should be commenced to attain an undetectable viral load during pregnancy[19]
2 Neonatal antiretroviral therapy
3 Avoidance of breastfeeding (in resource-rich countries where safe artificial formula is available)
4 Elective caesarean delivery — this remains of benefit in women with high viral load.
5 Where maternal viral load is less than 1000 copies/mL, the added benefit of elective caesarean delivery is unclear, with transmission rates less than 2%.[19]

REFERENCES

1 Mak T, Mangtani P, Leese J, et al. Influenza vaccination in pregnancy: current evidence and selected national policies. Lancet Infect Dis 2008;8:44–52.

2 Centers for Disease Control and Prevention. Evaluation of rapid influenza diagnostic tests for detection of novel influenza A (H1N1) virus. Morb Mort Wkly Rep 2009;58(30):826.

3 Siston A, Rasmussen S, Honein M, et al. Pandemic 2009 influenza A (H1N1) virus illness among pregnant women in the United States. JAMA 2010;303(15):1517–25.

4 Zaman K, Roy E, Arifeen S, et al. Effectiveness of maternal influenza immunization in mothers and infants. N Engl J Med 2008;359(15):1555–64.

5 Smaill F, Vazquez J. Antibiotics for asymptomatic bacteriuria in pregnancy. Cochrane Database Syst Rev 2007;(2).

6 Antibiotic Guidelines Expert Group. Therapeutic Guidelines: Antibiotics. 14th ed. Melbourne: Therapeutic Guidelines; 2010.

7 Miller E, Cradock-Watson J, Pollock T. Consequences of confirmed maternal rubella at successive stages of pregnancy. Lancet 1982;320(8302):781–4.

8 McCarthy F, Giles M, Rowlands S, et al. Antenatal interventions for preventing the transmission of cytomegalovirus (CMV) from the mother to fetus during pregnancy and adverse outcomes in the congenitally infected infant. Cochrane Database Syst Rev 2011;(3).

9 Khandaker G, Marshall H, Peadon E, et al. Congenital and neonatal varicella: impact of the national varicella vaccination programme in Australia. Arch Dis Child 2011;96(5):453–6.

10 Watson B, Civen R, Reynolds M, et al. Validity of self-reported varicella disease history in pregnant women attending prenatal clinics. Public Health Rep 2007;122(4):499–506.

11 Jones C, Palasanthiran P, Starr M, Australasian Society for Infectious Diseases, editors. Management of perinatal infections Sydney: Australasian Society for Infectious Diseases. 2002.

12 Enders M, Weidner A, Zoellner I, et al. Fetal morbidity and mortality after acute human parvovirus B19 infection in pregnancy: prospective evaluation of 1018 cases. Prenatal Diagnosis 2004;24(7):513–18.

13 Panaretto K, Lee H, Mitchell M, et al. Prevalence of sexually transmitted infections in pregnant urban Aboriginal and Torres Strait Islander women in northern Australia. Aust N Z J Obstet Gynaecol 2006;46(3):217–24.

14 Schrag S, Gorwitz R, Fultz-Butts K, et al. Prevention of perinatal group B streptococcal disease. Revised guidelines from CDC. Morb Mort Wkly Rep Reccom Rep 2002;51(RR-11):1–22.

15 Brown Z, Wald A, Morrow R, et al. Effect of serologic status and cesarean delivery on transmission rates of herpes simplex virus from mother to infant. JAMA 2003;289(2):203–9.

16 Shatrov J, Birch S, Lam L, et al. Chorioamnionitis and cerebral palsy: a meta-analysis. Obstet Gynecol 2010;116(2 Pt 1):387–92.

17 O'Sullivan B, Gidding H, Law M, et al. Estimates of chronic hepatitis B virus infection in Australia, 2000. Aust N Z J Public Health 2004;28(3):212–16.

18 Giles M, Visvanathan K, Lewin S, et al. Chronic hepatitis B infection and pregnancy. Obstet Gynecol Surv 2012;67(1):37–44.

19 Australasian Society for HIV Medicine, Giles M, Edmiston N, Fisken R. Antenatal testing and blood-borne viruses (BBVs). Darlinghurst: Australasian Society for HIV Medicine; 2011.

MCQS

Select the correct answer.

1   A woman who consults her doctor after discovering that she was immunised against rubella 3 weeks after conceiving should be offered:

A   termination of pregnancy.
B   paired rubella IgM and IgG antibody titres 2 weeks apart.
C   chorionic villous sampling.
D   reassurance and standard antenatal care.
E   varicella serology.

2   Which is the most accurate statement?

A   Most fetal infections in pregnancy are diagnosed by screening programs that detect changes in paired IgG and IgM titres.
B   Most mother-to-child (perinatal) transmission of hepatitis B, C and HIV occurs antenatally, through placental transmission prior to labour and birth.
C   Most maternal infections in pregnancy will not result in the birth of a baby with congenital abnormalities or illness.
D   Most rubella infection in the first trimester results in severe maternal illness.
E   CMV is always benign to the fetus.

3   Which of the following statements about GBS is **false**?

A   All neonatal GBS is preventable by intrapartum chemoprophylaxis.
B   GBS is an important cause of maternal UTI, endometritis, and sepsis.
C   Maternal screening for GBS is best performed at 35–37 weeks gestation.
D   Universal screening and treatment prevents more neonatal GBS than selective screening and treatment.
E   GBS stands for group B streptococcus.

4   Which of the following diseases can both cause serious maternal illness in pregnancy and a fetal malformation syndrome?

A   hepatitis C
B   varicella (VZV)
C   group B streptococcus
D   toxoplasmosis
E   listeriosis

OSCE

Linda Chen is a 34-year-old G1P0 who comes for her first antenatal visit at 15 weeks gestation. She brings the following antenatal screening results:

- Hb 121
- MVC 85.2
- WCC 9.5
- Plt 320
- Blood group O+ve, nil antibodies detected
- Rubella IgG 8 (>15=adequate immunity in this laboratory's reference range)
- RPR non-reactive
- HBsAg positive
- HbsAb negative
- HBeAg positive
- HbeAb negative
- HCV antibody negative
- HIV antibody negative
- MSU no growth

First trimester screen (nuchal translucency ultrasound and biochemistry): Low risk (adjusted risk Trisomy 21 1:1300, adjusted risk for Trisomy 18 1:3500, adjusted risk for Trisomy 13 1:4500). Fetal size consistent with dates.

Outline your history and examination appropriate to this case, and discuss the results, including any appropriate further investigation and management, with the patient.

Chapter 14

Medical disorders in pregnancy

Sandra Lowe

KEY POINTS

Medical disorders unique to pregnancy include:

- hyperemesis gravidarum
- preeclampsia
- eclampsia.

Preeclampsia is de-novo hypertension after 20 weeks gestation with organ involvement.

Gestational diabetes occurs in up to 10% of all pregnancies in Australia.

Venous thromboembolism is up to five times more common in pregnancy than in non-pregnant women.

The dose of radiation received from one chest X-ray is roughly equivalent to that received during half a long haul flight from Australia to Europe.

Women may enter pregnancy with a preexisting medical problem, or a woman may experience a medical disorder during pregnancy that is incidental to or specifically related to pregnancy. These conditions may affect any one organ or multiple systems, and may impact on mother, fetus, or both. Understanding these conditions requires recognition of both the effects a medical disorder may have on the pregnancy and the effects of the pregnancy on the medical condition.

A number of medical conditions in pregnancy represent an exaggeration of normal physiological changes, for example hyperemesis gravidarum and iron deficiency anaemia, while others such as preeclampsia are unique to pregnancy. Some conditions such as venous thromoembolism occur more commonly in pregnancy, while pregnancy may uncover a preexisting susceptibility to other conditions such as gestational diabetes.

In this chapter we discuss some of the more common and important medical disorders that may impact on pregnancy.

NAUSEA AND VOMITING OF PREGNANCY

Nausea and vomiting are common in early pregnancy and are referred to as morning sickness, but symptoms are restricted to the morning in only 2% of women. Up to 85% of pregnant woman are affected, and symptoms are commonly experienced from the 4th to the 12th week of pregnancy. Although the symptoms may be troublesome, they rarely require investigation or drug therapy. In general, first-trimester nausea has no adverse effect on the mother or fetus.

HYPEREMESIS GRAVIDARUM

Hyperemesis gravidarum (HG) is excessive pregnancy-related nausea and/or vomiting that prevents adequate food and fluid intake and is associated with weight loss of more than 5% of body mass. It occurs in fewer than 3% of pregnancies. Symptoms usually begin at 4–6 weeks' gestation and peak between 9 and 13 weeks. In 10–20% of cases, symptoms may last the entire pregnancy. The inability to retain food and fluids leads to dehydration, nutritional deficiency and metabolic imbalance.

If inadequately treated, HG may lead to severe maternal and fetal complications. Management is directed at correction of both fluid and electrolyte imbalance and nutritional and vitamin deficiencies, antiemetic therapy and general supportive care.

Etiology

The cause of HG is not well understood although hormonal, mechanical and psychological factors have been implicated. It is associated with female embryos, molar pregnancies, multiple gestations and *Helicobacter pylori* infection. Human chorionic gonadotrophin (hCG), which rises to a peak at 12 weeks' gestation and falls thereafter, has been held responsible. However, the total hCG level is not significantly higher in women with HG. These women may have an excess sensitivity to hCG or elevated levels of free beta chain hCG.

HG is commonly associated with elevated serum thyroxine levels due to cross-reactivity between HCG and thyroid-stimulating hormone (TSH). Hyperthyroidism usually resolves early in the second trimester, subsiding along with the hyperemesis. Psychosocial stress is not a cause of hyperemesis but can aggravate it, and should be taken into consideration in the overall management of the woman with HG.

Women who have experienced HG in a previous pregnancy or who have experienced nausea while taking oral contraceptives are more likely to suffer from HG.

Clinical picture

Prolonged vomiting and poor oral intake may cause hypokalaemia, hyponatraemia, hypochloraemic alkalosis and reduced extracellular fluid volume. This results in thirst, malaise, dizziness when standing and, rarely, syncope. Severe hyponatraemia (<125 mmol/L) may cause listlessness or even convulsions. Urine output is reduced. This occurs by hyperosmolar stimulation of antidiuretic hormone secretion and reduced glomerular filtration, associated with reduced ECF volume.

Physical examination may reveal signs of weight loss and dehydration such as a dry, furry tongue, loss of skin elasticity, tachycardia and postural hypotension. Hyperemesis is also associated with excessive salivation (ptyalism), causing constant and distressing spitting in many women.

Sign of hyperthyroidism are similar to those of normal pregnancy (tachycardia, sweating), but the presence of goitre, tremor and signs of eyelid lag or exophthalmos should alert to the possibility of 'true' thyroid disease.

Severe hyponatraemia or its too rapid correction may result in central pontine myelinolysis, a localised osmotic demyelination in the brain. Prolonged or violent vomiting may cause Mallory-Weiss tears of the oesophagus, presenting as haematemesis or rarely oesophageal rupture. If prolonged, anaemia and peripheral neuropathy may occur as a result of cyanocobalamin (vitamin B12) and pyridoxine (B6) deficiency. The most commonly reported serious complication is Wernicke's encephalopathy, which is due to thiamin (B1) deficiency. The prognosis for this condition is poor, as irreversible neurological damage occurs. Death is rare in Western society, as medical help is readily available. In former times, however, it was not a rare cause of maternal death.

Diagnosis

The diagnosis of HG is made by exclusion of other causes of vomiting including urinary tract infections, gastroenteritis, acute appendicitis or biliary tract disease. Rare causes of nausea and vomiting such as Addisons disease (hypocortisolaemia) should also be considered as this may be life-threatening. In the second half of pregnancy, nausea and vomiting may be symptoms of labour, preeclampsia or, rarely, acute fatty liver of pregnancy.

Investigations

A urine dipstick is used to check for specific gravity and ketones as inadequate oral intake is associated with high specific gravity and the production of ketones. Urinary tract infection should be excluded by microscopic examination of a midstream urine sample. The haematocrit is increased as a result of a concentrated blood volume. There are blood electrolyte changes, for example decreased sodium, potassium, chloride and magnesium are common, as well as elevated liver enzymes such as aspartate transaminase (AST), alanine transaminase (ALT) or bilirubin. Overt jaundice is rare. Thyroid function tests should be checked in women with clinical signs of hyperthyroidism, in which an increased T4 concentration and reduced TSH may be found. An ultrasound should be performed to identify a twin or molar pregnancy.

Treatment

Most HG resolves spontaneously by 16 weeks gestation. Treatment consists of supportive care with correction of both fluid and electrolyte imbalance and nutritional and vitamin deficiencies. The woman and her family will also need social and emotional support through this very distressing time.

With less severe degrees of HG, outpatient management through a pregnancy day facility may be preferable. Hospitalisation is necessary in severe cases. First-line management includes intravenous rehydration with normal saline or Hartmann's solution with potassium chloride supplementation. It is important not to correct severe hyponatraemia too rapidly. A woman who has been unable to eat sufficiently for weeks is at risk of significant malnutrition. Vitamin supplementation, especially of the water-soluble vitamins such as thiamin (100 mg oral or IV), is important to prevent development of Wernicke's encephalopathy. Oral intake should be given as tolerated. Small carbohydrate-rich meals are often better tolerated. Any oral fluid is encouraged to maintain hydration. Drugs that may aggravate nausea and vomiting should be discontinued, for example iron supplements.

A stepwise approach to pharmacotherapy should be used. Over the counter agents such as ginger (500–1000 mg daily) and vitamin B6 (75 mg daily) have been shown to be effective. Antiemetics, either oral, rectal or parenteral, are indicated for symptoms that are intractable despite adequate hydration. Although there is no randomised trial data available, dopamine antagonists (metoclopramide, domperidone), phenothiazines (prochlorperazine) and antihistamines (promethazine, doxylamine, cyclizine) are all commonly used and have not been associated with teratogenic effects. Ondansetron, a highly selective 5-HT3 antagonist, is also used with success, although it was no better than metoclopramide in a comparative study and there is less data about its safety in the first trimester. A randomised,

placebo trial of corticosteroids demonstrated a trend to reduced nausea, vomiting and dependence on intravenous fluids but was not statistically significant. Corticosteroids are associated with a possible increased risk of clefting when used prior to 10 weeks gestation. Treatment for excess gastric acidity, for example histamine 2 blockers, should also be given. Enteral feeding or even total parenteral nutrition may occasionally be required.

It is important to remember that a woman who has been hospitalised for a prolonged period with HG, who is dehydrated and confined to bed, is at increased risk of venous thromboembolic disease, and thromboprophylaxis (low molecular weight heparin and compression stockings) should be commenced. Milder cases of nausea and vomiting in pregnancy have not shown a long-term adverse outcome for the fetus. In severe cases with prolonged maternal nausea, vomiting and weight loss, the fetus is at risk of growth restriction, which may lead to preterm delivery and its complications.

HYPERTENSION

The hypertensive disorders of pregnancy include chronic hypertension, gestational hypertension and preeclampsia.[1] The most important of these is preeclampsia, which affects up to 5% of women in pregnancy. It is a multisystem disease unique to humans that impacts on both maternal and fetal wellbeing.

Definitions

Hypertension occurs in up to 10% of pregnancies and is defined as an absolute blood pressure greater than or equal to systolic ≥ 140 and/or diastolic ≥ 90 mmHg. As described in Box 14.1, it is classified as:

- gestational hypertension
- preeclampsia
- chronic hypertension
- preeclampsia superimposed on chronic hypertension.

Preeclampsia

In developing countries, preeclampsia remains one of the most common causes of maternal death and is a common cause of death in young women.[2] (See Figure 14.1.) Death may occur from acute hypertensive crisis, eclampsia, acute pulmonary oedema, acute renal failure, liver failure, haemorrhage, or coagulopathy. In the developed world, maternal

---

Box 14.1 Classification system for hypertension in pregnancy

Preeclampsia

De novo hypertension arising after 20 weeks' gestation, returning to normal within 3 months postpartum, plus evidence of dysfunction in at least one other organ:

- Kidney: proteinuria, raised plasma creatinine, oliguria
- Liver: raised AST or ALT, epigastric/right upper quadrant pain
- Neurological: convulsions (eclampsia); hyper-reflexia with clonus; severe headaches, visual disturbance, stroke
- Haematological: thrombocytopenia, haemolysis, disseminated intravascular coagulation
- Fetal: intrauterine growth restriction, stillbirth, placental abruption

Gestational hypertension

De novo hypertension after 20 weeks' gestation without any other feature of preeclampsia, returning to normal within 3 months postpartum.

Chronic hypertension

- Essential: hypertension in the first half of pregnancy, without an apparent secondary cause or evidence of 'white-coat' hypertension.
- Secondary: hypertension due to renal or endocrine disease.

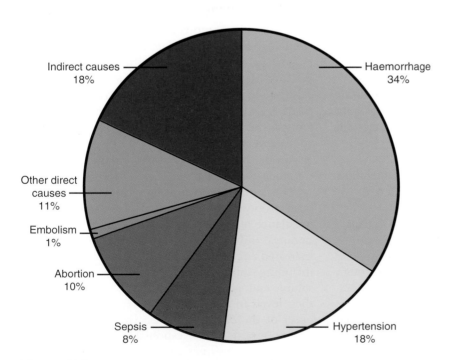

Figure 14.1
The causes of maternal death globally.

(World Health Organization. The World Health Report 2005: Making every mother and child count. Geneva: World Health Organization, 2005.)

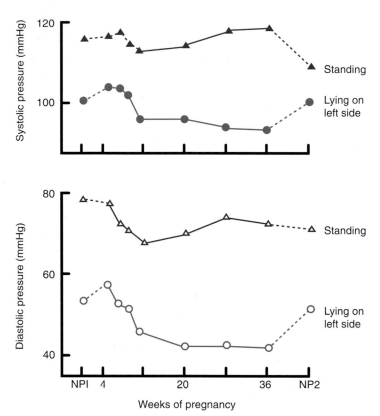

Figure 14.2

Longitudinal changes in blood pressure with normal pregnancy.

(Medical Disorders in Obstetric Practise. Ed De Swiet, M. Blackwell Scientific Publications 1989, 2nd ed. p. 250)

mortality is now uncommon, but preeclampsia is the major cause of iatrogenic premature delivery.

Pathophysiology

In normal pregnancy, physiological changes occur that cause a fall in maternal blood pressure (Figure 14.2).[3] In preeclampsia, these adaptive changes fail to occur and the result is:
- vasoconstriction
- platelet activation with intravascular coagulation (usually local but occasionally disseminated)
- maternal plasma volume contraction
- endothelial dysfunction in a variety of vascular beds.

This leads to impairment of blood flow through the placenta as well as through the maternal kidneys, liver and brain. The clinical presentation of pre-eclampsia will depend upon the extent to which different maternal organ systems and the placenta have been affected by this process, but once pre-eclampsia has begun it runs a progressive course until delivery.

Preeclampsia is a placental disorder that manifests in symptoms and signs in both the mother and fetus. It occurs most commonly in primigravid women, but other risk factors include a previous pregnancy with preeclampsia, a family history of this disorder, multiple pregnancies, diabetes, pre-existing hypertension, renal disease, connective tissue disorders, obesity, membership of some ethnic groups, and possibly thrombophilias. Smoking appears to reduce the likelihood of developing pre-eclampsia, but babies of smokers tend to be small for gestational age.

The cause of preeclampsia remains elusive. It has been proposed that abnormal placentation and an imbalance of angiogenic factors lead to the clinical findings and complications seen in preeclampsia. Increased circulating levels of antiangiogenic factors including soluble fms-like tyrosine kinase-1 and soluble endoglin are secreted from the placenta and their levels in maternal blood rise, even before the onset of the clinical disease. These antiangiogenic factors appear to be responsible for the maternal endothelial dysfunction. Genetic susceptibility, excessive oxidative stress and immune maladaptation may exacerbate the condition and may explain how preexisting disorders increase the risk of preeclampsia.

Clinical assessment

Preeclampsia is detected initially in most cases by the presence of hypertension arising after the 20th week of pregnancy. It does not occur before the 20th week, except in the rare case of hydatidiform mole. Symptoms are not always present but may comprise non-specific headaches, visual scintillations (like migraine aura), epigastric or right upper quadrant pain radiating into the back as a reflection of hepatic ischaemia, oliguria, lower abdominal pain and bleeding caused by placental abruption, or reduced fetal movements.

In most cases, however, clinicians must search for the other systemic features that characterise pre-eclampsia. Clinical assessment may reveal hepatic tenderness or enlargement, hyper-reflexia or clonus, pulmonary oedema, or signs of fetal growth restriction and/or distress. Oedema is not included in the diagnostic features of preeclampsia as it is common even in normal pregnancy.

Full assessment of preeclampsia should include:
- urine dipstick testing for proteinuria, with quantitation by laboratory methods if > '1+' (30 mg/dL)
- full blood count. If there is thrombocytopenia or a falling haemoglobin, add investigations for haemolysis and disseminated intravascular coagulation
- urea, creatinine, electrolytes, uric acid
- liver function tests.

Blood test abnormalities should be interpreted using pregnancy-specific ranges, some of which are gestation-dependent. The aim of these investigations is to distinguish preeclampsia from chronic hypertension and gestational hypertension, and to determine the extent and severity of the disease. In the latter the blood tests should be normal unless preexisting renal disease is causing proteinuria or a raised serum creatinine. Fetal assessment will usually include CTG and ultrasound assessment of fetal growth, amniotic fluid volume and umbilical artery flow. It should be stressed that none of the assessments of fetal wellbeing provide any long-term certainty about fetal outcome.

Eclampsia

Eclampsia (convulsions) associated with preeclampsia is now uncommon in developed countries, with a prevalence of around 0.3% of hypertensive pregnancies. It is much more common in developing countries. Eclampsia is not directly related to the level of blood pressure, and it has been reported in the absence of proteinuria. Importantly, about half the cases of eclampsia occur after delivery, although rarely more than 5 days postpartum.

Prevention

Unfortunately no set of tests has reliably predicted the development of preeclampsia, although measurement of antiangiogenic factors looks promising. Low-dose aspirin and supplemental calcium commenced in early pregnancy reduce the risk of developing preeclampsia. Although these are safe, they are best reserved for women considered at highest risk, such as those who have experienced previous preeclampsia or women with diabetes.

Treatment

Preeclampsia is a progressive disorder that will inevitably worsen if pregnancy continues. The only definitive treatment for preeclampsia is delivery of the placenta. Indications for delivery include:
- progressive evidence of maternal organ dysfunction: worsening renal or hepatic function, worsening thrombocytopenia, development of neurological symptoms or signs
- inability to control blood pressure
- concerns for fetal wellbeing.

Antihypertensive medications should be given if the systolic blood pressure is persistently ≥160 mmHg and/or diastolic pressure ≥100 mmHg because of the risk of intracerebral haemorrhage and eclampsia (Figure 9.3).[4] The agents used are the same as those used for preexisting hypertension. Drugs that are considered safe and have been widely used in pregnancy include methyldopa, oxprenolol, labetalol and clonidine as first-line agents. When additional treatment is required, hydralazine, nifedipine or prazosin may be added. Angiotensin-converting enzyme (ACE) inhibitors, angiotensin II (AII) receptor antagonists and diuretics are generally avoided: the first two groups are considered teratogenic and nephrotoxic, while diuretics reduce an already impaired maternal blood volume.

Blood pressure ≥170/110 mmHg constitutes severe, urgent hypertension in pregnancy and is considered a medical emergency. The blood pressure should be lowered promptly but with care not to impair placental perfusion further. The fetus should be carefully monitored during acute blood pressure

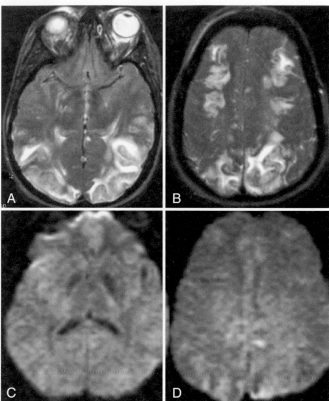

Figure 14.3
MRI of the brain in eclampsia: patient with hypertensive encephalopathy secondary to eclampsia with HELLP (haemolysis, elevated liver enzymes, and low platelets) syndrome. A: T2-weighted magnetic resonance imaging (MRI) showing the extensive cerebral oedema in the posterior white matter regions with less involvement of the grey matter. B: A higher level of the same scan sequence as in A, showing some frontal lobe involvement. C and D: Diffusion-weighted images (DWI) with only one small area of involvement. The lack of DWI changes is consistent with this being a vasogenic type of oedema, and the patient had a good recovery without residual deficit.

(Daroff: Bradley's Neurology in Clinical Practice, 6th ed. 2012 Saunders; 9781437704341; Figure 59.7A to D)

lowering. Intravenous hydralazine or labetalol as well as oral nifedipine may be used to lower the blood pressure over 30–60 minutes.

Intravenous magnesium sulfate rather than anticonvulsant drugs is the drug of choice for prevention of eclampsia. Eclampsia is characterised by significant localised areas of hypoperfusion in the brain (Figure 14.3). Magnesium sulfate probably acts to improve cerebral blood flow in vasoconstricted areas and is administered to those women who have already had a convulsion or are considered at high risk of eclampsia.

Postpartum management

Resolution of preeclampsia commences following delivery of the placenta but may take days, weeks or even months. Assessment of the preeclamptic woman several months postpartum is mandatory. Blood pressure should have returned to normal within 3 months. If it does not, this should prompt a search for underlying essential or secondary hypertension. Urinalysis and urine microscopy should be normal, certainly by 12 months postpartum, if not before. If this is not the case, a primary underlying renal disease should be sought.

As a general rule, preeclampsia or gestational hypertension will recur in about 15% of women in a subsequent pregnancy. Women who have presented at or before 28 weeks of gestation may have a higher risk of recurrence. Women with preeclampsia are at increased risk of cardiovascular disease, venous thromboembolism and hypertension within the 15 years following their pregnancy. These associations are likely to reflect a common cause for preeclampsia and cardiovascular disease, or an effect of preeclampsia on vascular disease development, or both. Women who have had preeclampsia should therefore be encouraged to exercise, eat sensibly, and have their cardiovascular risk factors assessed regularly.

Gestational hypertension

New-onset hypertension after 20 weeks gestation is a relatively benign disorder with good maternal and fetal outcomes. Blood pressure is controlled with the same medications as described above for preeclampsia.

Women with gestational hypertension have a 10% risk of progressing to develop preeclampsia if they present after 36 weeks' gestation, but a greater than 1 in 3 risk if they present before 32 weeks' gestation. It may be that gestational hypertension is the very earliest clinical phase of preeclampsia, or it may be a separate disorder.

Chronic hypertension

In most cases, chronic hypertension is due to essential hypertension and, unlike preeclampsia or gestational hypertension, it is apparent in the first half of pregnancy. It is important to exclude 'white-coat' hypertension with 24-hour ambulatory home blood pressure monitoring before making a certain diagnosis of essential hypertension.

The main risks of chronic hypertension in pregnancy are:

- fetal growth restriction
- accelerated maternal hypertension
- superimposed preeclampsia (in about 25% of cases).

The same antihypertensives are used as for preeclampsia. Regular reviews are required to monitor fetal growth and detect changes of preeclampsia.

DIABETES

Epidemiology

Gestational diabetes mellitus (GDM) is defined as carbohydrate intolerance of variable severity with onset or first recognition during pregnancy. It was first recognised retrospectively, when parous women with diabetes were noted to have had an excess number of both macrosomic infants and perinatal deaths.

In Australia GDM is found in 6–8% of all pregnancies, and this percentage is increasing as the population becomes more obese. There is an increased risk in women with a family history of type 2 diabetes, a personal history of GDM, carbohydrate intolerance, or polycystic ovarian syndrome (PCOS), elevated body mass index before pregnancy, older maternal age, a previous macrosomic infant, or unexplained fetal demise. Some ethnic groups (e.g. Indigenous Australians, Polynesian and Indian women) are at particularly high risk of developing GDM.

Pathophysiology

Normal pregnancy is characterised by hyperplasia of pancreatic beta cells, increased insulin secretion and insulin sensitivity in early pregnancy, followed by a progressive increase in insulin resistance. Placental diabetogenic hormones, such as human placental lactogen, growth hormone, progesterone and corticotrophin, as well as increased levels of free fatty acids and tumour necrosis factor-alpha, lead to changes in maternal carbohydrate metabolism during pregnancy. These hormones rise linearly during the second and third trimesters in order to supply the growing fetus with sufficient nutrients. The mother switches from carbohydrate to fat metabolism, utilising free fatty acids, triglycerides and ketones for fuel.[5]

In normal pregnancies, blood glucose levels fall by 10–20% owing to increased storage of tissue glycogen, increased peripheral glucose utilisation, decreased hepatic glucose production, and increased fetal glucose consumption.

Women with preexisting diabetes have an increased risk of fetal congenital abnormalities, in particular cardiac defects and neural tube defects (Figure 14.4).[6] In the early part of pregnancy

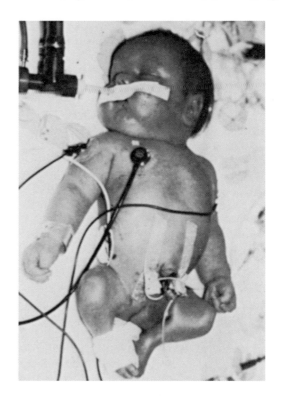

Figure 14.4
Newborn with caudal regression syndrome — the most specific but rare congenital anomaly in pregnancies complicated by diabetes.

(Gleason: Avery's Diseases of the Newborn, 9th ed. 2011 Saunders; 9781437701340; Figure 9.1; From Creasy RK, Resnik R, editors: Maternal-fetal medicine: principles and practice, ed 2, Philadelphia, 1989, WB Saunders.)

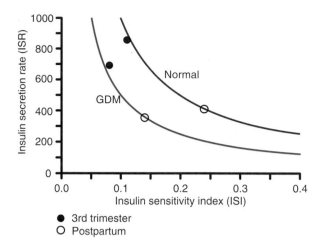

Figure 14.5
Insulin sensitivity index.

(Gabbe: Obstetrics: Normal and Problem Pregnancies, 5th ed. 9781437719352 Figure 39.10. Copyright © 2007 Churchill Livingstone, An Imprint of Elsevier)

(<14 weeks), the fetus has no insulin production and maternal hyperglycaemia leads to fetal hyperglycaemia, which is teratogenic. Later influences (>14 weeks) on the fetus depend on the degree of fetal hyperinsulinism induced by placental transfer of excess maternal glucose.

In GDM, there is greater insulin resistance and impaired insulin secretion from the maternal pancreas (Figure 14.5).[7] Hyperglycaemia is associated with an increase in maternal and fetal complications. The maternal sequelae of GDM include an increased risk of preeclampsia, premature delivery, and caesarean delivery.

Fetal hyperglycaemia stimulates hyperinsulinaemia, which leads to storage of excess energy and accelerated growth. This is manifested as macrosomia, with resulting increased rates of shoulder dystocia and birth trauma. Polyhydramnios is caused by hyperosmolar fetal polyuria and may precipitate preterm labour. The increased fetal metabolic rate and oxygen requirements may partly explain the increased risk of intrauterine asphyxia. They also lead to the development of raised haematocrit and neonatal hyperbilirubinaemia.

Admissions to neonatal intensive care units occur more often, and perinatal mortality is increased. Neonatal complications include hypoglycaemia and hypocalcaemia, the latter being attributed to reduced parathyroid hormone synthesis. Compared with infants of similar gestational age,

infants of mothers with diabetes have less surfactant production and are at increased risk of respiratory distress syndrome.

Despite good glycaemic control in pregnancy, there is a persisting increased risk of stillbirth in pregnancy complicated by maternal diabetes, both preexisting and GDM requiring hypoglycaemic treatment. The cause of late stillbirth is likely to be multifactorial. Fetal hypoxia and acidosis have been implicated, as has hypokalaemia leading to fetal cardiac dysrhythmias, as well as placental dysfunction. This increased risk of stillbirth has led to a generally accepted policy of induction of labour at around 38–39 weeks to avoid late fetal loss, which has invariably contributed to the higher caesarean delivery rate experienced by women with diabetes. Identifying the fetus at risk of late intrauterine death remains a challenge.

There is good evidence that the incidence of childhood obesity, insulin resistance and adult diabetes is increased in the offspring of women with diabetes in pregnancy, particularly if the fetus is macrosomic.

Maternal signs and symptoms

A woman with GDM is usually asymptomatic and diagnosed after screening for the condition. Alternatively, she may have symptoms of hyperglycaemia (polyuria, polydipsia) or an elevated fundal height secondary to polyhydramnios and/or macrosomia.

Screening for GDM

The Australian Carbohydrate Intolerance Study in Pregnant Women[8] demonstrated that identifying and treating women with hyperglycaemia in late pregnancy resulted in a significant reduction in pregnancy complications such as preeclampsia and adverse perinatal outcomes. What remains controversial is what degree of hyperglycaemia matters and how to identify these women. A review of the screening criteria for GDM demonstrated there is a continuum of risk, with no clear threshold that could divide women into those with gestational diabetes and those without.[9]

Most guidelines recommend universal screening of pregnant women, usually at 24–28 weeks' gestation, when insulin resistance increases. A two-step screening regime is currently used comprising:

- An oral glucose challenge test after a morning non-fasting 50 g glucose load

- If the plasma blood sugar level (BSL) is ≥7.8 mmol/L, proceed to fasting 75 g oral GTT. GDM is diagnosed if fasting BSL ≥5.5 mmol/L and/or 2-hour BSL ≥8.0 mmol/L. A 2-hour cut-off level of 9 mmol/L is used in New Zealand.

Therapy

In women with preexisting diabetes, optimal therapy requires preconceptual counselling to achieve euglycaemia prior to conception. End-organ involvement such as retinal disease, renal disease and cardiovascular disease should be assessed and optimised. Irrespective of the type or timing of diabetes, the objective is maternal euglycaemia. Ideally, a team comprising an obstetrician, diabetes physician, diabetes educator, dietician and midwife should care for the woman with abnormal glucose tolerance. Education and frequent self-monitoring of capillary glucose levels is standard. Recommended target glucose concentrations are: fasting capillary glucose <5 mmol/L, 1-hour postprandial glucose of <8 mmol/L and 2-hour postprandial glucose <7 mmol/L.

Treatment comprises an appropriate diabetic diet and daily exercise in all women and, if these blood sugar targets are not met, insulin with or without oral hypoglycaemic agents (short acting sulfonylureas or metformin) will be required. The choice of insulin versus oral hypoglycaemic will depend on the type of diabetes, the severity of hyperglycaemia, and the patient's preference. Insulin has the benefit of flexibility, individualised dosing and fetal safety, as it does not cross the placenta. However it is administered by subcutaneous injection between one and four times daily, and may cause maternal hypoglycaemia. Oral hypoglycaemics, although convenient, do cross the placenta, but they are not believed to be harmful to the fetus.

Fetal monitoring

An ultrasound examination at 18–20 weeks' gestation should identify significant congenital abnormalities in babies of women with prepregnancy diabetes. In all women with abnormal glucose tolerance in pregnancy, fetal growth should be assessed clinically and by regular ultrasound to identify growth restriction or accelerated growth. Monitoring of these fetuses is problematic because, unlike hypertensive pregnancies, CTG and ultrasound monitoring have not been proven to predict poor

outcomes. Delivery is often considered after 38 weeks' gestation in women with poorly controlled diabetes or those with evidence of fetal involvement. There is no evidence that perinatal mortality is increased in the presence of well-controlled GDM.

Good glycaemic control should be maintained in labour. Lower insulin requirements are common in labour for reasons that are not well understood, and hypoglycaemia should be avoided. Close fetal monitoring is advisable.

Close neonatal follow-up is important, particularly for the detection of hypoglycaemia, jaundice, and respiratory distress syndrome. Breastfeeding is actively encouraged.

Prognosis

Most women become euglycaemic within 24 hours after delivery, as the diabetes-inducing factors produced by the placenta have a short half-life. Women who develop GDM have a lifetime risk of developing type 2 diabetes of 40%.[10] All women should, therefore, be advised of the symptoms of hyperglycaemia and offered lifestyle advice that includes weight control, diet and exercise in order to reduce this risk of developing type 2 diabetes. They should be screened regularly, particularly in subsequent pregnancies. GDM is therefore an important, modifiable risk factor for diabetes with a significant impact on community health status.

Contraceptive advice should be given in the puerperium, and women should be advised to plan future pregnancies with careful attention to good pre-conception blood glucose control.

THROMBOEMBOLISM

Thromboembolic disease encompasses thrombotic events such as deep vein thrombosis (DVT) and superficial thrombophlebitis as well as embolic phenomena such as pulmonary emboli (PE). Thrombosis of the cerebral sinuses is a rare condition that usually presents postpartum as headache, seizure or focal neurological deficit. Strokes due to paradoxical emboli that have crossed into the arterial circulation via a cardiac right–left shunt are even rarer.

All components of 'Virchow's triad' are present in pregnancy. Venous stasis is induced by venous dilation and obstruction to venous return. Procoagulant factors are increased while physiological anticoagulants are reduced, and vessel wall injury may occur during labour and following caesarean delivery. This prothrombotic state is aggravated

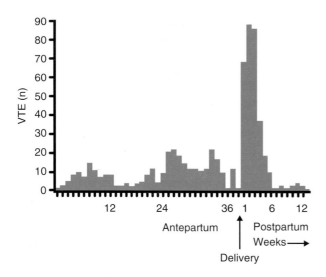

Figure 14.6
Distribution of VTE in pregnancy and puerperium: number of VTEs per week.

(Jacobsen AF, Skjeldestad FE, Sandset PM. Incidence and risk patterns of venous thromboembolism in pregnancy and puerperium — a register-based case-control study. Am J Obstet Gynecol 2008;198:233 e1–7)

immediately after delivery and resolves gradually over the 6 weeks postpartum. The majority of women who develop venous thromboembolism (VTE) in association with pregnancy have personal or pregnancy-specific risk factors for thrombosis that were either untreated or unrecognised.

Incidence
Although there is a four- to five-fold increased risk compared to that in non-pregnant women of the same age, the absolute risk of VTE is low at no more than two episodes per 1000 pregnancies. One-third to one-half of VTE occur postpartum (Figure 14.6), most within the first 6 weeks.[11] At least half of the antepartum events occur in the first two trimesters. Only one-quarter of events are pulmonary embolism (PE), of which 1 in 40 are fatal. Despite these low numbers, pulmonary embolism remains one of the most common causes of maternal mortality in the developed world.

Clinical assessment
Thrombosis often starts in the calf but only thrombosis above the knee produces clots large enough to create a significant risk of pulmonary embolism. Alone, superficial thrombophlebitis in the leg or thigh is unlikely to generate a PE. Most DVTs occur

in the left leg or bilaterally. The signs and symptoms include pain, swelling, heat, and redness. As swelling is a common symptom in late pregnancy, it has poor sensitivity as a sole symptom. The signs and symptoms of PE include chest or back pain (commonly pleuritic), breathlessness, tachycardia, tachypnoea, apprehension and haemoptysis. Chest auscultation may demonstrate reduced air entry, a friction rub or crepitations. If the pulmonary emboli are large, the woman may collapse with syncope or have signs of acute right heart strain.

Investigations and the use of diagnostic radiation in pregnancy
In pregnancy and postpartum, there should be a low threshold for excluding DVT. Diagnostic investigations are the same as for non-pregnant patients, except the D-dimer has no role as it is physiologically elevated. Doppler compression ultrasound is the diagnostic test most commonly used in pregnancy. It is very useful for thigh thrombosis, less so for calf, and of no use for pelvic vein thrombosis. If DVT is confirmed or PE suspected, an ECG, arterial blood gases and often a chest X-ray will be required.

When pulmonary embolism is suspected, some form of diagnostic imaging involving radiation is usually required. This always raises concerns for both the woman and her doctor. Unequivocally, the benefit of performing these important investigations far outweighs the risk, even in pregnancy. For practical purposes, no specific counselling is required for women undergoing diagnostic imaging with a predicted fetal absorbed dose of less than 10 mGy. This includes all X-ray and CT scanning not involving the abdomen. For direct exposures or nuclear scanning with a potential exposure >10 mGy, the woman should be counselled on a risk–benefit basis. The specific risk appears to be childhood malignancy. For each 10 mGy exposure, theoretical projections suggest a maximum risk of 1 additional cancer death per 1700 exposures. Balanced with this is the benefit of the imaging in terms of management of the maternal condition.

CTPA (CT pulmonary angiography) is generally accepted as the recommended initial lung imaging modality for non-massive pulmonary embolus. Ventilation–perfusion scanning may be considered as an alternative when the chest X-ray is normal and there is no intercurrent cardiac or pulmonary disease. This is often the case in the pregnant or postpartum woman with suspected pulmonary embolus. Numerous attempts have been made to compare the fetal radiation dose from CTPA versus ventilation–perfusion scanning for the detection of pulmonary embolus during pregnancy. Most recent estimates indicate a fetal absorbed dose of <0.01 mGy for CTPA versus 0.12 mGy for low-dose perfusion scanning. Both these doses would be considered negligible and of no risk to the fetus. However, the absorbed dose to the maternal breast was 10 mGy for CTPA and only 0.28 mGy from perfusion scanning. This can be reduced by the use of appropriate shielding. The risk of breast cancer is increased by radiation, with an estimated addition risk of 18 per million per mGy. It is likely that the breast in pregnant women might be especially sensitive to such radiation, and the selection of the most appropriate imaging for the detection of pulmonary embolus needs to take into account maternal as well as fetal risks. If MRA (magnetic resonance angiography) is available, it is an option that should be considered in this setting.

Treatment

The treatment of VTE is the same as in the non-pregnant state, except that warfarin is not used until postpartum as it crosses the placenta and may cause teratogenesis or haemorrhage. Initial treatment of DVT is usually with therapeutic doses of heparin (which does not cross the placenta), rest, and analgesia. Once clinical improvement is seen, the woman is encouraged to ambulate and wear compression stockings. The treatment is continued with subcutaneous low-molecular-weight heparin (LMWH). Therapy is required for the duration of pregnancy and 6 weeks postpartum. Around the time of delivery, the anticoagulation will need to be suspended because of the risk of haemorrhage. The woman may change to warfarin postpartum. Breastfeeding is not contraindicated with either heparin or warfarin.

Next pregnancy and contraception

Testing for underlying thrombophilias is generally performed after delivery as a number of these factors are altered by pregnancy. This will help determine the risk of future thrombosis, and assist with management of any future pregnancy. Patients with a pregnancy-related VTE are generally advised to have LMWH prophylaxis commencing in early pregnancy and continuing until 6 weeks

postpartum. The dose will depend on the estimated risk, with most patients able to use prophylactic dose therapy while very high-risk women may need more intensive treatment. In general, women with previous VTE should not receive oestrogen-containing contraceptives or hormone replacement therapy, and alternative contraception such as an IUD should be considered.

Prophylaxis for VTE

Thromboprophylaxis with LMWH during pregnancy may be offered to women with a previous history of VTE, or those with a high-risk thrombophilia. At delivery, risk assessment should be performed on all women, and postpartum prophylaxis considered based on the risk assessment.[12]

ANAEMIA

Low haemoglobin (Hb) concentrations are a part of normal pregnancy. Plasma volume increases by about 1.2 L by term and causes a dilutional anaemia despite an associated increase in red cell mass. Hb levels fall from early pregnancy, reaching a nadir at 36 weeks, 20–25 g/L below pre-pregnancy ranges. A haemoglobin <110 g/L in the first trimester or <100 g/L in late second and third trimesters should be considered as anaemia and investigated further. Following delivery, there is an auto-transfusion of approximately 500 mL of blood from the uteroplacental vessels.

The most common pathological cause of anaemia in pregnancy is iron deficiency. Rare causes include haemolytic anaemia and haemoglobinopathies such as thalassaemia. It is rare today, with food fortification and vitamin supplementation for prevention of neural tube defects, to see folic acid deficiency or the haematological manifestations of vitamin B12 deficiency.

Clinical features of anaemia

Anaemia in pregnancy may aggravate fatigue, shortness of breath or palpitations; common symptoms of normal pregnancy. When the haemoglobin is 60–70 g/L, the mother is at risk for high-output cardiac failure and extreme fatigue. At these levels, the fetus is at the lower limit of adequate oxygenation.

Investigation of anaemia

A full blood count (FBC) estimates haemoglobin concentration, platelet and white blood cell counts.

In addition, the red cell size (mean corpuscular volume, MCV) and the red cell Hb concentration (mean corpuscular Hb concentration, MCHC) are calculated.

Microcytic anaemia (MCV <80 fL) is commonly found in iron deficiency anaemia and thalassaemia. Provided the platelet and white blood cell count are normal, the first investigation of microcytic, hypochromic (low MCHC) anaemia is directed at identifying iron deficiency, by estimating serum ferritin concentration. Ferritin is an acute phase reactant, and elevated levels may occur during intercurrent disease states such as infection. If the serum ferritin is normal (especially when the MCHC is very low, with a mildly depressed MCV), haemoglobin electrophoresis is performed to identify carrier states of haemoglobinopathies. If these are identified, further investigation of the partner may be required.

A macrocytic anaemia (MCV >100 fL) is associated with folic acid and vitamin B12 deficiencies. Anaemia associated with macrocytic red blood cells and hypersegmented polymorphs should be investigated to determine erythrocyte folate levels. Serum B12 levels are difficult to interpret in pregnancy and are commonly physiologically low in the second half of gestation.

Iron deficiency in pregnancy

The fetus requires about 280 mg of iron and a further 400–500 mg is required for the expansion of maternal red cell mass. If iron intake does not meet increased requirements, iron deficiency with or without anaemia can occur. The use of routine iron supplements in pregnancy remains controversial. In women eating an adequate diet, the decrease in Hb is rarely significant enough to cause a serious clinical problem. The risk of iron deficiency is increased in women with low socioeconomic status, vegetarians, women with multiple gestations, and in women with a history of iron deficiency or menorrhagia. In these women, prophylactic iron supplementation should be considered.

Iron supplementation

Oral iron is absorbed in the stomach and duodenum, in a mildly acidic medium. Thus enteric-coated or sustained-release iron preparations are inefficient. Iron absorption is inhibited by antacids and enhanced by ascorbic acid, and therefore iron is best taken on an empty stomach. The iron available for absorption is termed the elemental iron. Different iron preparations contain variable quantities of elemental iron as well as different salts. For example, ferrous sulfate 300 mg contains 60 mg elemental iron, of which only 10% actually gets absorbed. The side effects of iron supplementation include upper gastrointestinal discomfort and constipation. If oral iron is ineffective or not tolerated, parenteral iron may be required, for example intravenous iron sucrose.

Iron is actively transported across the placenta. The fetus takes iron from the mother at a very efficient rate, and the placenta becomes more efficient in removing iron, even as the mother becomes more anaemic. In states of extreme maternal iron deficiency, the fetus, although having normal haemoglobin, may not have sufficient iron stores and so becomes anaemic within the first year of life.

REFERENCES

1 Lowe SA, Brown MA, Dekker G, et al. Guidelines for the management of hypertensive disorders of pregnancy. Australian and New Zealand Journal of Obstetrics and Gynecology 2009;49(3):242–6.

2 World Health Organization. The World Health Report 2005: Making every mother and child count. Geneva: World Health Organization; 2005.

3 Medical Disorders in Obstetric Practice. Ed De Swiet, M. 2nd ed. Oxford, UK: Blackwell Scientific; 1989. p. 250.

4 Bradley: Neurology in Clinical Practice. 5th ed. Philadelphia: Butterworth-Heinemann; 2008.

5 Lain KY, Catalano PM. Metabolic changes in pregnancy. Clin Obstet Gynecol 2007;4:938.

6 Gleason: Avery's Diseases of the Newborn. 9th ed. Philadelphia: Saunders; 2011.

7 Gabbe: Obstetrics: Normal and Problem Pregnancies. 5th ed. New York: Churchill Livingstone; 2007.

8 Crowther CA, Hiller JE, Moss JR, et al. Effect of treatment of gestational diabetes mellitus on pregnancy outcomes. N Engl J Med 2005;352:2477–86.

9 Waugh N, Royle P, Clar C, et al. Screening for hyperglycaemia in pregnancy: a rapid update for the National Screening Committee. Health Technology Assessment 2010;14(45):1–183.

10 Lauenborg J, Hansen T, Jensen DM, et al. Increasing incidence of diabetes after gestational diabetes: A long-term follow-up in a Danish population. Diabetes Care 2004;27:1194–9.

11 Jacobsen AF, Skjeldestad FE, Sandset PM. Incidence and risk patterns of venous thromboembolism in pregnancy and puerperium — a register-based case-control study. Am J Obstet Gynecol 2008;198(233):e1–7.

12 McLintock C, Brighton T, Chunilal S, et al. Recommendations for the prevention of pregnancy-associated venous thromboembolism. Aust N Z J Obstet Gynaecol 2012;52(1):3–13. doi: 10.1111/j.1479-828X.2011.01357.x.

MCQS

Select the correct answer to complete the sentence.

1   Preeclampsia:

    A   should be treated with aspirin in all patients.
    B   is diagnosed by oedema.
    C   is more common in women with chronic hypertension.
    D   is always associated with growth restriction of the fetus.
    E   can be safely treated with ACE inhibitors.

2   Gestational diabetes:

    A   will not recur in subsequent pregnancies.
    B   decreases the risk of preeclampsia.
    C   if treated, improves maternal survival.
    D   occurs more frequently in young women.
    E   results from insulin resistance in pregnancy.

3   Deep vein thrombosis in pregnancy:

    A   is diagnosed with D-dimer.
    B   is more common in pregnancy than in the non-pregnant woman.
    C   never occurs in the first trimester.
    D   is always associated with a thrombophilia syndrome.
    E   can be safely treated with warfarin.

OSCE

Mary is a 28-year-old primigravid woman who has been sent in for assessment at 35 weeks pregnancy with a blood pressure of 165/105 and 2+ proteinuria. What information will you seek on history and examination? What would be your expected investigation and management plan?

Chapter 15

Labour and delivery

Rajit Narayan and Jonathan Hyett

KEY POINTS

Normal birth begins with the spontaneous onset of labour at 37–42 weeks gestation.

The first stage of labour is the period from the commencement of regular painful contractions to full cervical dilatation.

The second stage of labour is the period from full cervical dilatation to the delivery of the infant.

The third stage of labour is the interval between delivery of the baby and delivery of the placenta and membranes.

Assisted vaginal delivery involves use of the forceps or the vacuum extractor to facilitate delivery of the fetus.

Caesarean delivery involves a laparotomy and incision into the uterus to deliver the fetus.

Perineal tears are classified as:

- first degree: injury to vaginal or perineal skin only
- second degree: injury to perineal muscles in addition to skin as above
- third degree tear: second degree plus injury to anal sphincter
- fourth degree tear: third degree plus injury to rectal mucosa.

INTRODUCTION

Labour is a natural process that culminates in the delivery of one or more infants. The process of birth is one of the most significant events in a woman's life, one of the riskiest in an infant's life and one of the most poignant affecting humanity. Obstetricians and midwives are privileged to be involved in the birth of the next generation and need to respect the significance of labour and delivery to the family.

The World Health Organization defines normal birth as involving the spontaneous onset of labour at term (37–42 weeks gestation). Labour is defined by progressively more painful and more frequent uterine activity that results in progressive effacement and dilatation of the cervix. In normal situations, the woman is regarded as being low risk at the onset of labour and continues to be low risk through to delivery, which is spontaneous, with an infant presenting in the vertex position. After birth, mother and infant are in good condition.[1]

Labour can be regarded as a physiological process, but it is associated with significant risks of both maternal and fetal mortality and morbidity. While a birth attendant has an important role supporting women through labour, they must also be able to recognise deviation from the process of normal birth, allowing appropriate intervention to improve outcomes for both mother and child. We discuss the physiology of labour, the normal process of birth, and options for management when complications arise.

THE PHYSIOLOGY OF NORMAL LABOUR

Throughout most of pregnancy, the uterus, which is a smooth muscle, is maintained in a state of quiescence. During the last few weeks of pregnancy, a series of changes occur that affect the structure and function of the myometrium, decidua, and uterine cervix. At a cellular level, myocytes change in character, with alterations in ion channels and gap junctions that make the cell highly responsive to endogenous stimulants. These changes allow coordinated myometrial contraction, starting at the uterine fundus and sweeping down over the lower segment, drawing the lower segment up over the presenting part and pushing the fetus down into the pelvis during labour. The constitution of the cervix changes, with decreasing collagen content, a change in proteoglycan concentration, and an increase in water content.

It is not clear what triggers labour. A number of autocrine and paracrine pathways have been implicated, involving hormones such as oestrogen, progesterone, prostaglandins and oxytocin. The final common pathway for initiation of labour appears to be activation of the fetal hypothalamic–pituitary–adrenal axis.

The three Ps

There are three variables that can affect progress in spontaneous labour. These are known as the 'three Ps': the fetus (passenger) is driven through the maternal pelvis (passage) by uterine contractions (powers), to be born.

Passenger

The fetus (the passenger) is not a passive agent that slips through the maternal pelvis driven by forces of uterine contraction (Figure 15.1). Fetal variables

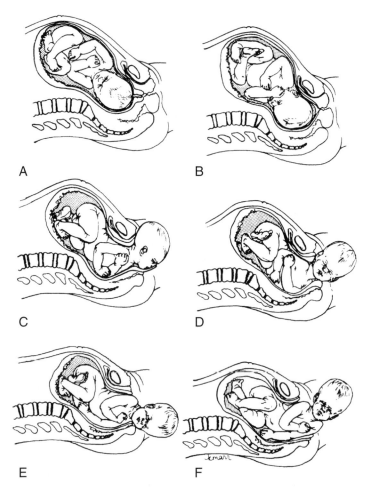

A B C D E F

Figure 15.1

Descent of the fetus through the pelvis during the course of labour. **A**: The fetus presents in a longitudinal lie, presenting cephalically by the vertex. The head is engaged transversely and is flexed. **B**: As the head descends through the birth canal there is internal rotation so that the occiput is anterior. **C**: The head extends for delivery. **D**: The head then returns to the transverse position, through external rotation. **E, F**: This is followed by delivery of the anterior and posterior shoulders.

(Based on on Figure 14-4, Ratcliffe: Family Medicine Obstetrics, 3rd ed. Copyright © 2008 Mosby, An Imprint of Elsevier; 9780323043069)

that play significant roles in the labour process include:

- lie: relationship of the long axis of the fetus to the long axis of the mother
- presentation: the fetal pole that lies over the pelvic inlet
- attitude: relation of fetal parts with each other. The basic attitudes are flexion and extension
- denominator: a fixed bony point on the presenting part of the fetus that is used to describe position (e.g. the occiput)
- position: the relationship of the denominator to the front, back and sides of the maternal pelvis.

The fetus normally presents at the onset of labour in a longitudinal lie with cephalic presentation. The head is normally flexed, presenting the smallest diameter to the maternal pelvis, which is defined as the vertex — the area lying between the anterior and posterior fontanelles and bounded by the parietal eminences.

Passage

The passage consists of the maternal bony pelvis and the pelvic floor musculature which offers resistance to the fetus. The passage is commonly assessed at four different levels, or planes: the obstetric inlet, plane of greatest dimensions, plane of least dimensions, and the obstetric outlet (Figure 15.2).

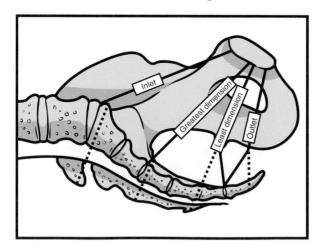

Figure 15.2
The pelvic planes.

(Based on Figure 72-1 'The obstetric planes of the pelvis and forceps classification: 1, Plane of inlet. 2, Plane of greatest pelvic dimension. 3, Plane of least pelvic dimension. 4, Plane of outlet. James: High Risk Pregnancy, 4th ed. Copyright © 2010 Saunders, An Imprint of Elsevier; 9781416059080)

Power

The power (frequency, intensity and duration) of uterine contractions can be assessed subjectively by palpation of the uterine fundus or mechanically using a tocometer that is attached to the maternal abdomen. Recordings of the fetal heart rate and maternal uterine activity can be made simultaneously (cardiotocography; CTG) and can be used to determine how the fetus responds to uterine contraction during labour. A frequency of 3–5 contractions in a 10-minute period is considered to be adequate to effect cervical change in labour. Fewer, or asynchronous, contractions may prevent cervical dilatation, while an increase in uterine activity, hyperstimulation, is associated with fetal distress.

Stages of labour

Although labour is a continuous process, it is traditionally divided into three stages that allow assessment of progress.

First stage

The first stage of labour describes the period from commencement (progressively more painful and more frequent contractions with progressive effacement and dilatation of the cervix) to full cervical dilatation. This can be subdivided into latent and active phases, the former describing the period prior to the establishment of regular contractions and cervical dilation and the latter where contractions become established with cervical dilatation.

Progress through the first stage of labour can be documented graphically using a partogram (Figure 15.3). This is usually started once the active phase of the first stage of labour has been defined (through abdominal palpation and vaginal examination). The partogram can be marked so that both the anticipated rate of progress, and a rate at which intervention would be required, are defined. These points can then be compared to the actual rate of progress observed as labour advances. The rate of cervical dilatation increases as labour progresses; with a median of 1.2 hours/cm dilation at 3–4 cm dilation and 0.4 hours/cm dilation at 7–8 cm dilatation.[2]

Second stage

The second stage of labour refers to the interval between full (10 cm) cervical dilatation and delivery of the infant. It can be split into a passive phase, allowing the presenting part to descend though the pelvis, and an active phase, where maternal effort is used to drive the presenting part through the birth canal. The mean length of second stage is around one hour for nulliparous women and 20 minutes for multiparous women.[3] The older the woman (>30 years of age) the longer the second stage. Use of narcotic and epidural analgesia also increases the length of the second stage. In the absence of fetal distress, the duration of the second stage is not significantly associated with the risk of low neonatal Apgar score or admission to neonatal intensive care, but there is an increased risk of maternal postpartum haemorrhage and pyrexia as time elapses, and the risk of postpartum infection is doubled after 4 hours. The active part of the second stage of labour is considered to be protracted, or 'arrested', if it exceeds 2 hours in a nulliparous woman or 1 hour in a multiparous woman. This limit is extended by one hour for women with epidural analgesia.[4]

Third stage

The third stage of labour refers to the interval between delivery of the baby and separation and expulsion of the placenta. Although the infant has been delivered, it is important to monitor progress through this stage as failure to deliver the placenta in a timely fashion can lead to significant maternal morbidity. The World Health Organization has stated that the third stage of labour should typically be complete within 60 minutes of delivery of the infant.[5]

Progress of the presenting part

There are six major components to advancement of the presenting part: descent, engagement, lateral flexion, internal rotation, extension and restitution (or external rotation) (Figure 15.1). In normal labour the fetus presents cephalically. Neither the fetal head nor the pelvis have regular diameters. The head is egg-shaped and the pelvis ovoid; the antero-posterior (AP) diameter is the narrowest diameter at the pelvic inlet and becomes the widest diameter at the pelvic outlet. At the onset of labour, the presenting part is located over the pelvic brim and is described as being engaged once the widest diameter has passed below the level of the pelvic inlet. The head is typically transverse at this point. As labour progresses, the head descends through the pelvis and is flexed as a result of the resistance offered by the soft tissues of the maternal pelvis. As it advances through the pelvis it undergoes a process of internal rotation into an AP position. Once the

cervix is fully dilated, the head continues to descend, following the course of the sacral curve. Once the head reaches the perineum and distends the introitus, the inferior border of the pubic symphysis acts as a fulcrum around which the fetal head extends, prior to birth. Once free of the mechanical forces associated with passage through the pelvic floor, the head rotates back into the transverse plane through a process called restitution.

Maternal physiological changes during labour

Active labour is hard work, and the systemic maternal changes reflect this. The maternal heart rate and respiratory rate rise, the cardiac output, peripheral vascular resistance and blood pressure rise, and catecholamine secretion increases. For some women with preexisting or acquired medical diseases, the superimposed demands of labour may be detrimental to their health and limitations may need to be imposed to prevent injury.

Fetal physiological changes during labour

The healthy fetus is able to tolerate the repetitive but intermittent interruption to oxygenation that occurs with uterine activity. In the healthy fetus, ultrasound reveals a dramatic reduction in breathing and limb movements during labour. Biochemically, the healthy fetus maintains a normal cord arterial pH until the second stage.

MANAGEMENT OF NORMAL LABOUR AND DELIVERY

The majority of low-risk women who labour spontaneously will make good progress through the first stage and continue to deliver both baby and placenta normally. In this circumstance the accoucheur provides support during labour and assists with delivery. In other circumstances, where normal progress in labour is not maintained and there is the potential for injury to either mother and/or baby, the accoucheur needs to be able to recognise complications as they arise and take appropriate steps to reduce these risks. This process of surveillance is best managed in a structured, systematic manner that involves taking a history, examining the woman and performing appropriate investigations, while recognising the specific risks and complications associated with different stages of labour and delivery.

The partogram and progress in labour

A partogram can be started, and this is a useful point to review the clinical history to define risk (low or high risk for labour) and to record basic findings related to maternal (temperature, pulse, blood pressure and urinalysis) and fetal (fundal height, lie presentation, position, engagement) examination. The findings of vaginal examination are also normally recorded on the partogram, including cervical dilatation, the station, position and attitude of the presenting part, and whether the membranes remain intact (Figure 15.3).

The process of risk assessment helps define the level of fetal surveillance needed through labour. Low-risk pregnancies do not need to be monitored continuously with a CTG, rather by intermittent auscultation during the first stage.[6]

Progress in the first stage of labour can be monitored by performing vaginal examination. In most circumstances, an interval of 4 hours between examinations is adequate to demonstrate appropriate cervical change. If slow progress is suspected due to poor uterine activity or if there is evidence of fetal distress, then earlier assessment may be necessary. Low-risk pregnancies may become high-risk during the first stage of labour for a number of reasons. Most commonly, this would be due to failure to make sufficient progress or due to evidence of potential fetal distress (the identification of meconium in amniotic fluid or the detection of heart rate abnormalities through intermittent auscultation). In this circumstance, continuous electronic fetal monitoring should commence and the ongoing management plan for surveillance and delivery should be redefined.

Labour and delivery of low-risk women who make normal progress in labour and have no evidence of fetal distress during labour is unlikely to be complicated. Many would advocate that this natural, physiological event should happen outside the hospital environment and that women are best supported, and therefore most likely to labour well, in their own homes. The rate of home birth is low in Australia, and our medical infrastructure does not readily lend itself to supporting this model of care.[7] Many centres do, however, offer facilities to birth in a low risk/low tech environment where transfer to more medically oriented care can be managed if complications develop.

Most women lose their appetite in labour, but should be encouraged to drink clear fluids as dehydration can affect uterine activity. Women should be encouraged to mobilise in labour and can adopt whatever position is comfortable for them. There is good evidence that continuous support from a birth partner(s) reduces the need for medical intervention in labour.

Pain management in labour

Labour can be painful and this is distressing when prolonged. Simple pain relief strategies include use of breathing and relaxation techniques, massage, and immersion in water. Transcutaneous electrical nerve stimulation (TENS) and Entonox (inhaled nitrous oxide and oxygen) are also easy to use, and in some studies appear to be more effective than intramuscular opioid analgesia. Systemic opioids are also often prescribed for pain in labour: side effects are those typical of opioid drugs, including nausea and sedation. Epidural analgesia involves the administration of intermittent or continuous infusion of opioids or local anaesthetic via a fine catheter placed in the lumbar epidural space, and is most effective in providing pain relief. The major disadvantages include maternal motor blockade, which limits or prevents ambulation, the need for continuous fetal monitoring, possible maternal hypotension causing non-reassuring fetal heart patterns, and the loss of bladder sensation, requiring an indwelling urinary catheter. Epidurals may also increase the duration of the second stage of labour, and the risk of having an instrumental birth.[8]

The second stage of labour: delivery

The second stage of labour commences at full cervical dilatation. If the fetal head is still at a high station then labour may be managed expectantly for 1–2 hours to allow descent of the head. Allowing time for passive descent significantly increases a woman's chance of having a spontaneous vaginal birth, and decreases her risk of having an instrument-assisted delivery. Women should then be guided by their own urge to push, and progress is judged by monitoring advancement of the presenting part. Intermittent auscultation should be performed more frequently during the active part of the second stage. Women may birth in a variety of positions, including lying prone (with some lateral support to prevent fetal distress), lying laterally, on all fours, standing, in a supported squat, or on the birth stool. The accoucheur can assist delivery but there is no

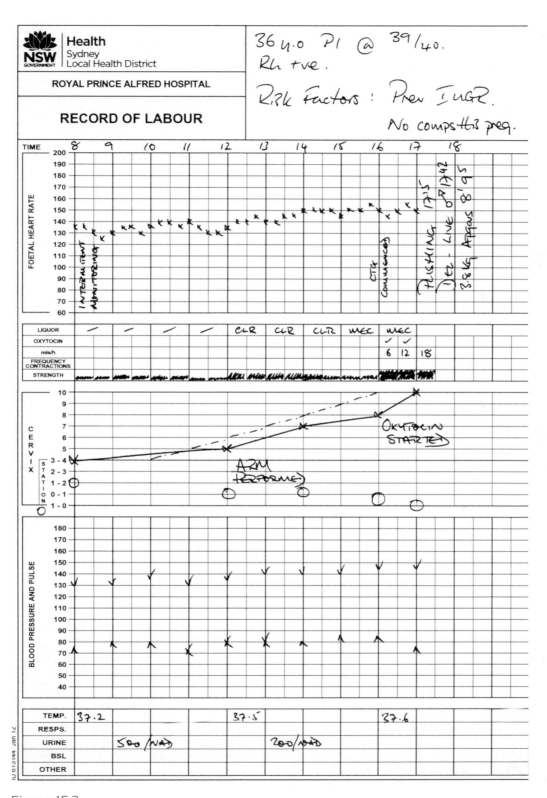

Figure 15.3

The partogram provides a graphical representation of progress in labour. This multiparous woman is defined as being in labour (4 cm dilated) at 8 a.m. Progress is recorded with further vaginal examinations (x) and progress is slow, falling behind the action line (_ _ _ _). An amniotomy (ARM) and oxytocin are used to improve the rate of progress. Delivery occurs soon after full dilatation is reached. Details of fetal and maternal wellbeing are also recorded.

evidence that either a 'hands-on' or 'hands-off' approach affects rates of perineal trauma. Routine episiotomy is not advocated.[9]

The third stage of labour: delivery of the placenta

The third stage of labour starts after delivery of the infant and the focus for risk shifts from the fetus to the mother. The major risk at this stage is one of haemorrhage — which is likely to be significant in 6% of cases managed expectantly. There is robust worldwide advice that active management of the third stage with oxytocin or oxytocin and ergometrine at the time of delivery of the anterior shoulder of the infant to cause uterine contraction reduces the risk of bleeding.[10] After the cord is clamped and cut, delivery of the placenta can be expedited by applying controlled cord traction. The placenta should be checked as being complete after delivery.

MANAGEMENT OF ABNORMAL LABOUR AND DELIVERY

Labour may deviate from normal for a number of reasons. There may be antenatal factors that suggest a higher risk of either maternal or fetal compromise. Labour may not progress normally, and may be described as dysfunctional. The fetus may not tolerate the intermittent periods of hypoxia caused by uterine contraction.

Failure to progress in labour

Slow progress in the active phase of the first stage of labour is typically defined as < 2 cm cervical dilatation over a 4-hour period. When slow progress is identified it is important to look for the underlying cause; it could be related to the passenger, the passage, or the powers. If the fetus is too big or the pelvis too small — which means the diameter of the presenting part is bigger than the diameter of the pelvis — then there may be cephalopelvic disproportion. Estimation of fetal weight and of the size of the pelvis are difficult, but malposition and deflection of the presenting part maybe defined through vaginal examination in labour and may be correctable. If vaginal examination finds the fetus is presenting by the vertex in an occipito-anterior position then this is unlikely to be the cause of slow progress. In this circumstance, attention may turn to the powers, with assessment of the effectiveness of uterine contraction.

Application of the head to the cervix and uterine contraction may improve once membranes are ruptured — amniotomy is the first intervention offered to a woman making slow progress. If a second examination continues to show failure to make progress, then an oxytocin infusion can be used to improve coordinated uterine activity (Figure 15.3). Care needs to be taken when oxytocin is used to augment labour in a multiparous patient as it is unusual for the uterus to be dysfunctional, and failure to progress is more likely to reflect a true obstruction. In this situation, augmentation with oxytocin may lead to uterine rupture. Cephalopelvic disproportion is normally considered to be a retrospective diagnosis where no progress is made through the first stage of labour despite interventions designed to rectify fetal presentation and improve uterine contraction.

In the second stage, progress is monitored by documenting advancement of the presenting part. Failure to advance in the second stage also needs careful assessment to consider the underlying cause, but there are occasions where augmentation with syntocinon is appropriate to try to achieve spontaneous vaginal delivery.

Fetal distress in labour

Intermittent fetal monitoring may show either an elevation of the fetal heart rate or identify periods of fetal bradycardia after contraction. If these occur, then continuous electronic fetal monitoring using a CTG is needed to help determine whether the fetus is distressed. The fetal heart rate is normally 110–150 beats per minute and has 5–10 beats per minute variability. An active fetus will have periods where the heart rate accelerates, although this feature may not be present during labour. An increase in the baseline heart rate, reduction in variability, periods of fetal heart rate deceleration or of prolonged bradycardia may be indicative of fetal distress. The CTG is highly sensitive for fetal acidosis, but has poor specificity, and the findings of CTG screening may need to be confirmed by taking a fetal scalp blood sample to determine whether the fetus is acidotic or not. If the fetus is acidotic then delivery needs to be effected immediately. If full dilatation has been reached, then this may best be achieved by assisted vaginal delivery using forceps or ventouse (see below). If fetal acidosis is diagnosed in the first stage of labour then delivery must be effected by caesarean delivery.

Assisted vaginal delivery

In most circumstances, vaginal delivery can be achieved once full cervical dilatation has occurred, but on some occasions assistance is required through either forceps or ventouse delivery. Approximately 12–15% deliveries in Australia are effected by instrumental procedures. Safe instrumental delivery requires that the cervix is fully dilated, the fetal head is fully engaged, the fetal station is at or below the maternal ischial spines (i.e. below the plane of least dimensions), and the exact position of the fetal head is known (so the instrument is applied correctly). Some instruments (e.g. Kiwi cup or Bird cup ventouse or Kiellands forceps) can be used to correct malposition or the attitude of presentation, and reduce the diameter of the presenting part during the process of delivery (Figure 15.4). Others (Silc cup or Neville-Barnes forceps) are simply applied to the vertex, allowing traction while the mother is pushing to expel the fetus (Figure 15.5).

Indications for instrumental delivery include failure to advance in the second stage (due to maternal exhaustion, difficulties in effective pushing with epidural analgesia, poor uterine activity), and evidence of fetal distress. Less commonly, in some maternal circumstances, instrumental delivery may be performed to reduce the amount of maternal effort required for delivery. Instrumental delivery carries risks of complication to mother and infant and should be performed with adequate analgesia.

Perineal trauma (e.g. episiotomy) is more likely and often more severe after instrumental delivery. Fetal injury such as retinal haemorrhage, cephalohaematoma and subgaleal haemorrhage may occur and can be life-threatening (Box 15.1). There may be a contraindication to instrumental delivery, such as a risk of haemophilia affecting the infant.

Perineal trauma

The perineum may be damaged during normal vaginal birth. The perineum may also be cut during the second stage of labour (episiotomy). Perineal trauma has been classified into the following groups:

- First-degree tear: injury to vaginal or perineal skin only.
- Second-degree tear: as above, plus injury to perineal muscles.
- Third-degree tear: second-degree injury, with additional involvement of anal sphincter muscles.
  - 3a: <50% of external anal sphincter torn
  - 3b: >50% of external anal sphincter torn
  - 3c: internal anal sphincter also torn.
- Fourth-degree tear: as third degree, with injury to the rectal mucosa (Figure 15.6).

There is no strong evidence to suggest that routine use of episiotomy reduces the risk of third- and fourth-degree perineal tears.

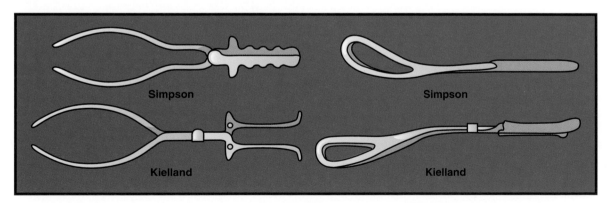

Figure 15.4

Examples of obstetric forceps. Simpson forceps are an example of a classic pair of forceps used for delivery of a fetus presenting in an occiput-anterior position. Kielland forceps are less frequently used, principally for rotational delivery (rotating from occiput-posterior to occiput-anterior before advancing through the birth canal). The Kielland forceps have less pelvic curve, allowing them to be used as a rotational instrument.

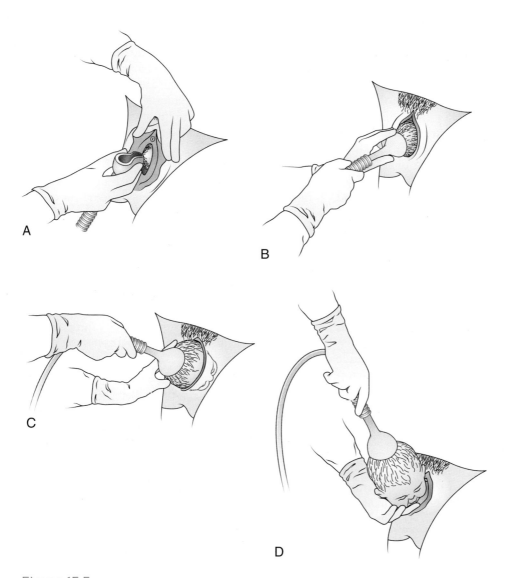

Figure 15.5

Effecting delivery with a ventouse (Silc cup). **A**: The cup is applied to the vertex, taking care not to traumatise the vaginal wall. Vacuum is applied and time allowed for the chignon to develop, providing a better seal. **B, C, D**: Traction is applied while the mother is pushing, in coordination with uterine contraction. As the head advances through the birth canal the accoucheur mimics the normal mechanics of labour. An episiotomy may be needed as the head crowns for delivery — the cup can be removed at this point.

(Copyright © 2010 Saunders, An Imprint of Elsevier. Taken from: James: High Risk Pregnancy, 4th ed. 9781416059080; Figure 72–3)

A perineal tear should be repaired as soon as possible after the delivery. A first-degree tear that is not bleeding may be allowed to heal by secondary intention, but all other tears should be repaired in layers. A rectal examination should be done after the repair to ensure the anal mucosa is free of suture material.

Unusual presentations

Persistent occipito-posterior or occipito-transverse position

Up to 30% of fetuses enter labour in an occipito-posterior (OP) or occipito-transverse (OT) position. The vast majority rotate spontaneously to occipito-anterior (OA) (Figure 15.1). Those that do not

Box 15.1 Potential maternal and fetal complications from instrumental delivery

Most complications have been reported for both methods of instrumental delivery, and are listed here under the mode of delivery associated with the higher prevalence of that complication.

Forceps

MATERNAL

- Vaginal laceration
- Perineal tear
- Damage to the anal sphincter
- Urinary and faecal incontinence
- Postpartum haemorrhage (related to vaginal/perineal trauma)

FETAL*

- Facial bruising / forceps marks (transitory)
- Facial nerve (VII) palsy (transitory)
- Skull fracture

Ventouse

MATERNAL

- Higher procedural failure rate

FETAL*

- Scalp abrasions
- Intracranial haemorrhage
- Cephalhaematoma
- Subgaleal haematoma
- Retinal haemorrhage

*There is evidence that the rate of severe neonatal injury is not significantly different for forceps, ventouse or caesarean delivery during labour.

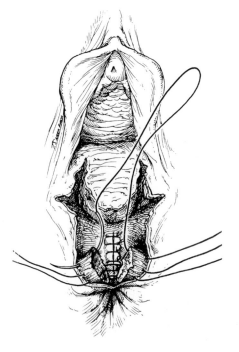

Figure 15.6

An example of a fourth-degree tear. The rectal mucosa has already been repaired (midline) and the external anal sphincter is now been repaired with a series of interrupted sutures. Bilateral tears in the vaginal wall can be seen and will be repaired next.

(Copyright © 2008 Mosby, An Imprint of Elsevier. Taken from: Ratcliffe: Family Medicine Obstetrics, 3rd ed. 9780323043069; Figure 14-17)

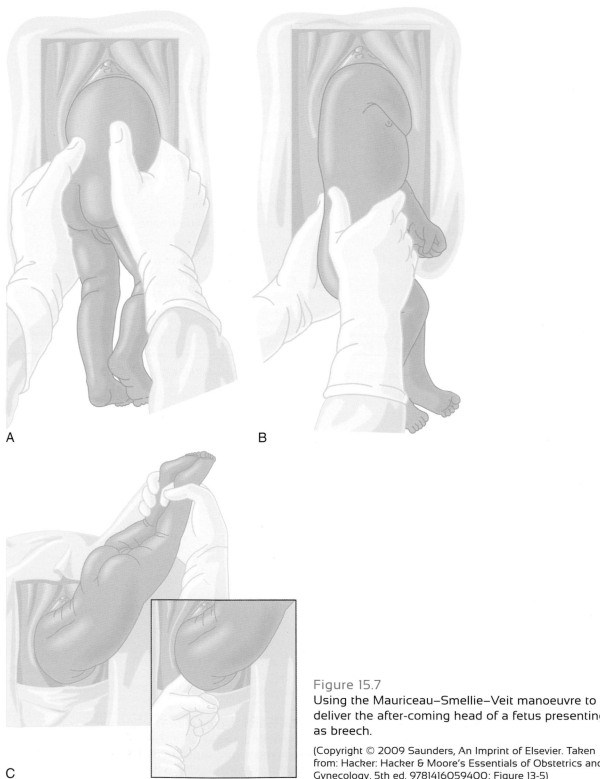

A

B

C

Figure 15.7
Using the Mauriceau–Smellie–Veit manoeuvre to deliver the after-coming head of a fetus presenting as breech.

(Copyright © 2009 Saunders, An Imprint of Elsevier. Taken from: Hacker: Hacker & Moore's Essentials of Obstetrics and Gynecology, 5th ed. 9781416059400; Figure 13-5)

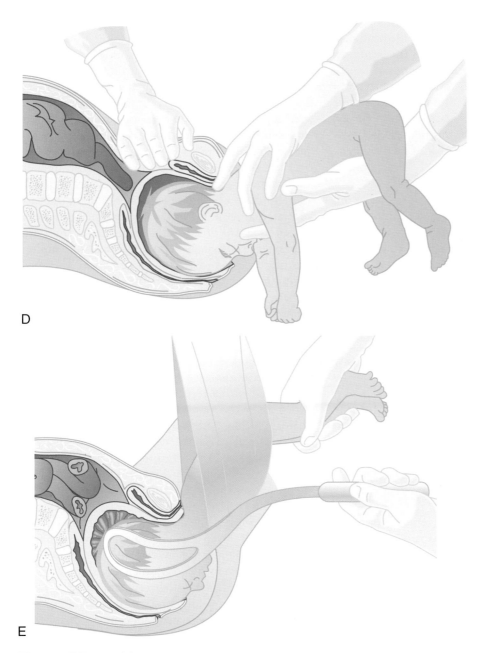

D

E

Figure 15.7, cont'd

present a wider diameter to the birth canal, increasing the risk of prolonged labour, perineal trauma, instrumental delivery, caesarean delivery and fetal birth trauma. A proportion of fetuses presenting in OP position will deliver spontaneously, but manual rotation of the fetal head may be used to effect this, or rotational instrumental delivery may be considered.

Face and brow presentations

Rarely, there is progressive extension rather than flexion of the head as the fetus descends into the pelvis and the fetus presents as a face (1 in 500 pregnancies) or brow (1 in 1500 pregnancies). Face and brow presentations are more common in premature deliveries and post-dates pregnancies, and are associated with macrosomia and cephalopelvic disproportion. The presenting diameter of a brow is too large to allow vaginal delivery and the head may either flex or become more extended (to become a face presentation) during labour. Diagnosis of these presentations is not typically made until cervical dilatation is quite advanced. The majority of these infants require delivery by caesarean delivery. Mento-anterior face presentations may deliver vaginally but there is an increased risk of fetal trauma.

Breech presentation

The prevalence of breech presentation reduces from 25% at 20 weeks' gestation to 3% at term. There is an increased incidence in women with uterine or fetal anomalies. Breech presentation is associated with a higher risk of perinatal mortality and morbidity, some of which may be attributed to delivery of the largest part of the fetus last. Although long-term data from the Term Breech Trial[11] is less definitive, the initial data led to consensus that breech presenting fetuses are best delivered by elective caesarean section. The consequence of this is that many accoucheurs have become less practised in the manipulations required for successful vaginal breech delivery. The role of the accoucheur is primarily supportive, although various manoeuvres (Løvset, Bracht, Mariceau–Smellie–Veit) that aid delivery of the shoulders, arms and head have been described (Figure 15.7).

Transverse or oblique lie

When the longitudinal axis of the fetus is not parallel to that of the mother, the fetus is deemed to be in transverse or oblique lie. This may reflect some obstruction in the pelvis (for example placenta praevia) that prevents descent of the head. It is more common in multiparous patients, where lie may be unstable, and it may be possible to stabilise the lie with a cephalic presentation and induce labour with amniotomy and oxytocin infusion. If the fetus remains transverse or oblique then it should be delivered by caesarean delivery as obstructed labour risks uterine rupture.

CAESAREAN DELIVERY

An alternative to vaginal delivery involves surgical incision of the abdomen and uterus. Caesarean delivery was originally performed after maternal death in pregnancy and has only become regarded as a relatively routine procedure since the mortality and morbidity associated with surgery have reduced.

Abdominal delivery is increasingly common, occurring in 28% of the obstetric population in Australia.

Caesarean delivery may be planned electively — before the onset of labour — or offered as an emergency procedure once labour has been diagnosed. Elective caesarean delivery is traditionally considered in circumstances where the process of labour and delivery may be detrimental for the mother or fetus. A small number of women now request caesarean delivery in circumstances where no medical indication exists, highlighting the ethics and risks of performing an unnecessary operation on the basis of maternal request. Once a woman has had a caesarean delivery, risks of uterine dehiscence and rupture in subsequent labours increase, so siblings are often delivered by the same route. The most common indications for emergency caesarean delivery are failure to progress through the first stage of labour, fetal distress, or an abnormal lie or malpresentation at the onset of labour.

In some circumstances, such as preterm delivery or after rupture of membranes with an abnormal lie, caesarean delivery may be difficult and is better performed with a vertical (classical) uterine incision rather than the transverse lower segment incision that is typically performed. The uterine scar formed after classical caesarean delivery is more likely to rupture (2% risk) in a future pregnancy, and these women would typically be advised that all subsequent fetuses should be delivered abdominally. The rate of uterine rupture also increases after two or more caesarean deliveries have been performed, and women with this history are typically advised to have an elective caesarean delivery for all future births.

Approximately 5% of women will suffer complications after caesarean delivery, and there is a risk of long-term morbidity and mortality.[12] Complication rates increase when abdominal delivery is repeated, and there is also an increased risk of morbid adherence of the placenta in future pregnancies, which can lead to significant haemorrhage requiring hysterectomy at the time of delivery. The recent increase in prevalence of caesarean delivery has not been accompanied by a reduction in perinatal mortality, and many jurisdictions are now developing strategies to place downward pressure on the caesarean delivery rate.

INDUCTION OF LABOUR

In circumstances where the risks associated with continuing pregnancy outweigh the risks associated

Table 15.1 Bishop score for cervical assessment prior to induction of labour

Indication	Score*		
	0	1	2
Cervical length	≥3 cm	1–2 cm	<1 cm
Cervical dilatation	<1 cm	1–2 cm	≥3 cm
Cervical consistency	Firm	Average	Soft
Cervical position	Posterior	Central	Anterior
Station of the presenting part	≥ 3 cm above spines	2 cm or 1 cm above spines	at/beyond the spines

*If the Bishop score is ≥6 then induction normally involves amniotomy + oxytocin augmentation. If the Bishop score is <6 then induction normally starts with cervical preparation using prostaglandin E_2.

with being delivered, induction of labour should be considered. Approximately 15% of labours are induced for a variety of maternal and fetal indications. One example is induction for postmaturity: the risk of stillbirth rises significantly after 42 weeks' gestation while delivery at this stage has no risk of prematurity. In addition, women who have not laboured by 42 weeks' gestation are more likely to have dysfunctional labour, and there is evidence that the caesarean delivery rate is not increased by inducing labour in this circumstance.[13]

Most induction policies aim to simulate the process of natural labour as closely as possible. Abdominal and vaginal examination are used to define how close the fetus is to being engaged and how the cervix has changed through the later part of pregnancy. The cervix is assessed digitally by vaginal examination using Bishop's score; based on length, dilatation, position, consistency and fetal station (Table 15.1). If the cervix is unfavourable (Bishop score <6) then it needs to be primed, either pharmacologically with prostaglandin E_2, or mechanically with a balloon catheter. If the cervix is favourable (Bishop score ≥6) then induction can move straight to amniotomy followed by uterine stimulation with oxytocin. The process of cervical preparation may take 1–2 days, but once amniotomy is performed delivery will normally occur within 16 hours.

Induction of labour involves the administration of drugs that cause uterine contraction, and can cause hyperstimulation and fetal distress. As induction is normally performed because of perceived risk to the pregnancy, the fetus should be monitored intermittently when these drugs are given and when there is significant uterine activity. In some circumstances continuous electronic fetal monitoring may be necessary. If the cervix cannot be primed and ARM is not possible, then the induction has failed and delivery necessitates caesarean delivery. Similarly, if induction and uterine activity stress the fetus, then caesarean delivery may be necessary to effect safe delivery. Caesarean delivery rates are generally 10% higher in nulliparous women having an induced labour compared to those who labour spontaneously.

DELIVERY OF MULTIPLE PREGNANCIES

Approximately 1 in 60 pregnancies in Australia are multiples. The prevalence has increased from the natural incidence of around 1 : 80 due to the increasing maternal age of the population and use of assisted reproductive technologies. Twins and specifically monochorionic twins (sharing the same placenta) have significantly higher rates of mortality and morbidity. Although they account for less than 2% of all deliveries they account for more than 20% of admissions to the neonatal intensive care unit. All potential complications of pregnancy are more prevalent in twin pregnancies — with the exception of postmaturity.

Twins are more likely to deliver preterm and to have intrauterine growth restriction; they are therefore more likely to be stressed in labour. Uterine activity is more likely to be dysfunctional, and the lie of the first twin may not allow the force of contraction to be appropriately applied to the cervix, resulting in a higher risk of failure to progress. In most circumstances the presenting twin is cephalic and larger than the second twin, factors that facilitate delivery. If the first twin is breech and the second cephalic, then the heads can lock during delivery, leading to hypoxic injury and death. Twins should be delivered by caesarean section if the presenting fetus is breech. If the second twin is larger, the cervix may not have dilated adequately during delivery of the first twin to allow delivery of the second infant.

Epidural analgesia is often recommended to mothers labouring with twins as effective analgesia may be needed for manipulation of the second twin. If the second twin turns to be an abnormal lie or presentation then external cephalic version or internal podalic version (locating a foot which is then pulled down into the vagina) may be used to deliver the second twin.

Monochorionic diamniotic twins may also be complicated by their communicating placental vasculature. Uterine contraction may cause an acute imbalance in the vascular anastamoses running between the two twins, and this may lead to acute twin–twin transfusion during labour. There is some evidence that this imbalance can become profound very rapidly, leading to death and injury of one or both infants. Some obstetricians therefore elect to deliver all monochorionic diamniotic twins by caesarean section, although this remains controversial. Preterm caesarean delivery of all monochorionic monoamniotic twins is more readily accepted due to the risk of cord entanglement during the third trimester or during vaginal delivery.

SUMMARY

The pinnacle of pregnancy is delivery. Midwives and obstetricians are privileged to play an important role in assisting women through labour and the process of birth, making sure that the risks to maternal and fetal health are minimised. Labour is a complicated process and surveillance needs to be structured so that any subtle deviation from the norm is recognised. Families anticipate an uncomplicated course and a normal outcome — and any perceived risks and necessary interventions need to be openly discussed so that the woman remains empowered during delivery.

REFERENCES

1 World Health Organization. Care in normal birth: a practical guide. Report of a Technical Working Group. WHO/FRH/MSM/96.24. Geneva: World Health Organization; 1999.

2 Zhang J, Troendle J, Mikolajczyk R, et al. The natural history of the normal first stage of labor. Obstet Gynecol 2010;115:705–10.

3 Albers LL. The duration of labor in healthy women. J Perinatol 1999;19:114.

4 Derham RJ, Crowhurst J, Crowther C. The second stage of labour: durational dilemmas. Aust NZ J Obstet Gynaecol 2003;31:31–6.

5 World Health Organization. Maternal and child health and family planning. The prevention and management of postpartum haemorrhage. Report of a Technical Working Group. WHO/MCH 1990;90(7):3.

6 RANZCOG. IntrapartumFetal Surveillance. Melbourne: Clinical Guideline; 2006.

7 RANZCOG College statement, Nov 2011 (C-Obs-2: Home births) http://www.ranzcog.edu.au/womens-health/statements-a-guidelines/college-statements/425-home-births-c-obs-2.html

8 Leighton BL, Halpern SH. The effects of epidural analgesia on labor, maternal and neonatal outcomes: a systematic review. Am J Obstet Gynecol 2002;186:S69–77.

9 Aasheim V, Nilsen A, Lukasse M, et al. Perineal techniques during the second stage of labour for reducing perineal trauma. Cochrane Database Syst Rev 2011;CD006672.

10 Begley CM, Gyte GM, Devane D, et al. Active versus expectant management for women in the third stage of labour. Cochrane Database Syst Rev 2011;CD007412.

11 Hannah ME, Hannah WJ, Hewson SA, et al. Planned caesarean section versus planned vaginal birth for breech presentation at term: a randomised multicentre trial. Term Breech Trial Collaborative Group. Lancet 2000;356:1375.

12 Häger RM, Daltveit AK, Hofoss D, et al. Complications of cesarean deliveries: rates and risk factors. Am J Obstet Gynecol 2004;190:428–34.

13 Hannah ME, Hannah WJ, Hellmann J, et al. Induction of labor as compared with serial antenatal monitoring in post-term pregnancy. A randomized controlled trial. The Canadian Multicenter Post-term Pregnancy Trial Group. N Engl J Med 1992;326:1587–92.

MCQS

Select the correct answer.

1   The onset of labour is defined by:

   A   A cervix that is 2 cm dilated in the presence of some irregular uterine activity.
   B   50% effacement of the cervix in the presence of regular uterine activity.
   C   Progressive effacement and dilatation of the cervix in the presence of progressively more frequent and more painful uterine contractions.
   D   A cervix that is 4 cm dilated with no uterine activity.
   E   Rupture of membranes with some irregular uterine activity.

2   Epidural analgesia:

   A   does not affect the rate of instrumental delivery.
   B   may be associated with a low-grade maternal pyrexia.
   C   should not be offered once the cervix is 8 cm dilated.
   D   is almost as effective as pethidine in providing pain relief for labour.
   E   does not impact on the method of fetal monitoring.

3   Dysfunctional labour in nulliparous women:

   A   is most frequently associated with an abnormally shaped pelvis.
   B   is most frequently associated with fetal macrosomia.
   C   is most frequently associated with poor or incoordinate uterine activity.
   D   describes failure of the presenting part to advance in the second stage.
   E   is primarily judged through descent of the head through labour.

4   Which one of these statements about operative delivery is correct?

   A   5% of low-risk nulliparous women require an instrumental delivery.
   B   Simpson forceps can be used for a rotational delivery.
   C   Ventouse is less likely to cause maternal complications than forceps.
   D   Low-risk nulliparous women should be allowed to push for 30 minutes before proceeding to instrumental delivery.
   E   Ventouse is contraindicated for rotational delivery.

5   Which of the following statements about inducing labour is correct?

   A   Cervical ripening should always precede amniotomy.
   B   Amniotomy is an ineffective method of inducing labour.
   C   Cervical ripening with prostaglandin is recommended if the Bishop score is 3.
   D   Induction of labour reduces the caesarean section rate.
   E   Intermittent auscultation is recommended for women on an oxytocin infusion.

OSCE

Angela, a 27-year-old woman who is 37+6 weeks gestation in her first ongoing pregnancy, attends the delivery suite with a 3-hour history of lower abdominal pain and a small amount of PV bleeding.

Describe how you would assess Angela on admission.

On examination you find the following:

- lie: cephalic, 2/5 palpable
- cervix 3 cm dilated, fully effaced, soft, central os. Station −2, no PV bleeding seen

Through your assessment you find that Angela has increasingly frequent and painful contractions, now spaced every 2–3 minutes. The contractions can be palpated and the uterus is relaxed between times. The fetus is appropriately grown, longitudinal lie, cephalic presentation and the head is engaged. The cervix is effaced and dilated on examination. What is your diagnosis?

Chapter 16

Obstetric emergencies

Tanya Nippita, Kirsty Foster and Jonathan Morris

KEY POINTS

Maternal and perinatal mortality rates are much lower in rich than in poor countries.

Maternal mortality is defined as the a death of a woman while pregnant or within 42 days of pregnancy.

Postpartum haemorrhage is defined as greater than 500 mL of blood loss within 24 hours after vaginal delivery.

Placental abruption occurs when bleeding causes premature separation of the placenta from the wall of the uterus.

Shoulder dystocia occurs when the fetal shoulders become impacted in the maternal pelvis after delivery of the fetal head.

Cord prolapse is the descent of the umbilical cord alongside or beyond the presenting part in the presence of ruptured membranes.

INTRODUCTION
Maternal and perinatal mortality

It is important to remember that the birth of a baby, an experience which can be the most wonderful and joyous in life, can also be the most deadly. Every day, one thousand women die from causes related to pregnancy and birth. Ninety-nine per cent of these deaths occur in developing countries,[1] and almost all are preventable. A determination to tackle this shocking statistic at a global level was formed by the United Nations 5th Millennium Development Goal: to reduce the maternal mortality ratio (MMR) by 75% between 1990 and 2015.

There is a major inequity between rich and poor countries. The most recent 'Maternal Deaths in Australia' report 2003–2005, quotes the maternal mortality rate (MMR) as 8.4 per 100 000 women giving birth.[2] This is comparable to the MMR of other developed countries, but the mortality rate in some developing countries is several hundred times greater (Table 16.1).

Even within Australia there is discrepancy: the maternal mortality for Aboriginal or Torres Strait Islander women is more than two and a half times higher than for the rest of the Australian population, with 21.5 deaths per 100 000 for Indigenous women giving birth compared to 7.9 per 100 000 for non-Indigenous women.[2]

The World Health Organization (WHO) definition of a maternal death is: 'The death of a woman while pregnant or within 42 days of termination of pregnancy, irrespective of the duration and site of the pregnancy, from any cause related to or aggravated by the pregnancy or its management, but not from accidental or incidental causes.'

Direct deaths are those that result from obstetric complications of the pregnant state, see Table 16.2. Indirect deaths result from preexisting disease or

Table 16.1 Maternal mortality rates across the world[3]

Country or region	MMR (deaths per 100 000)
United Kingdom	8
United States of America	11
Oceania	430
South Asia	490
Sub-Saharan Africa	900

Table 16.2 Causes of direct maternal deaths, Australia 2003–2005[2]

Cause of death	Number
Amniotic fluid embolism	8
Hypertensive disorders of pregnancy	5
Thrombosis and thromboembolism	5
Obstetric haemorrhage	4
Cardiac conditions	3
Infections	1
Deaths associated with anaesthesia	1
Non-genital tract haemorrhage	1
Thrombotic thrombocytopenic purpura	1
TOTAL	29

Table 16.3 Causes of indirect maternal deaths, Australia 2003–2005[2]

Cause of death	Number
Cardiac	10
Psychiatric causes	6
Non-obstetric haemorrhage	5
Infection	4
Hypertension	1
Other indirect causes	10
TOTAL	36

disease that developed during pregnancy and was not due to direct obstetric causes, but which was aggravated by the physiological effects of pregnancy, see Table 16.3. Incidental deaths result from conditions occurring during pregnancy where the pregnancy is unlikely to have contributed significantly to the death, for example road accidents and some malignancies.

The leading causes of indirect maternal deaths are shown in Table 16.3.

Four categories accounted for almost half of all maternal deaths in Australia between 1997 and 2005:
- cardiac disease (32 deaths, 15% of deaths)
- amniotic fluid embolism (25 deaths, 12% of deaths)
- psychiatric illness (23 deaths, 11% of deaths)
- genital tract haemorrhage (22 deaths, 10% of deaths).

Babies and fetuses die more commonly than mothers. Worldwide, the perinatal mortality rate (PNMR) is used as an indicator of the general health status of a community. Variations across the world in the definitions of the PNMR make comparison between countries challenging. The Australian Bureau of Statistics and other countries with a low PNMR use a wider definition than the WHO, as can be seen in Table 16.4. Thus in Australia a birthweight of 400 g or more, or if birth weight is unavailable, a gestational age of at least 20 weeks, counts as a fetal death (stillbirth). However, if the birth weight is not known, death before 20 weeks gestation is classed as a miscarriage; death less than 28 days after birth is a neonatal death but death at age 28 days or more becomes an infant death.

Table 16.4 Perinatal mortality definitions[4]

Institution	Perinatal deaths		
	FETAL DEATHS		NEONATAL DEATHS
	Birth weight (g)	Gestational age	
WHO: international comparison	≥1000	28 weeks (only if birth weight unavailable)	<7 days
WHO: national reporting	≥500	22 weeks (only if birth weight unavailable)	<7 days
Australian Bureau of Statistics	≥400	20 weeks (only if birth weight unavailable)	<28 days
NHDD and NPESU	≥400	20 weeks	<28 days

NHDD: National Health Data Dictionary.
NPESU: AIHW National Perinatal Epidemiology and Statistical Unit.

The most recent Australian Mothers and Babies report 2010[4] reports 9.3 perinatal deaths per 1000 births, of which almost 80% were fetal deaths. Again, Aboriginal and Torres Strait PNMR was almost twice that of babies born to non-Indigenous women. Perinatal death rates were highest in babies of mothers at the extremes of reproductive age: those 40 years and over (13.5 per 1000 births) and teenage mothers (13.3 per 1000 births).

In order to improve these statistics and progress towards the 5th Millennium Development Goal, it is crucial that obstetricians, midwives and others involved in the care of women of childbearing age are vigilant for complications arising in pregnancy, labour and the puerperium. They also require the knowledge, skills and understanding to manage complications should they arise.

GENERAL OBSTETRIC COMPLICATIONS
Maternal collapse

This can occur at any time over the gestational cycle and, like any adult collapse, treatment of the cause should be instigated as part of the acute life support algorithm. Maternal resuscitation is performed along guidelines for adult resuscitation according to the Australian Resuscitation Council guidelines, which include basic and advanced life support (BLS and ALS); see Figures 16.1 and 16.2.

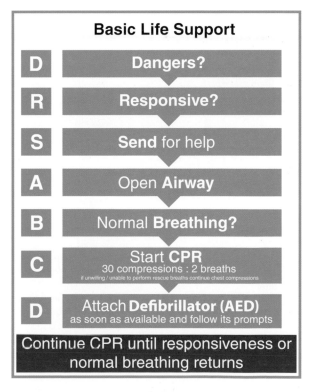

Figure 16.1
Basic life support.

(Australian Resuscitation Council.)

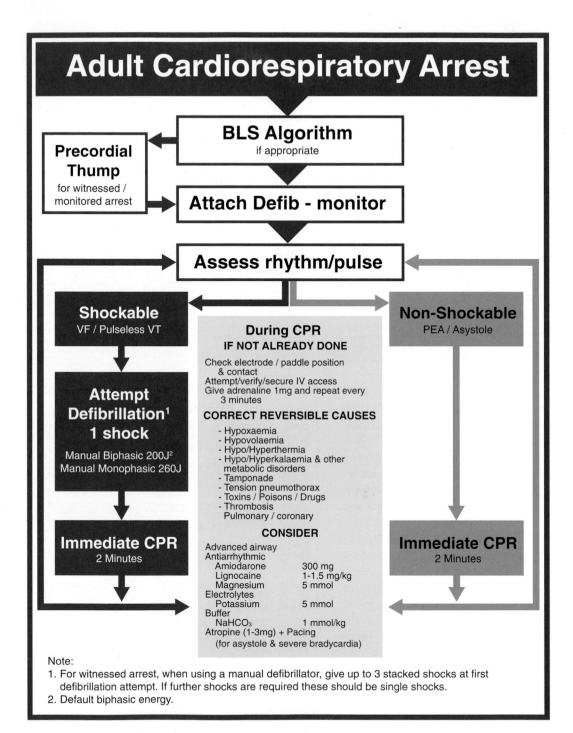

Adult Cardiorespiratory Arrest

BLS Algorithm
if appropriate

Precordial Thump
for witnessed / monitored arrest

Attach Defib - monitor

Assess rhythm/pulse

Shockable
VF / Pulseless VT

Non-Shockable
PEA / Asystole

Attempt Defibrillation[1] 1 shock
Manual Biphasic 200J[2]
Manual Monophasic 260J

Immediate CPR
2 Minutes

During CPR
IF NOT ALREADY DONE
Check electrode / paddle position & contact
Attempt/verify/secure IV access
Give adrenaline 1mg and repeat every 3 minutes

CORRECT REVERSIBLE CAUSES
- Hypoxaemia
- Hypovolaemia
- Hypo/Hyperthermia
- Hypo/Hyperkalaemia & other metabolic disorders
- Tamponade
- Tension pneumothorax
- Toxins / Poisons / Drugs
- Thrombosis
  Pulmonary / coronary

CONSIDER
Advanced airway
Antiarrhythmic
  Amiodarone   300 mg
  Lignocaine   1-1.5 mg/kg
  Magnesium   5 mmol
Electrolytes
  Potassium   5 mmol
Buffer
  $NaHCO_3$ 1 mmol/kg
Atropine (1-3mg) + Pacing
  (for asystole & severe bradycardia)

Immediate CPR
2 Minutes

Note:
1. For witnessed arrest, when using a manual defibrillator, give up to 3 stacked shocks at first defibrillation attempt. If further shocks are required these should be single shocks.
2. Default biphasic energy.

Figure 16.2
Adult cardiorespiratory arrest.

(Australian Resuscitation Council.)

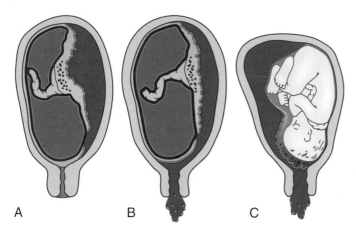

Figure 16.3

Degrees of placental abruption. **A**: Concealed abruption; **B**: Revealed abruption; **C**: Complete placental separation.

(Miller: Miller's Anesthesia, 7th ed. 2009 Churchill Livingstone; 9781416066248; Figure 69.16A to C. Redrawn from Bonica JJ, Johnson WL: Placenta previa, abruptio placentae or rupture of the uterus. In Bonica JJ (ed): Principles and Practice of Obstetric Analgesia and Anesthesia, vol 2, 1st ed. Philadelphia, FA Davis, 1969, p 1164.)

Dosages of resuscitation drugs and energy levels with defibrillation are unchanged by pregnancy.

During resuscitation from 20 weeks gestation onwards, the mother needs to be positioned with a left lateral tilt to reduce aortocaval compression by the gravid uterus. Aortocaval compression reduces cardiac output by 30% and in itself can cause collapse through hypotension.

Perimortem caesarean delivery

Pregnant women develop anoxia faster than non-pregnant women and can suffer irreversible brain damage within 4–6 minutes after cardiac arrest. Delivery of the fetus and placenta reduces oxygen consumption, increases venous return and cardiac output, and facilitates ventilation and cardiac compressions.[5] Thus, perimortem caesarean delivery should be performed to aid maternal resuscitation, not only for neonatal survival. Ideally caesarean delivery should begin within 4 minutes of cardiac arrest and delivery should be accomplished by 5 minutes.

ANTENATAL OBSTETRIC COMPLICATIONS

Antepartum haemorrhage

Antepartum haemorrhage (APH) is defined as bleeding from the genital tract after 20 weeks of gestation, and occurs in approximately 2–6% of pregnancies. The most important causes of APH are placental abruption, placenta praevia and placenta accreta. Other causes include vasa praevia, cervicitis, and lower genital tract infections and malignancy. APH is largely unpredictable and is a major contributor to maternal and perinatal morbidity in the developed world, but even more so in the developing world. Women should be advised to seek the attention of a healthcare professional should they experience an APH.

All women that experience antepartum haemorrhage are at significantly increased risk of postpartum haemorrhage.

Placental abruption

Placental abruption is caused by premature separation of the placenta from the uterus (Figure 16.3). Concealed abruption occurs when there is no evidence of vaginal bleeding, and may only be diagnosed by the presence of abdominal pain. Abruption occurs in approximately 1% of pregnancies and is the cause of 10% of preterm births. Risk factors include hypertensive disorders of pregnancy, previous abruption, cigarette or cocaine use, trauma, preterm premature rupture of membranes, overdistension of the uterus such as with multiple pregnancy or polyhydramnios, placental anomalies, uterine manipulation (such as external cephalic version), and thrombophilias.

The diagnosis is made according to symptoms and the presentation can vary widely. The classical presentation is of per vaginal (PV) bleeding, continuous abdominal pain, and tenderness on palpation of the uterus. The presence of bleeding causes the uterus to contract in a sustained, tonic fashion. This is recognised clinically by increased uterine tone, or, at its most extreme, a wooden hardness. Placental abruption is a clinical diagnosis since ultrasound fails to detect 50% of cases.

The management of abruption depends on its severity and the gestational age at which it presents. Expectant management may be considered where the fetus is preterm (<37 weeks gestation), with no signs of fetal heart rate abnormality, the mother is haemodynamically stable, and has mild bleeding and minimal pain. If there is ongoing bleeding, the obligation to deliver becomes stronger the heavier the bleeding, particularly in the context of maternal haemodynamic compromise. Any woman who is seriously compromised should be resuscitated and delivered.

If the abruption occurs intrapartum, vaginal birth is possible if there is no serious fetal compromise and the mother is haemodynamically stable. The mother should be carefully monitored, have an IV line in-situ with an assessment made of her haematological and cardiovascular status, and continuous electronic fetal monitoring. Blood products may become necessary depending on the amount of bleeding. An assessment of feto-maternal haemorrhage should be made by sending a Kleihauer test. Haemorrhagic shock, coagulopathy, ischaemic necrosis of the distal organs, in particular the kidney, are all complications of abruption, especially when the abruption is severe is enough to cause fetal death.

Placenta praevia

Placenta praevia is defined by implantation of the placenta in the lower segment of the uterus. It is classified into four grades, as shown in Figure 16.4.

In an Australian cohort the incidence of placenta praevia was 4.3 per 1000,[6] which is similar to other developed countries. The incidence of placenta praevia increases with age, multiparity, smoking, IVF, uterine surgery, and history of caesarean delivery. The likelihood of placenta praevia increases in a dose-response fashion: the greater the number of caesarean deliveries the greater the relative risk. Risk of placenta praevia after one caesarean delivery is 4.5 (95% CI 3.6–5.5), increasing tenfold to 44.9 (95% CI 13.5–149.5) after four caesarean deliveries.[7]

The diagnosis is usually made during routine morphology ultrasound in the second trimester in asymptomatic women. The placenta is described as 'low lying', but more than 90% of these placentas will appear to move away from the cervix and out of the lower uterine segment as the pregnancy progresses. This has been attributed, first to the hypertrophy of the lower uterine segment in the third trimester,[7] and second to the placenta growing preferentially towards the better vascularised fundus, whereas the placenta overlying the less well-vascularised cervix may undergo atrophy.

Malpresentation of the fetus is more common in cases of placenta praevia since the placental site prevents fetal head engagement.

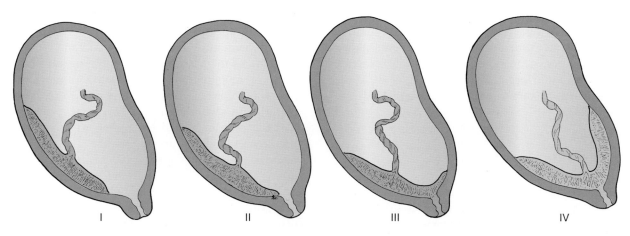

I   II   III   IV

Figure 16.4

Grades of placenta praevia. Grade I: low lying placenta: extends into the lower uterine segment but does not reach the internal os; Grade II: marginal placenta praevia: reaches the internal os but does not cover it; Grade III: partial placenta praevia: the placenta partially covers the internal os; Grade IV: complete or total placenta praevia: the placenta completely covers the internal os.

Classically the clinical presentation is of painless vaginal bleeding in the third trimester. However, pain may occur if there is additional uterine activity or abruption. Digital vaginal examination should be deferred until ultrasound has excluded the diagnosis, since it can cause excessive bleeding. Perinatal morbidity is related to the gestational age at delivery. Most episodes of vaginal bleeding are small and self-limiting, in which case at preterm gestations expectant management is reasonable without compromise to the fetus or the mother. However, as with placental abruption, serious maternal compromise will indicate delivery regardless of gestation.

Caesarean delivery is advised, since vaginal birth would risk major haemorrhage compromising the mother and the fetus, except in the case of grade I placenta praevia where the placenta is more than 2 cm away from the cervical os, when vaginal delivery can be offered. In terms of the timing of delivery, there is an increased risk of bleeding as gestational age increases, and it is safer to perform the caesarean delivery electively rather than as an emergency. Thus, elective delivery may be planned earlier than 39 weeks gestation if there have been prior episodes of APH. In the case of major placenta praevia, a large population study has indicated that neonatal mortality is lowest when elective caesarean delivery is planned at 37 weeks gestation.[8] Regional anaesthetic techniques are recommended for the caesarean delivery since they are associated with less blood loss and reduced blood transfusion requirements.

Placenta accreta

The condition of placenta accreta is potentially more serious and unfortunately more common as caesarean delivery rates have risen. Placenta accreta occurs when the placenta is morbidly adherent to the uterine wall; placenta increta where the placenta invades into the myometrium; and placenta percreta where the placenta invades through the myometrium and the serosa of the uterus and may invade other body organs. The incidence is quoted to be 1 in 2500 deliveries. The risk of placenta accreta is related to the number of prior caesarean deliveries.

In the presence of placenta praevia or multiple previous caesarean deliveries one should always be suspicious of the presence of placenta accreta, since it is associated with life-threatening haemorrhage and significant morbidity and mortality to the mother. Delivery should involve multidisciplinary care in a tertiary centre with intensive care facilities, a blood bank, and interventional radiology. Options for delivery include caesarean hysterectomy, caesarean delivery with the placenta left in-situ, with additional procedures such as embolisation of the internal iliac vessels.

Vasa praevia

Vasa praevia is a rare condition in which the fetal blood vessels run in the amniotic membranes below the presenting part of the fetus in front of the cervix, with no placenta or umbilical cord present. Thus vaginal bleeding, should it occur, is fetal rather than maternal, and is likely to be fatal. Rupture of membranes, either artificial or spontaneous, can lead to rapid fetal demise due to exsanguination. The fetal blood volume at term is approximately 100 mL/kg, so a mild to moderate amount of vaginal loss may be equivalent to the total fetal blood volume. There is minimal maternal risk, aside from the risk of rapid obstetric intervention on behalf of the fetus.

The diagnosis may be made incidentally on Doppler ultrasound (Figure 16.5), clinically on palpation of fetal vessels over the membranes, or classically when rupture of the membranes is accompanied by vaginal bleeding followed by acute fetal bradycardia. The recommended management of vasa praevia is caesarean delivery prior to the onset of labour (Figure 16.6). If there has been bleeding

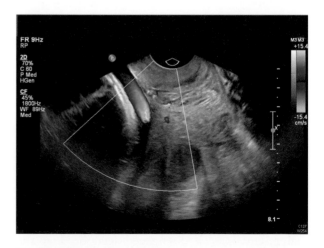

Figure 16.5

Transvaginal ultrasound demonstrating the fetal head on the left, and the large umbilical vein (coloured in red) coursing over the internal os of the cervix (to the right).

(Image courtesy of author.)

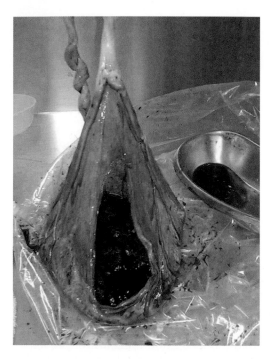

Figure 16.6

At caesarean delivery for the vasa praevia in figure 16.5, placenta showing fetal blood vessels within the amniotic membrane consistent with the diagnosis of a velamentous cord insertion, which is necessary for vasa praevia to occur.

(Image courtesy of author.)

from fetal blood vessels, a swift emergency delivery is required.

PERIPARTUM EMERGENCIES
Cord prolapse

Cord prolapse is the descent of the umbilical cord alongside or past the presenting part in the presence of ruptured membranes. This should be distinguished from a cord presentation, a less urgent condition in which the umbilical cord presents in front of the fetal presenting part with or without membrane rupture.

The incidence of cord prolapse overall is less than 1 in 200, although it is more common with breech presentation. Cord prolapse is associated with other malpresentations, a disengaged fetal head at the beginning of labour, multiple pregnancy, grand multiparity, preterm labour, polyhydramnios, and instrumental delivery. When the membranes rupture the umbilical cord can slip past the presenting part of the fetus and present at the cervix, or prolapse into the vagina. Without rapid action perinatal

mortality is high. Morbidity and mortality relates to birth asphyxia as the umbilical cord is directly compressed against the presenting part of the bony pelvis, or there is umbilical arterial vasospasm, depriving the fetus of oxygen.

Once the diagnosis is made, an emergency call for assistance should be initiated, summoning obstetric, midwifery, operating theatre, anaesthetic and neonatal staff. The prolapsed umbilical cord should be replaced into the vagina and if possible above the presenting part. If it is not possible, the presenting part should be dislodged to relieve pressure on the cord. To assist this, the mother is placed in a steep Trendelenburg position or knee–chest position to relieve pressure on the presenting part. Once the cord is replaced in the vagina, the examiner's hand should exert pressure on the presenting fetal part to prevent cord compression. If cord pulsations are palpable and the fetus is at a viable gestational age, the fetus should be delivered immediately. If vaginal delivery is possible it should be performed immediately. Where immediate vaginal delivery is not possible, the woman should be transferred to an operating theatre for an emergency caesarean delivery. Senior neonatal personnel skilled in resuscitation should be in attendance. The person responsible for preventing cord compression should remove their hand from the vagina only as the baby is being delivered.

Shoulder dystocia

Shoulder dystocia is infrequent, occurring in 0.2–3% of all deliveries,[9] but all healthcare workers providing obstetric services need to be prepared to handle this often unpredictable emergency. Shoulder dystocia occurs when there is a size discrepancy between the fetal shoulders and the pelvic inlet. The fetal shoulders become impacted on the maternal bony pelvis after delivery of the head, with the anterior shoulder wedged under the maternal pubic symphysis (Figure 16.7). In this situation further maternal expulsive efforts and traction on the fetal head become futile and specialised manoeuvres are necessary in order to deliver the infant.

Risk factors and complications

Maternal risk factors for shoulder dystocia are:
- shoulder dystocia with a previous birth
- diabetes
- instrumental vaginal delivery
- prolonged first and second stage of labour
- maternal obesity.

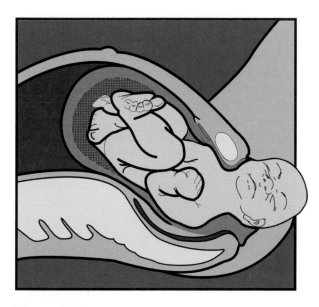

Figure 16.7
Shoulder dystocia where the fetal shoulders are impacted on the maternal bony pelvis.

(Taken from Lanni SM, Seeds JW. Malpresentations. In: Gabbe SG, Niebyl JR, Simpson JL. Obstetrics: normal and problem pregnancies, 5th ed. Philadelphia, Churchill Livingstone, 2007, pp 428–55.)

Fetal risk factors are:
- fetal macrosomia
- post-date pregnancy
- fetal anomalies.

When shoulder dystocia occurs, the umbilical cord is compressed between the body of the fetus and the maternal pelvis. During this time the fetal pH falls rapidly by 0.04 units per minute, so that delivery of the baby must occur within a few minutes to avoid asphyxia and death. The baby is at increased risk of fracture of the humerus or clavicle, or damage to the brachial plexus during delivery. However, fewer than 10% of children have permanent brachial plexus injury. Maternal associated complications include soft tissue injury or damage to the perineum, rectum, bladder and urethra, and post-partum haemorrhage.

Management

If risk factors are present and the possibility is anticipated, senior medical and midwifery personnel should be in attendance at the birth. In more than half of cases, however, there are *no* risk factors and shoulder dystocia occurs unexpectedly. Slow delivery of the fetal head over the perineum, delay of shoulder restitution, or the fetal head retracting against the perineum (the 'turtle' sign) are all warning signs.

A multidisciplinary team, involving obstetric, paediatric and anaesthetic staff, should be called immediately. The woman should be transferred to a dorsal lithotomy position, an episiotomy performed (to assist manoeuvres) and downward traction applied to the fetal head. If this fails the following manoeuvres can be employed:
- McRoberts position: this involves sharp flexion of the mother's thighs against her abdomen (See Figure 16.8.)
- Suprapubic pressure, usually applied in conjunction with the McRoberts manoeuvre in order to disimpact the anterior shoulder from the symphysis pubis.
- Wood's corkscrew manoeuvre to abduct the posterior shoulder.
- Delivery of the posterior arm.
- Moving the mother to all-fours position.

Most cases of shoulder dystocia can be resolved within 4 minutes of identification using the above manoeuvres.

AMNIOTIC FLUID EMBOLISM

Amniotic fluid embolism (AFE) is one of the leading causes of maternal mortality in developed countries. In the 2008 Maternal Deaths in Australia Report,[2] AFE accounted for 12% of all maternal deaths and was the leading cause of direct maternal death. Case fatality is high, and in survivors there is significant maternal (6–50% neurological impairment)[10] and perinatal (24–50%) morbidity.

The diagnosis of AFE is one of exclusion, but it is characterised by acute maternal collapse with one or more of the following features:
- acute fetal compromise
- cardiac arrest
- cardiac arrhythmias
- coagulopathy
- hypertension
- haemorrhage
- seizures
- shortness of breath
- premonitory symptoms such as restlessness, agitation.

Sadly the diagnosis is often made postmortem, with fetal squames found in the maternal lungs.

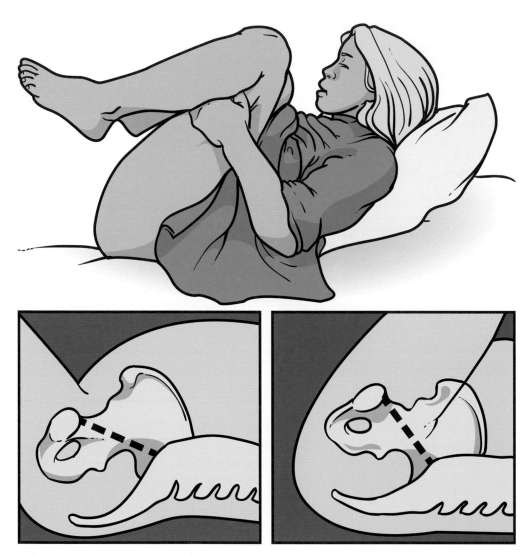

Figure 16.8
McRoberts position.

(Taken from Lanni SM, Seeds JW. Malpresentations. In: Gabbe SG, Niebyl JR, Simpson JL. Obstetrics: normal and problem pregnancies, 5th ed. Philadelphia, Churchill Livingstone, 2007, pp 428–55.)

Risk factors include induction of labour, in particular with prostaglandins, caesarean delivery, older maternal age, and placental pathology (including abruption, manual removal of placenta).

POSTPARTUM HAEMORRHAGE

Primary postpartum haemorrhage (primary PPH) is defined as >500 mL of vaginal blood loss during the third stage of labour or in the first 24 hours after delivery. Secondary PPH is excessive vaginal bleeding from 24 hours to 6 weeks after birth.

PPH is a major cause of maternal morbidity and is the major cause of maternal death worldwide. It occurs in 5–15% of deliveries in Australia. The incidence of postpartum haemorrhage is increasing in Australia over the past decade, but the reasons for this are unclear.[11] All staff attending births should be trained in dealing with this common life-threatening event.

Prevention

Prevention of anaemia: dietary advice about foods high in iron and iron supplementation are important preventive strategies and health professionals should ensure that women are suitably informed.

Active management of the third stage of labour: this includes administering a prophylactic uterotonic such as oxytocin, controlled cord traction and then fundal massage of the uterus immediately after delivery of the placenta. Compared to physiological (or expectant) management of the third stage, active management is associated with a 34% reduction in the risk of PPH, maternal blood transfusion and anaemia.[12] However, it is associated with increased vomiting, raised diastolic blood pressure and analgesic use postpartum. Oxytocin administered after the delivery of the anterior shoulder is the uterotonic agent of choice as it is associated with fewer maternal side effects than oxytocin–ergometrine, for which risks include vomiting, nausea, headache, cardiac arrhythmias and hypertension.

Management

1 Early recognition and call for help. Particular vigilance should be applied to women with risk factors as per Table 16.5.
   It is important to monitor women closely in the third stage of labour and in the puerperium. If significant PPH occurs a multidisciplinary team of obstetric, anaesthetic, midwifery, operating theatre, haematology and intensive care staff should be involved.
2 Rapid replacement of fluid loss.
   Immediate intravenous access via two large bore cannulae is needed for intravenous fluid resuscitation. Bloods should be sent for FBC, cross-match of 4 units of packed cells, UEC, LFT and coagulation screen.
3 Consider the cause of the PPH (the 4 'T's – see Table 16.5) and treat accordingly.
   • TONE (70%) — atonic uterus accounts for the vast majority of cases of PPH. See below for treatment.
   • TRAUMA (20%) — vaginal lacerations should be identified and sutured to achieve haemostasis.
   • TISSUE (10%) — recognised or unrecognised retained placental tissue and/or membranes may be the cause.
   • THROMBIN (1%) — abnormalities of clotting may also be a causative factor in PPH.
4 Facilitate uterine tone:
   Fundal massage is the initial step. Bimanual compression of the uterus (Figure 16.9) may be necessary in the unresponsive atonic

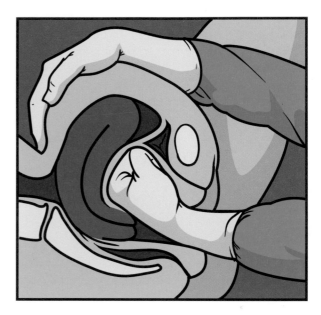

Figure 16.9
Bimanual compression of the uterus.

(Taken from Lanni SM, Seeds JW. Malpresentations In: Gabbe SG, Niebyl JR, Simpson JL. Obstetrics: normal and problem pregnancies, 5th ed. Philadelphia, Churchill Livingstone, 2007, pp 428–55.)

uterus. Uterotonics including ergometrine, oxytocin infusion and prostaglandin F2-alpha are used in that order. Rectal misoprostol and PGF2-alpha can be used to control severe PPH when the uterus is atonic despite ergometrine and oxytocin. Side effects include cardiac arrest and bronchospasm, so anaesthetist assistance should be available; ideally PGF2-alpha should be given in an operating theatre.
   An indwelling catheter is also inserted as a full bladder will counteract compression of the uterus.
5 Check for trauma to the vagina and perineum and repair appropriately.
6 Exclude retained products of conception: check the placenta and membranes are complete.

Surgical management

If haemorrhage continues despite these measures, the patient must be taken to theatre for a systematic exploration of the genital tract. Initially the uterine cavity is manually explored for retained placental tissue and membranes. Then the cervix is systematically checked for cervical lacerations, and finally the vagina is rechecked for any lacerations.

Table 16.5 Risk factors for postpartum haemorrhage

Cause	Aetiology	Clinical risk factors
Abnormal uterine contraction (Tone) 70%	Atonic uterus	Physiological management of the third stage Prolonged third stage (>30 minutes)
	Over-distended uterus	Polyhydramnios Multiple pregnancy Macrosomia
	Uterine muscle exhaustion	Rapid or incoordinate labour Prolonged labour (first or second stage) Labour dystocia High parity Labour augmented with oxytocin
	Intra-amniotic infection	Pyrexia Prolonged ruptured membranes (>24 hours)
	Drug-induced uterine hypotonia	Magnesium sulfate, nifedipine, salbutamol General anaesthesia
	Functional or anatomical distortion of the uterus	Fibroid uterus Uterine anomalies
Genital tract trauma (Trauma) 20%	Episiotomy or lacerations (cervix, vagina or perineum)	Induced labour Augmented labour Abnormal labour (dystocia) Malposition Precipitous birth Instrumental birth (forceps or vacuum)
	Extensions or lacerations at caesarean delivery	Malposition Deep engagement
	Uterine rupture	Previous uterine surgery
	Uterine inversion	Strong cord traction in third stage (especially with fundal placenta) Short umbilical cord High parity Uterine relaxation Placenta accreta (especially with fundal placenta) Congenital uterine anomalies or weakness Antepartum use of magnesium sulfate or oxytocin
Retained pregnancy tissue (Tissue) 10%	Retained products Abnormal placenta Retained cotyledon or succenturiate lobe	Incomplete placenta at birth Placenta accreta Previous uterine surgery High parity Abnormal placenta on ultrasound

Table 16.5 (Continued)

Cause	Aetiology	Clinical risk factors
Abnormalities of coagulation (Thrombin) 1%	Retained blood clots	Atonic uterus
	Coagulation disorders acquired during pregnancy Idiopathic thrombocytopenia purpura (ITP) von Willebrand's disease Haemophilia Thrombocytopenia with preeclampsia Disseminated intravascular coagulation (DIC) Preeclampsia Retained dead fetus Severe infection Placental abruption Amniotic fluid embolism	Bruising Elevated blood pressure Fetal death Fever Antepartum haemorrhage Sudden collapse
	Therapeutic anticoagulation	History of thromboembolism

From http://www.health.nsw.gov.au/policies/pd/2010/pdf/PD2010_064.pdf

Advanced surgical techniques

If haemorrhage persists despite the above efforts, there are other surgical techniques that can be used to achieve haemostasis. These include the insertion of an intrauterine balloon, B-Lynch or other type of brace sutures, bilateral ligation of the uterine arteries or internal iliac arteries, embolisation of internal iliac arteries, activated VIIa, and lastly hysterectomy. When these advanced techniques are required, the patient is often coagulopathic and correction of coagulopathy is essential.

A patient who has experienced a major PPH will require intensive postpartum care for a period of at least 24 hours.

PRETERM BIRTH

Definition

Preterm birth refers to delivery prior to 37 weeks gestation or 257 days of pregnancy.

Incidence

The incidence of preterm birth in 2010 in Australia was 8.3%,[4] which includes spontaneous preterm births and iatrogenic deliveries for a maternal or fetal condition. The incidence of preterm delivery has frustratingly remained constant over the past decade. Spontaneous preterm births accounted for 22.9% of perinatal deaths in Western Australia, South Australia, Queensland, Tasmania, Australian Capital Territory and Northern Territory (the six jurisdictions to provide cause of death) in 2010.[4]

Risk factors

Previous preterm birth is a major risk factor, with the risk of recurrence increasing the earlier the gestational age of delivery and the greater the number of previous preterm births. Numerous epidemiological studies have indicated an association with poverty, smoking, poor antenatal care, young maternal age and being black. Previous cervical surgery, such as cold knife cone biopsy or large loop excision of the transformation zone of the cervix is a recognised risk factor for preterm birth, as it may cause cervical incompetence. Chorioamnionitis is a recognised risk factor for preterm birth, but in many cases of preterm labour, infection is subclinical and diagnosed only on histopathology with inflammation of the membranes, cord and placenta.

Forty per cent of preterm births are preceded by preterm premature rupture of the membranes

(PPROM), which complicates 2–3% of all pregnancies. Although in most women birth occurs within a few days of membranes rupturing, in some circumstances the latency interval can be several weeks. The risk of ascending infection, cord prolapse and abruption are greater after PPROM. Oral erythromycin taken by the mother may increase latency and reduce newborn sepsis. Antibiotics seem to confer no long-term benefits and in those women with intact membranes and threatened preterm labour may increase the risk of cerebral palsy. There is no good evidence to guide inpatient or outpatient care for women with PPROM. There are large randomised controlled trials underway to establish whether expectant management of planned early birth is associated with better maternal and newborn outcomes following PPROM close to term.

Prevention

Unfortunately few treatments have been demonstrated to be effective in the prevention of preterm birth.

Cervical cerclage (the placement of a cervical suture), has been demonstrated to be effective for women with a previous preterm birth who have demonstrated cervical shortening of less than 15 mm at less than 24 weeks gestation.[13] However, cerclage has never been demonstrated as an effective way of preventing preterm birth in the general population. The benefits of potentially prolonging gestation must be balanced against the risks of insertion of cerclage — in particular infection, which in itself can increase the risk of preterm birth.

Progesterone

There is considerable interest in the use of progesterone to prolong pregnancy in those women at risk, with many trials being performed with conflicting results. One study concluded that for women with a previous spontaneous preterm birth, progesterone was associated with a significant reduction in preterm birth prior to 34 weeks, but no difference in perinatal death rates. Progesterone was also associated with a reduction in preterm birth prior to 34 weeks in women with a short cervix (defined as less than 15 mm).[14] As studies have indicated a decrease in preterm birth but no improvement in newborn health, a number of randomised studies are currently underway to address this issue.

Smoking cessation

Pregnant women may be more receptive to smoking cessation programs, which can reduce the risk of preterm birth.

Bed rest

There is *no* evidence that bed rest reduces the risk of preterm labour. It may cause harm by increasing the risk of thromboembolic disease and reducing maternal muscle mass.

Antibiotics

There is conflicting evidence about the use of antibiotics for women with a prior preterm birth and bacterial vaginosis. Secondary analyses suggests that the use of antibiotics may reduce risk of recurrent preterm birth if abnormal flora is present.[15] Treatment of asymptomatic bacteriuria in pregnancy reduces the risk of urinary tract infections, and possibly reduces the risk preterm birth and low birth weight infants.[16] Periodontal treatment is safe for pregnant women but does not reduce the risk of preterm birth.

Diagnosis

The clinical diagnosis of preterm labour is based on a careful history and examination. It is dependent on the presence of uterine activity in combination with effacement and dilatation of the cervix. Cervical change and PPROM are diagnosed on speculum examination, as digital examination is avoided to reduce the risk of infection.

Often uterine activity may be accompanied by little cervical change, and the diagnosis is unclear. A fetal fibronectin test may be useful in this situation. Fetal fibronectin is a glycoprotein found in amniotic fluid and placental tissue, and can be thought of as a biological 'glue' that binds the fetal sac to the uterine wall. The test is more useful for its negative predictive value, as the negative predictive value is 99% in determining the risk of preterm delivery within 7–10 days, whereas the positive predictive value in determining the risk of preterm delivery is poor at only 20%.

Management
Steroids

Respiratory distress syndrome (RDS) is the primary cause of neonatal mortality and morbidity. A Cochrane review in 2006[17] of 21 studies found that antenatal corticosteroids administered to the mother reduce neonatal death, RDS, cerebroventricular haemorrhage, necrotising enterocolitis, infectious morbidity, the need for respiratory support and neonatal intensive care admission, with a wide gestational age benefit from 26–34+6 weeks gestation. The benefit wanes with time after administration in infants delivered more than 7 days after the first dose, but there is benefit even when infants are born less than 24 hours after the first dose has been given.

Tocolysis

Overall, tocolytics are associated with a reduction in the rate of delivery within 24 hours, but no reduction in preterm birth less than 37 weeks or perinatal morbidity. No tocolytic has been shown to be successful in the prevention of preterm labour. There are a variety of agents for tocolysis, including calcium channel blockers (e.g. nifedipine), beta-mimetics (e.g. terbutaline), cyclo-oxygenase (COX) inhibitors (e.g. indomethacin), nitric oxide donors (e.g. nitroglycerin), oxytocin receptor antagonists (e.g. ritrodrine). The calcium channel blockers such as nifedipine are preferred due to a lower side effect profile, cheapness, ease of oral administration and availability. Historically beta-mimetics such as salbutamol were used for tocolysis, however these had to be given parenterally and were associated with more side effects.

Within Australia, tocolytic administration may facilitate transfer of the pregnant preterm woman to a specialised tertiary care facility that has neonatal intensive care facilities. Tocolytics may also allow time for steroids administration.

Antibiotics

The routine use of antibiotics as an adjunct to tocolysis for women in preterm labour with intact membranes is not recommended after the publication of the ORACLE II trial, which showed no neonatal benefit and raised concerns about increased neonatal mortality.[18] However, antibiotics are indicated if there is preterm premature rupture of membranes or clinical evidence of chorioamnionitis.

Transfer to a tertiary unit

It has been well established that delivery of a preterm infant outside a tertiary centre is associated with increased neonatal mortality or pre-discharge death, thus patients who are likely to deliver preterm should be transferred to an appropriate tertiary centre as long as this does not risk the safety of the mother or the fetus. In such cases, trained neonatal retrieval teams should attend the birth and transfer the infant ex-utero to the appropriate tertiary centre.

Prognosis

The prognosis for the preterm infant depends on the gestational age. This means accurate measurement of the gestational age is important so that appropriate neonatal counselling can take place.

REFERENCES

1 WHO fact sheet No 348. Maternal mortality. Nov 2010. Available from: www.who.int/mediacentre/factsheets/fs348/en/index.html
2 Sullivan, EA, Hall B, King JF. Maternal deaths in Australia 2003–2005. Maternal deaths series no 3. Cat. No. PER42. Sydney: AIHW National Perinatal Statistics Unit; 2008.
3 WHO. Maternal mortality in 2005: estimates developed by WHO, UNICEF, UNFPA, and the World Bank. WHO 2007. Available from: http://whqlibdoc.who.int/publications/2007/9789241596213_eng.pdf.
4 Li Z, Zeki R, Hilder L, et al. Australia's mothers and babies 2010. Perinatal statistics series no. 27. Cat. no. PER 57. Canberra: AIHW National Perinatal Epidemiology and Statistics Unit; 2012.
5 Johnston TA, Grady K, for the Guidelines and Audit Committee of the Royal College of Obstetricians and Gynaecologists. Green-top Guideline No. 56. Maternal collapse in pregnancy and the puerperium. London: RCOG; 2011.
6 Olive EC, Roberts CL, Algert CS, et al. Placenta praevia: maternal morbidity and place of birth. Aust N Z J Obstet Gynaecol 2005;45(6):499–504.
7 Oyelese Y, Smulian JC. Placenta previa, placenta accreta, and vasa previa. Obstet Gynecol 2006;107(4):927–41.
8 Ananth C, Smulian J, Vintzileos A. The effect of placenta previa on neonatal mortality: a population-based study in the United States, 1989 through 1997. Am J Obstet Gynecol 2003;188:1299–304.
9 Gherman RB, Chauhan S, Ouzounian JG, et al. Shoulder dystocia: the unpreventable obstetric emergency with empiric management guidelines. Am J Obstet Gynecol 2006:195(3):657–72.
10 Tuffnell DJ. United Kingdom amniotic fluid embolism register. Br J Obstet Gynaecol 2005;112:1625–9.
11 Knight M, Callaghan WM, Berg C, et al. Trends in postpartum hemorrhage in high resource countries: a review and recommendations from the International Postpartum Hemorrhage Collaborative Group. BMC Pregnancy & Childbirth 2009;9:55.

12 Begley CM, Gyte GML, Devane D, et al. Active versus expectant management for women in the third stage of labour. Cochrane Database Syst Rev 2011;11:CD007412. doi: 10.1002/14651858.CD007412.pub3.

13 Owen J, Hankins G, Iams JD, et al. Multicenter randomized trial of cerclage for preterm birth prevention in high-risk women with shortened midtrimester cervical length. Am J Obstet Gynecol 2009;201:375.e1–8.

14 Dodd JM, Flenady V, Cincotta R, et al. Prenatal administration of progesterone for preventing preterm birth in women considered to be at risk of preterm birth. Cochrane Database Syst Rev 2006;1:CD004947. doi: 10.1002/14651858.CD004947.pub2.

15 Brocklehurst P, Gordon A, Heatley E, et al. Antibiotics for treating bacterial vaginosis in pregnancy. Cochrane Database Syst Rev 2013;1:CD000262. doi: 10.1002/14651858.CD000262.pub4.

16 Villar J, Gulmezoglu AM, de Onis M. Nutritional and antimicrobial interventions to prevent preterm birth: an overview of randomized controlled trials. Obstet Gynecol Surv 1998;53(9):575–85.

17 Roberts D, Dalziel SR. Antenatal corticosteroids for accelerating fetal lung maturation for women at risk of preterm birth. Cochrane Database Syst Rev 2006;3:CD004454. doi: 10.1002/14651858.CD004454.pub2.

18 Kenyon SL, Taylor DJ, Tarnow-Mordi W. Broad-spectrum antibiotics for spontaneous preterm labour: the ORACLE II randomised trial. Lancet 2001;357:991–6.

MCQS

Select the correct answer.

1   Tocolytics are associated with:

   A   ability to administer the full course of steroids for prevention of RDS.
   B   reduction of perinatal mortality.
   C   reduction of preterm delivery prior to 34 weeks.
   D   reduction of perinatal morbidity.
   E   All of the above.

2   Postpartum haemorrhage:

   A   is increased in smokers.
   B   is increased with prolonged labour.
   C   is increased if there is shoulder dystocia.
   D   is not increased if there has been an antepartum haemorrhage.
   E   is not associated with induction of labour.

3   With respect to preterm birth:

   A   Bed rest reduces the risk of preterm birth.
   B   Intensive antenatal surveillance reduces the risk of preterm birth.
   C   Periodontal treatment in pregnancy reduces the risk of preterm birth.
   D   Smoking cessation reduces the risk of preterm birth.
   E   Ovarian cystectomy increases the risk of preterm birth.

4   With respect to shoulder dystocia:

   A   Is easy to predict.
   B   Is not increased with well-controlled gestational diabetes.
   C   Incidence is 7% of all births.
   D   Shoulder dystocia drills should be practised regularly.
   E   Incurs a 10% risk of brachial plexus injuries.

5   What is the main cause of perinatal mortality in developed countries?

   A   non-accidental injury
   B   unexplained stillbirth
   C   congenital anomalies
   D   preeclampsia
   E   spontaneous preterm birth

OSCE

PART 1

You are called to the delivery suite. Mrs Jones, who delivered a male infant 20 minutes ago, has collapsed and is unresponsive. She is lying in a large pool of blood. Describe how you would assess and manage the situation.

PART 2

The uterus is atonic. Describe how you would manage this situation.

Chapter 17

Routine care of postpartum women

Marjorie Atchan and Caroline SE Homer

KEY POINTS

The puerperium refers to the first 6 weeks after having a baby.

Breastfeeding is initiated during this time.

Mother and baby bond together.

THE PUERPERIUM

The puerperium refers to the 6 weeks during which a woman physiologically returns to her prepregnant state. These changes are a result of the withdrawal of pregnancy hormones. The puerperium continues the significant transition that pregnancy has begun. For many couples, it is not until these early days and weeks after their baby's birth that they begin to fully understand their new role as parents.

The midwife, family medical practitioner and the child and family health nurse (also known as a maternal and child health nurse or health visitor) are the primary care-givers during the puerperium. They support the woman to transition into motherhood, establish breastfeeding and develop parenting skills. Supporting and assessing her emotional wellbeing and mental health are as important as the physiological changes that occur through this time.

PHYSIOLOGICAL CHANGES IN THE PUERPERIUM
Involution

Involution refers to the gradual return of the uterus to its prepregnant state. The term uterus weighs approximately 1000 g, but involutes to 50–60 g by 6 weeks post-birth. This involves contraction and reduction in size of the myometrial muscle, thrombosis and hyaline degeneration of blood vessels, with consequent shedding of the decidua and later regeneration of the endometrium. Involution is assessed by the progressive descent of the uterine fundus (Figure 17.1). On the first day after the birth, the fundus can be palpated just below the woman's umbilicus. After 5–7 days, it is firm and non-tender, extending midway between the symphysis pubis and umbilicus. By 2 weeks, it is no longer palpable abdominally. By 6 weeks the uterus has returned to close to its pre-pregnant size. Uterine contractions under the influence of oxytocin are often painful (afterpains) and may require simple analgesia.

The woman's internal cervical os is closed by the second week. The vagina, ligaments of the uterus, muscles of the pelvic floor and separated rectus muscles return to close to their prepregnant state with time and exercise. The decidua is shed and appears as lochia (postpartum blood flow). Lochia consists of blood, leucocytes and decidual fragments. It is usually bright (lochia rubra) for 3 or 4 days, changing over the next 10–12 days to pale

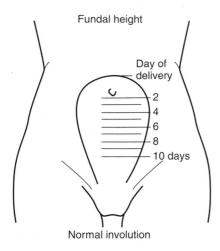

Figure 17.1
Normal involution: fundal height by days after birth.

brown (lochia serosa) and finally to yellowish white (lochia alba). Typically, between days 7 and 14 postpartum there may be a transient increase in vaginal blood loss, due to shedding of the placental site scar. In general, postpartum blood flow ceases by 4–5 weeks postpartum (median 30 days). External sanitary pads should be worn after the baby is born to absorb the lochia. Excessive loss, clots or malodorous discharge may indicate infection or retained products of conception.

Ovarian function

Ovarian function returns after about 10 weeks to the woman who is not breastfeeding, but may return as early as 4–5 weeks postpartum. In breastfeeding women, ovulation may be delayed for 8–10 months. All women need to consider contraception from 4 weeks postpartum. Recent guidelines for postpartum contraception advise postpartum women not to use combined hormonal contraceptives during the first 21 days after birth because of a high risk for venous thromboembolism (VTE).[1]

Perineal trauma

Perineal damage such as tears or episiotomies usually heal within 2–3 weeks. The woman needs to be advised to keep her perineum clean and dry, to shower frequently and to avoid constipation. Increasing pain, vaginal discharge or malodour may be signs of infection.

Many women are reluctant or fearful about having sexual intercourse after childbirth as it may initially be painful or uncomfortable. Additional lubrication will frequently be necessary for sexual intercourse since breastfeeding reduces the amount of vaginal lubrication. Pelvic floor exercise assists in the healing and reduction of pain and carries long-term benefits in terms of continence.[2]

Urinary and bowel function

There is a marked diuresis in the 24–48 hours after the birth. Bladder function needs to be monitored due to the possibility of urethral damage and an overstretched bladder. Urinary retention can commonly be seen after a caesarean delivery or an instrumental vaginal delivery. An over-distended bladder is also a risk factor for a postpartum haemorrhage in the first few hours after birth. The physiological dilatation of the urinary tract gradually resolves. Constipation is common in the early puerperium, due to inhibition of defecation associated with a painful perineum. Encouraging fluids and a high-fibre diet may help the woman's bowel function return to normal.

Cardiovascular system

The cardiovascular system goes through significant changes in the puerperium. In the first 24 hours, the woman's baseline pulse rate drops by about 10–15 bpm and her temperature may be slightly elevated. There is an increase in the leucocyte count during labour and in the first 24 hours postpartum. Evaluation of the haemoglobin concentration is important if there has been significant postpartum blood loss. The physiological hypercoagulable state of pregnancy persists up to 6 weeks postpartum and increases the risk of thromboembolic disease. During the puerperium, the woman's blood volume decreases and viscosity increases to prepregnant levels. Smooth muscle tone of vessel walls also improves and cardiac output reduces.

SOCIAL AND EMOTIONAL CHANGES IN THE PUERPERIUM
Supporting the transition into motherhood

An important component of postpartum care is to facilitate and support the transition to parenthood. Factors that influence a woman's adjustment to parenthood include her past experiences of parenting, health status, her experience of birth, and her expectations as a mother. Other factors influencing the parent–infant relationship include the level of support available to the mother from her partner, family, friends and community, Indigenous and cultural influences, social background, financial position, and physical home environment. These factors should be considered in a holistic approach for each new mother and her partner.

In the early days after the birth, the care provider (usually the midwife) provides support, anticipatory guidance and information, as required. One of the most common complaints in this period is the conflicting information received from different healthcare providers. The woman should be asked what she already knows about the subject under discussion and be provided with guidance and support, rather than offered completely different advice. Many women find going home early with midwifery support reduces the amount of conflicting advice they receive. It is also important to encourage the woman to discuss her experience of pregnancy, labour and birth and to identify any issues of concern.

Supporting mother–baby attachment

Attachment is defined as the deep and enduring connection established between a child and caregiver in the first several years of life. It profoundly influences every component of the human condition — mind, body, emotions, relationships and values. Attachment has received significant interest in the past decade as knowledge about neurobiological pathways has increased. It is now well established that the architecture of the brain is influenced by genetics, environment and experience. The neural circuits develop rapidly in-utero and in the first years of life, and experiences in the first weeks and months of life shape these circuits. Influences in the first 3 years have a major impact as the neural circuits are maturing. Attachment theory comes from these neurological developments and is critical for all babies. A baby's primary attachment can be with any person, and although capable of multiple attachments the primary and most important early interaction is usually with the mother.

Consistent, responsive and empathetic parenting occurs when parents have the necessary love and affection to prioritise their child. It is the role of care providers to support the new family and facilitate this process of attachment. The provision of consistent advice, relevant information and practical support are all tangible ways in which care providers can assist.

Addressing perinatal mental health issues

The puerperium is a time of great change in a woman's life, and it is common to experience a wide range of emotions. Feelings of worry and stress most commonly resolve by themselves, but pregnancy and early parenthood can trigger symptoms of more serious mental health problems that need to be addressed. Risk factors for postpartum depression and anxiety include mental health problems in the past, inadequate support at home, and recent traumatic major life events. Women who feel isolated by either distance, culture or both, including Aboriginal and Torres Strait Islanders and women from culturally and linguistically diverse backgrounds, have a greater likelihood of experiencing mental health problems.[3]

There is considerable evidence that up to one-fifth of women experience depression in the first 3 months postpartum. In addition, it has been identified that severe postpartum depression or psychosis is a significant cause of direct maternal deaths. Recent clinical guidelines recommend an approach based on routine assessment of emotional health and wellbeing, during both pregnancy and the following year, that can be integrated into a woman's regular health checks. The assessment uses the Edinburgh Postnatal Depression Scale (EPDS) and includes questions about psychosocial factors that may increase a woman's likelihood of mental health problems, and symptoms of depression or anxiety experienced in the previous week. Puerperal psychosis is rare and usually presents with delusions, hallucinations and impaired perception of reality.

LACTATION
Why is breastfeeding important?

Breastfeeding is the biological norm for feeding human babies. The World Health Organization (WHO) recommendations include exclusive breastfeeding until 6 months,[4] with the introduction of complementary foods and continued breastfeeding well into the second year. Benefits of breastfeeding include a reduction in infant respiratory tract infections, gastrointestinal illnesses, diabetes, obesity and cardiovascular disease, while maternal benefits include a reduction in premenopausal breast cancer, ovarian cancer and osteoporosis.[5] Community benefits include decreased healthcare costs, increased workplace productivity due to decreased parental

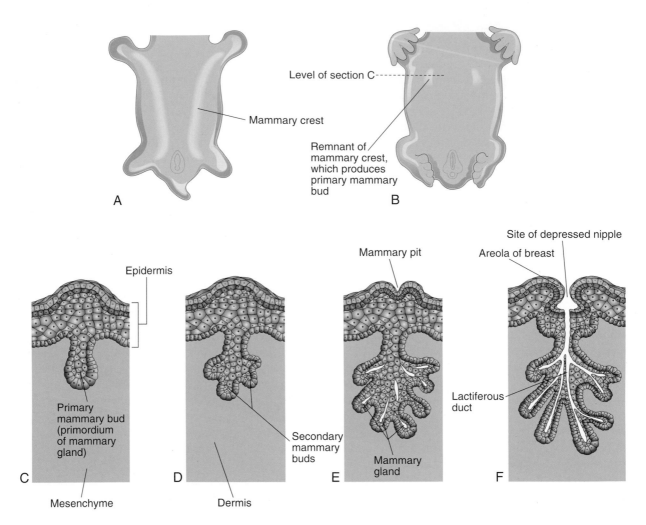

Figure 17.2

The development of mammary glands. **A**: Ventral view of an embryo of approximately 28 days showing the mammary crests; **B**: Similar view at 6 weeks showing the remains of these crests; **C**: Transverse section of a mammary crest at the site of a developing mammary gland; **D–F**: Similar sections showing successive stages of breast development between the 12th week and birth.

(Moore: The developing human, 9th ed. 978-1-4377-2002-0; Figure 19.7A to F. Copyright © 2011 Saunders, An Imprint of Elsevier)

absenteeism, and a positive impact on family income and lifestyle.

An understanding of the normal anatomy and physiology of the breast and how breastfeeding works is essential to understand normal lactation. It is important to review the developmental stages a woman's breast goes through to reach this point. It is during lactation that the human breast reaches its full functional capacity; it does not go through all developmental stages unless a woman experiences pregnancy and childbirth.

Breast developmental stages

The human breast in the fetal stage develops from a thickened ectodermal ridge which runs from the axilla to groin, as seen in Figure 17.2. The milk streak appears in the fourth week of gestation when the embryo is approximately 2.5 mm long. It becomes the milk line, or milk ridge, during the fifth week of gestation (2.5–5.5 mm). This ridge rapidly regresses till only the pectoral region remains, which forms the basis for the mammary gland.[6]

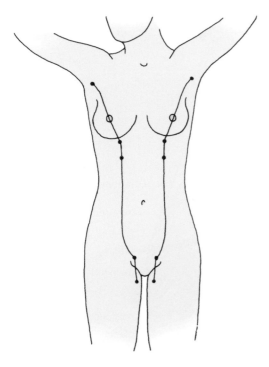

Figure 17.3
Mammary milk line indicating where accessory nipples or glands may form.

(Bland: The Breast, 4th ed. Figure 9.2. 2009 Saunders)

In 2–6% of women the structure fails to undergo its normal regression and accessory nipples (polythelia) or accessory mammary glands (polymastia) may occur along the original mammary ridges or milk lines, as shown in Figure 17.3. Excision can be considered, but glandular tissue may regrow with subsequent pregnancies.

The breasts of the newborn are rudimentary and there is little growth until puberty. The increase in breast size is mainly caused by the deposition of adipose tissue, but the ductal network also becomes more extensive. These maturational changes are associated with increased plasma concentrations of oestrogen, prolactin, luteinising hormone, follicle stimulating hormone and growth hormone. Figure 17.4 identifies the normal breast development that occurs from infancy to lactation. The breast of an adult woman is composed of glandular and adipose tissue and supported by a loose framework of connective tissue (Cooper's ligaments). The glandular tissue is composed of 15–20 lobes, each comprised of lobules containing 10–100 alveoli. The breast does not mature further until pregnancy occurs.

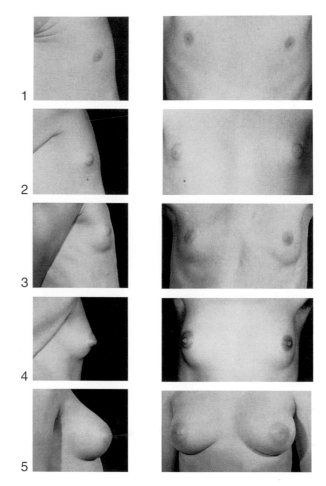

Figure 17.4
Normal female breast development from prepubertal to adult.

(Moshang: Pediatric Endocrinology: Requisites, 1st ed 2004 Mosby; 9780323018258, Plate 4.2. From Wales JKH, Wit JM, Rogol AD: Pediatric Endocrinology and Growth, 2nd ed, Philadelphia, 2003, Saunders.)

The breast in pregnancy

During the first half of pregnancy the effects of a number of hormones including oestrogen and progesterone, prolactin, growth hormone and various growth factors cause extension and branching of the ductal system, as well as intense lobular and alveolar growth. Growth of glandular tissue during pregnancy is believed to occur via its invasion of the adipose tissue, with the lactating breast becoming predominantly full of glandular tissue. From 16 weeks of pregnancy there is secretory activity with the commencement of colostrum production, otherwise known as Lactogenesis I.

In the last trimester there is a further glandular development. Glandular luminal cells begin actively synthesising milk fat and proteins near term; only small amounts are released into the lumen. The areola also darkens in colour and the Montgomery glands increase in size. The secretion from these glands acts as a protectant from sucking-related stress and pathogens. The odour produced may also act to attract babies and increase their latching speed and sucking activity. The woman should be advised not to wash her nipples with soap or use heavily perfumed products, as these will wash away the natural oils and mask their unique smell.

There is considerable variation of breast growth during pregnancy: some women may experience most of the growth by 22 weeks, some in the last trimester, and others in the early postpartum period (first month). Mammary blood flow also increases significantly during pregnancy and remains elevated in the lactating breast and until about 2 weeks after weaning has occurred. It is worth noting that women who miscarry from 16 weeks' gestation will almost certainly lactate and will require counselling and support to deal with this aspect of their loss.

The lactating breast

The greatest amount of glandular tissue relative to adipose tissue occurs within a 30 mm radius of the base of the nipple. There is great variability in the amount of adipose tissue in the breast. The amount of fat situated between the tissues is also highly variable. See Figure 17.5. Secretory lactocytes line the alveoli; lactocytes synthesise breastmilk that is then stored in the alveoli. There are approximately 5–9 milk ducts (range 4–18) in each lactating breast.

The glandular tissue located directly beneath the nipple is drained by branches that merge into the main collecting duct very close to the nipple. The amount of functioning glandular tissue, *not* breast size, is an indicator of how much milk the breast is able to store. Left and right breasts rarely produce the same volume of milk; the difference between them may be negligible or quite noticeable.

The composition of breastmilk

Breastmilk contains a variety of proteins including caseins and immunoglobulins, fats (triglycerides and fatty acids) and carbohydrates (e.g. lactose, glucose, galactose), minerals, electrolytes, vitamins and water.[7] Milk composition changes depending on the stage of lactation. Colostrum has high

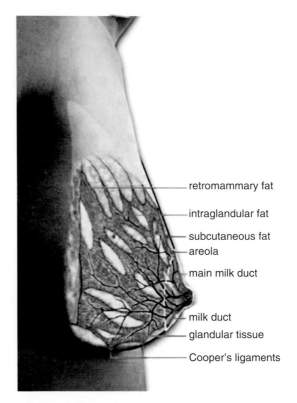

Figure 17.5
The lactating breast.

(Ramsey et al, 2006 Anatomy of the lactating human breast redefined with ultrasound imaging. Journal of Anatomy 206:525-534. Figure 7 p531.)

concentrations of proteins (immunoglobulins, lactoferrin and lysozyme), sodium and chloride, and low concentrations of casein and lactose. As the volume increases there are increases in the lipid content and concentrations of casein and lactose and decreases in the concentrations of total protein, sodium and chloride. The changes in the concentration of lactose, citrate, protein and sodium have been used as biochemical markers of the onset of copious milk secretion. The concentration of lactose does not change throughout lactation but there are changes in the total fat content and concentration of protein and calcium at various stages.[8]

How breastfeeding works

Lactogenesis II, or the onset of copious milk production, occurs after the withdrawal of circulating progesterone and placental lactogen. The subsequent rise in serum prolactin levels occurs usually around 30–70 hours postpartum, with the average around 60 hours, but it may not occur until 102 hours in some women. Adequate levels of insulin, adrenal cortisol and thyroid hormone are also required. The prolactin response to suckling is very important at this stage. Lactogenesis II may be delayed in women with diabetes due to a transient impairment in lactose synthesis.

Throughout lactation, whenever the baby feeds, prolactin is released from the anterior pituitary gland, reaching a peak after 45 minutes.[7] Once the supply is established (around 4 weeks), autocrine factors influence milk synthesis via the feedback inhibitor of lactation (FIL). The FIL acts in response to how much milk has been removed from the breast. As prolactin uptake from the blood by the lactocyte is dependent on the fullness of the breast, its uptake may be inhibited by full alveoli. If the woman uses breast fullness as her main indicator of when to feed, this may have a negative impact on her supply.

At each feed oxytocin is also released into the circulation from the posterior pituitary gland, stimulating the myoepithelial cells surrounding the alveoli. This causes their contraction and ejection of milk (MER — milk ejection reflex). Ultrasound imaging has demonstrated that the vacuum exerted by the baby on the breast during feeds also plays an integral part in milk transfer.

The rate of breastmilk synthesis is greatest when the breast is most fully drained (late evening), with higher serum levels of prolactin occurring between 2 a.m. and 6 a.m.

It is important for the woman to feed her baby according to need (demand feed) rather than try to impose a schedule.

Transmission of drugs in breastmilk

It is generally agreed that medications penetrate milk more during the first 4 weeks than in mature milk, although there are exceptions. In the breastfed newborn, the infant must also metabolise and eliminate the drug. In the case of many antibiotics, the oral bioavailability is such that generally less than 1% of the maternal dose will ultimately find its way into the milk and subsequently be transferred to the infant (although there are wide variations). The infant may suffer adverse effects such as diarrhoea and constipation, due to the action of antibiotics on the neonatal gastrointestinal tract. A comprehensive assessment is required to ascertain if it is safe for a mother who is breastfeeding to take a specific medication.[9]

Complications of lactation

Women's infant feeding decisions and practices are contextual and influenced by many personal and societal factors. The reality of the birthing experience may not match the ideal. There are a number of breastfeeding challenges that may also influence practice. Accurate health provider knowledge and appropriate support and respect validates women's experiences.

Mastitis

Mastitis occurs where the breast becomes inflamed or infected, most commonly by a staphylococcal organism acquired from the skin. Mastitis often presents as a hot red tender area or lump in the breast, with pain, fever, and sometimes symptoms of systemic infection. The mother should be encouraged to continue to drain the breast by feeding. If the symptoms are unresolved within 12 hours (or if she is systemically unwell) she should be treated with antibiotics. Some women require admission to hospital and treatment with intravenous antibiotics. In this case a breastmilk culture is required to determine sensitivities.

Breast abscess

Breast abscess usually occurs as a consequence of unresolved mastitis. It is diagnosed with ultrasound and requires drainage either by aspiration or surgically.

SIX-WEEK POSTPARTUM VISIT

Each woman is referred to her local child and family health or maternal health nurse 1–2 weeks after going home, and to her family medical practitioner, midwife or obstetrician 6 weeks after birth. The process of involution is checked, as well as the woman's continence, the integrity of her pelvic floor and perineal healing, and a cervical smear performed if necessary. The mother–partner relationship is discussed, the need for contraception explored, and any medical condition clinically evaluated. The baby's growth and development is assessed, immunisation schedules are planned, and the parent–infant relationship is discussed.

COMPLICATIONS OF THE PUERPERIUM
Infections and sepsis

Wound infection is more commonly seen in caesarean delivery wounds 1–2 weeks postdelivery but infection may also occur at the site of episiotomy and perineal tears. Infections usually present with fever, and reddening, inflammation and discomfort around the wound. The wound will appear inflamed and there may be associated offensive lochia. A swab and smear of the wound should be sent to microbiology and antibiotic therapy commenced.

Puerperal sepsis is any febrile condition in a woman where a temperature of 38°C or more is maintained or recurs within 14 days of birth. Genital tract sepsis has become the leading cause of direct maternal death in the United Kingdom for the first time since Confidential Enquiries into Maternal Deaths commenced in 1952.[10] In particular, community-acquired group A streptococcal disease was a major contributor to sepsis. Women who have recently given birth need to be informed of the risks, signs and symptoms of genital tract infection, and how to prevent transmission. Advice should include the importance of good personal hygiene. The increased incidence of group A streptococcal disease highlights the need for women to take particular care when around family or close contacts with a sore throat or upper respiratory tract infection.[11] See Box 17.1.

Women who have recently given birth may present with fever and malaise, offensive lochia that may be purulent or bloody, and a painful, tender uterus that is slow to involute.

Ureteric dilatation and vesico-ureteric reflux physiologically associated with pregnancy make urinary tract infection common in the postpartum period, so symptoms of dysuria, fever and cloudy, malodorous urine should be treated with suspicion. Other sources of infection that should be considered include chest infection and infection of the intravenous or epidural site. Endocervical smears and cultures should be taken on women who present with signs of infection. Other investigations may include blood cultures.

Any woman presenting with sepsis in the puerperium should be treated rapidly with intravenous antibiotics and intravenous fluid replacement. A midstream or catheter specimen of urine should be collected. The management of postpartum women who present with sepsis requires a multidisciplinary team approach with early consultation and referral to hospital, and involvement from anaesthetic and critical-care services.[11]

One of the major findings from the 2011 Confidential Enquiry into Maternal Deaths in the United Kingdom was that delays in recognising sepsis, prescribing antibiotics and seeking consultant help were common.[11] Antibiotics were sometimes prescribed in inadequate doses, were given orally rather than intravenously, were given too late, or were discontinued too soon. Immediate aggressive treatment in the first 'golden hour' or so offers the best hope of recovery, as each hour of delay in achieving administration of effective antibiotics is associated with a measurable increase in mortality.

Venous thromboembolism

Venous thromboembolism (VTE) is a leading cause of maternal death during pregnancy or postpartum and therefore requires particular consideration.[12] While VTE is up to ten times more common in pregnant women than in non-pregnant women of the same age and can occur at any stage of pregnancy, the puerperium is the time of highest risk.[13]

Any woman with signs and symptoms suggestive of VTE — most commonly this is a swollen erythematous leg — should have objective testing performed expeditiously: a compression duplex Doppler ultrasound investigation of blood flow in the venous system of the leg, or a pulmonary ventilation–perfusion scan or CTPA (computerised tomography of the pulmonary artery), where a pulmonary embolus (PTE) is suspected.

Treatment with low molecular weight heparin (LMWH) should be commenced until the diagnosis is excluded. If leg ultrasound is negative and there is a low level of clinical suspicion, anticoagulant treatment can be discontinued.

Box 17.1 Risk factors for puerperal sepsis

- Prolonged rupture of membranes resulting in an ascending infection
- Frequent use of urinary catheters
- Prolonged labour, with increased intervention and more vaginal examinations
- Assisted birth (vacuum or forceps delivery with episiotomy)
- Vaginal lacerations
- Postpartum haemorrhage
- Caesarean delivery.

Secondary postpartum haemorrhage

Secondary postpartum haemorrhage (PPH) is defined as excessive vaginal bleeding occurring between 24 hours and 6 weeks after the birth.[14] As the blood loss is difficult to quantify, the diagnosis is usually subjective and based on clinical findings. In developed countries, 2% of postnatal women are admitted to hospital with this condition, half of them undergoing uterine surgical evacuation.[15] Blood transfusion is required in 20% of women with secondary PPH. The main causes of a secondary PPH are infection (usually endometritis) or retained fragments of the placenta or membranes, or both, remaining in the uterus. Such retained fragments either cause infection or prevent the uterus from contracting, thus causing bleeding.[15]

Subinvolution or abnormalities of involution are clinically recognised by a large soft uterus and a patulous cervix, and may result from retained placental tissue or uterine infection. Attention to the signs of endometritis such as offensive lochia and fever is important. Clinical symptoms of secondary PPH are fresh vaginal bleeding of greater than 100 mL and cramping abdominal pain. The necessary investigations include a full blood count, blood group, and vaginal swabs for culture and sensitivity. It may be necessary to cross-match blood, depending on the degree of blood loss.

Ultrasound allows visualisation of the uterine cavity. Organised blood clots may resemble placental tissue sonographically, and in 10–15% of cases ultrasound will be incorrectly reported as retained placental tissue within the uterus (false-positive rate). The false-negative rate for ultrasound in this setting, however, is very low. An atonic uterus, without retained placental tissue, usually has an enlarged endometrial cavity on ultrasound (>2.5 cm antero-posterior diameter). Ultrasound may identify uterine fibroids or arteriovenous fistulae, which may be associated with secondary PPH.

There are three basic strategies in the management of secondary PPH:
- resuscitate in cases of excessive blood loss
- ascertain the aetiology of the bleeding
- instigate a medical or surgical management plan to treat the bleeding.

It is important to take the whole clinical picture into account to avoid overdiagnosis of retained tissue as a cause of secondary PPH and thus to minimise unnecessary surgery. Infection without retained placental tissue is optimally managed medically with antibiotics. If the woman experiencing a secondary PPH gave birth by caesarean delivery, retained placental tissue is unlikely, as the endometrial cavity should have been surgically checked and emptied. Severe secondary PPH usually occurs if retained placental tissue becomes necrotic and infected, preventing involution.

If the vaginal loss is mild and the clinical condition stable without the need for oxytocin, oral antibiotics such as amoxicillin/clavulanic acid and outpatient management may be adequate. If the vaginal loss is moderate, intravenous oxytocin is considered, and if there is evidence of retained placental tissue surgical evacuation of this tissue should be attempted. If the uterine cavity is empty on ultrasound assessment, antibiotics should be the first-line therapy. Iron and folate supplementation is indicated if there is evidence of anaemia.

Intravenous broad-spectrum antibiotics must be given perioperatively, as retained placental tissue is usually infected. The vulva, vagina and cervix must be inspected visually for evidence of trauma (e.g. ruptured vulval haematoma, vaginal haematoma, cervical laceration). Suction curettage with ultrasound imaging is best used to evacuate the uterus, as this technique minimises the risk of uterine perforation and of subsequent development of Asherman's syndrome. Intravenous oxytocin and bimanual compression usually will control intraoperative bleeding, once the retained tissue has been evacuated. Occasionally, additional agents will be required to achieve a firm contracted uterus (e.g. ergometrine, misoprostol or intramyometrial PGF_2). Rarely, laparotomy with internal iliac artery ligation, hysterectomy or uterine artery embolisation will be required to control the bleeding, particularly in the case of morbidly adherent placenta (placenta accreta). Evacuated placental tissue should be sent for histologic examination to exclude rare trophoblastic disease.

CONCLUSION

The puerperium is a period of considerable changes, physical as well as social and emotional. The woman recovers from the physical effects of labour and birth and establishes a feeding program with the additional impact of sleep interruption and the social changes that the new addition brings to the family. It is the role of the healthcare provider to assist the woman and her family with appropriate support, advice and guidance while ensuring that any physical or psychological complications are addressed in a timely manner.

REFERENCES

1 Centers for Disease Control and Prevention. Update to CDC's US Medical Eligibility Criteria for Contraceptive Use, 2010: Revised recommendations for the use of contraceptive methods during the postpartum period. MMWR 2011;60(26): 878–83.

2 Hay-Smith J, Mørkved S, Fairbrother K, et al. Pelvic floor muscle training for prevention and treatment of urinary and faecal incontinence in antenatal and postnatal women. Cochrane Database Syst Rev 2008;4:CD007471. doi: 10.1002/14651858. CD007471.

3 Austin M-P, Highet N, Guidelines Expert Advisory Committee. Clinical practice guidelines for depression and related disorders — anxiety, bipolar disorder and puerperal psychosis — in the perinatal period. A guideline for primary care health professionals. Melbourne: beyondblue: The national depression initiative; 2011.

4 World Health Organization. Global strategy for infant and young child feeding. Geneva: WHO; 2003.

5 Ip S, Chung M, Raman G, et al. Breastfeeding and maternal and infant health outcomes in developed countries. Evid Rep Technol Assess (Full Rep). 2007;(153):1–186.

6 Geddes D. Inside the lactating breast: the latest anatomy research. Journal of Midwifery and Women's Health 2007;52(6):556–63.

7 Kent J. How breastfeeding works. Journal of Midwifery and Women's Health 2007;52(6):564–70.

8 Mitoulas L, Kent J, Cox D, et al. Variations in fat, lactose and protein in human milk over 24h and throughout the first year of lactation. British Journal of Nutrition 2002;88:29–37.

9 Hale T. Medications and mothers milk. 14th ed. Amarillo, TX: Hale Publishing; 2010.

10 Lewis G. Saving mothers' lives: reviewing maternal deaths to make motherhood safer — 2006–08. The Eighth Report of the Confidential Enquiries into Maternal Deaths in the United Kingdom. BJOG 2011;118(Suppl. 1):1–203.

11 Draycott T, Lewis G, Stephens I. Executive Summary: The eighth Report of the Confidential Enquiries into Maternal Deaths in the UK. BJOG 2011;118(Suppl. 1):e12–e21.

12 Blanco-Molina A, Rota L, Di Micco P, et al. Venous thromboembolism during pregnancy, postpartum or during contraceptive use. Thromb Haemost 2010:103(2):306–11.

13 RCOG. The acute management of thrombosis and embolism during pregnancy and the puerperium (Green-top Guideline No. 37b). London: Royal College of Obstetricians and Gynaecologists; 2010.

14 RCOG. Postpartum Haemorrhage, Prevention and Management (Green-top 52). London: Royal College of Obstetricians and Gynaecologists; 2009.

15 Alexander J, Thomas P, Sanghera J. Treatments for secondary postpartum haemorrhage. Cochrane Database Syst Rev 2002;(1):CD002867.

MCQS

Select the correct answer.

1 Which of the following influences the initiation of lactation?

    A length of labour
    B decreased levels of prolactin
    C size of the breast
    D using a nipple shield
    E decreased levels of placental lactogen and progesterone post delivery

2 The process of involution is usually monitored by which of the following?

    A the return of ovulation and menstruation, signifying the process is complete
    B palpation of the descent of the uterine fundus
    C ensuring the woman is able to pass urine post delivery
    D the transition of lochia rubra to lochia serosa
    E the closing of the internal cervical os

3 Which are the most common clinical signs of endometritis?

    A primary PPH
    B urinary retention
    C subinvolution
    D uterine tenderness and vaginal bleeding
    E lower abdominal pain and dysuria

OSCE

Miriam has just given birth to her first baby. She has been discharged home at her request the following day. She comes to see you, her GP, a week later because she thinks her bleeding may be excessive. What are the important history and examination points in helping you answer her question? How would you manage her?

Chapter 18

Abnormal uterine bleeding

Amanda Cuss and Jason Abbott

KEY POINTS

AUB is a very common presenting issue for women.

The PALM–COIEN classification system should be used for causes of AUB.

Consider local gynaecological and non-gynaecological causes of bleeding.

History and examination are integral in considering a diagnosis.

Simple investigations may include exclusion of pregnancy and anaemia, and ultrasound to help differentiate causes.

Management options will vary depending on the cause, from observation, to hormonal regulation, to surgical options and interventional radiology.

INTRODUCTION

Abnormal uterine bleeding (AUB) is a very common problem among women of reproductive age. AUB represents changes in the volume, frequency, intervals and duration of the menstrual cycle. These abnormalities may present as irregular flow (i.e. frequency and duration); an abnormal volume of flow; absent flow; or bleeding between cycles. In childbearing years, as opposed to peri- or post-menopausally, AUB includes amenorrhoea (no menses for >90 days); menorrhagia (excessive or prolonged but regular bleeding); polymenorrhoea (bleeding intervals <21 days); oligomenorrhoea (bleeding intervals >35 days); metrorrhagia (irregular intervals between bleeding); menometrorrhagia (prolonged and excessive bleeding or irregular intervals) and intermenstrual bleeding. Terminology has changed in this area and the previous term to describe many of these problems — dysfunctional uterine bleeding — is best avoided. The International Federation of Gynaecologists and Obstetricians (FIGO) has ratified a new classification system, denoted by the acronym PALM–COIEN, and we shall use this terminology to look at the causes, diagnosis and management of AUB for women.

BACKGROUND AND EPIDEMIOLOGY

Epidemiological studies indicate that 20–25% of premenopausal women have experienced AUB, and that it accounts for 25% of gynaecologic surgery — often despite normal anatomical findings on investigation. When AUB is suspected, it is imperative to first exclude pregnancy as a cause of bleeding, and to undertake appropriate investigations to diagnose live pregnancy, miscarriage, trophoblastic disease and ectopic pregnancy.

The pathophysiology of ovulation and menstruation is described in chapter 3 and the reader is recommended to refer back to this chapter.

There are many causes of AUB and the acronym PALM–COIEN is a useful way to remember many — but not all — of these. Box 18.1 shows the

Box 18.1 Differential diagnosis of AUB

Pregnancy

Live, miscarriage, ectopic, trophoblastic disease, retained products and lactation.

Structural

PALM

- Polyps
- Adenomyosis
- Leiomyoma (myoma or fibroid)
- Malignancy

as well as localised lesions, infections and cervical/vaginal neoplasms.

Systemic and iatrogenic

COIEN

- Coagulation disorders
- Ovulatory dysfunction (anovulation such as peri-menarchal, peri-menopausal, excess androgens (e.g. PCOS, CAH, androgen producing tumours), thyroid disorders, excess prolactin and hypothalamic disorders)
- Iatrogenic
- Endometrium
- Not yet classified.

Others

This includes trauma, endocrine and hepatic disorders, most of which are rare causes of AUB.

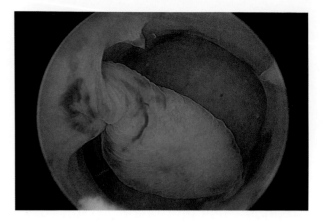

Figure 18.1
Pedunculated polyp attached to the right lower uterine wall. Note the vascularity on the polyp surface. The curved endometrial cavity can be seen at the top of the screen.

(Image courtesy of Jason Abbott)

(flat-based) or pedunculated (that is, have an elongated pedicle, or stalk). They contain dense stromal tissue, blood vessels and glandular epithelium. Figure 18.1 demonstrates a pedunculated polyp. Polyps are a common cause of AUB and are reported to occur in about 25% of women experiencing this problem. Polyps are thought to be influenced by hormone levels, in particular oestrogen, and cause AUB due to the fragile nature of the associated vasculature, which may undergo vasoconstriction, causing inflammation and eroding the tissue in the polyp, leading to bleeding symptoms.

Endometrial polyps are usually benign, but 0.5% of endometrial polyps contain malignant cells, commonly adenocarcinoma. This is not the main reason for removing polyps in premenopausal women, but rather because they lead to symptoms such as AUB. Polyps are most frequently and best identified by ultrasound, with constrast sonohysterography used on occasion. The more expensive imaging modalities of CT and MRI should not be used for diagnostic purposes. Hysteroscopy is a more invasive diagnostic modality that may also treat the lesion (see management below). Polyps may impact fertility and should be removed in this circumstance. Spontaneous regression of polyps is not uncommon, with a size of <8 mm being a postitive predictor for regression. Polyps larger than this are less likely to regress spontaneously.

extended version of this acronym and how we will address these problems further in this chapter.

DETAILED AETIOLOGY

Although the precise causative factors cannot always be identified, the most common are those listed below.

Polyps

Polyps are outgrowths of endometrial tissue found within the endometrial cavity. They may be sessile

Adenomyosis

Adenomyosis is defined as the presence of endometrial glandular tissue (both glands and stroma) occurring in the myometrium. The exact pathogenesis is unknown, but excess oestrogen levels may act as an induction agent. Bleeding is believed to result from the ectopic tissue inducing hyperplasia and hypertrophy of the surrounding myometrium, enlarging the uterus and increasing endometrial surface area, as well as initiating possible vascular changes.

The finding of the endometrial glands and stroma in the myometrium may indicate that adenomyosis is on the spectrum of endometriosis. Histologically this makes sense, although controversy continues around this assumption. The aetiology of adenomyosis has also been associated with uterine trauma that interferes with the barrier between myometrium and endometrium, such as caesarean delivery, tubal ligation, and termination of pregnancy.

Symptoms of this condition include pain, pressure in the pelvis, and an enlarged uterus clinically or symptomatically (symptoms such as urinary frequency or the finding of a mass). Ultrasound and MRI are both suitable and sensitive to make the diagnosis, and ultrasound is the most useful first-line imaging tool for excluding other pathology such as leiomyoma. Management of adenomyosis may be medical in the form of hormonal therapy (oral or local) or surgical (endometrial ablation is less effective compared with hysterectomy, which is definitive).

Leiomyoma (myoma, fibroid)

Uterine leiomyomas, also called myoma or fibroid, are benign smooth muscle tumours of the uterus. Up to one in two women will have a myoma at some time in her life, with half of these coming to clinical attention. Myoma growth has been demonstrated to be very variable, with oestrogen, progestogen or an absence of hormonal receptors found on their surface. Consequently, they have an unpredictable growth pattern. It was previously considered that oestrogen was a driving force in all myomas, but this does not appear to be the case and myomas do not always increase in size during pregnancy.

Myomas are be found in three structural locations within the uterus (Figure 18.2):
- myometrial or intramural: within the muscular layer of the uterine wall
- submucosal: directly underneath the endometrial layer

- subserosal: under the serosal layer of the uterine wall.

Myomas may be pedunculated (found on a stalk), either outside the uterus or within the cavity, and they may easily distort the shape and size of the uterus if multiple or large.

Myomas may be asymptomatic, but most commonly they will present with AUB. Common presenting features of myomas are:
- abnormal uterine bleeding
- pelvic pain
- subfertility
- mass effects (finding of lump, compression of bladder or bowel).

Clinical examination may distinguish myomas, where they may be palpated as irregular, smooth lumps on the uterus, or the entire uterus may be enlarged. Imaging is best undertaken by grey scale ultrasound, with other investigations including sonohysterography, hysteroscopy and MRI having a limited role in the diagnosis. Management of myomas may be medical or surgical, dependent primarily on patient symptomatology in conjunction with the size, number and position of the myomas, and other factors such as the preservation of fertility. Medical management includes oral hormones, NSAIDs, and other medications to reduce bleeding (such as tranexamic acid). There is no medical treatment available to date that will reduce the size of myomas in the long term. Interventional treatments include myoma ablation, myomectomy or hysterectomy, and radiological interventions including uterine artery embolisation (UAE) and magnetic resonance guided focused ultrasound (MRgFUS) (see below).

Malignancy

Refer to chapter 25 for details on endometrial hyperplasia and malignancy.

Localised causes

Bleeding from other lower genital tract and surrounding structures should also be excluded.

Cervix

Localised lesions including polyps and tumours may cause bleeding due to ulceration and inflammation. This may commonly present as postcoital bleeding. Investigations need to include a Pap smear

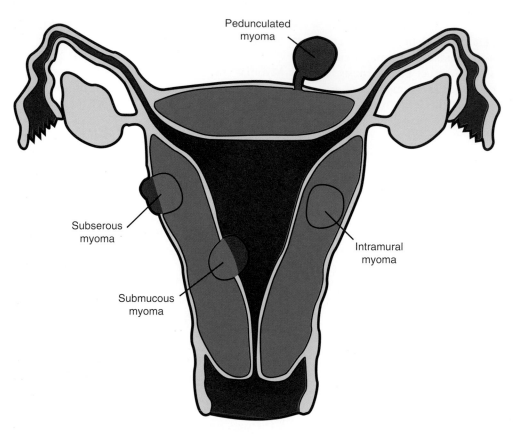

Figure 18.2
Typical location of myomas within the uterus.

(Image courtesy of Jason Abbott)

and biopsy if a lesion is seen on speculum or colposcopic examination.

Cervicitis is inflammation of the cervix which may be infectious in origin from bacteria including *Neisseria gonorrhoeae*, *Chlamydia trachomatis*; viruses like herpes simplex; or non-infectious from trauma, allergies, or devices such as IUDs and diaphragms.

Vagina

Look for localised lesions or tumours.

In vaginitis and vulvovaginitis, inflammation or infection of the vulva or vagina may present as bleeding. The infection may be bacterial (e.g. *Neisseria gonorrhoeae*), *Gardnerella* (causing bacterial vaginosis), *Chlamydia trachomatis*, viral (herpes simplex), fungal (*Candida albicans*) or parasites (trichomonas). Non-infectious causes of vaginitis may include chemical irritation or allergy, hormonal (atrophy from a lack of oestrogen), or irritation from foreign bodies.

Other

Other causes include urethral, lower urinary tract and gastrointestinal bleeding, or bleeding from the perineal skin.

Coagulopathy

In episodes of unexplained bleeding, coagulation defects must be considered and excluded. Von Willebrand disease is the most common inherited bleeding disorder in women with AUB. This disorder is a dysfunction or deficiency in von Willebrand factor, a protein necessary for platelet function and a cofactor to Factor VIII. It is characterised by excessive or prolonged bleeding under otherwise normal circumstances. A coagulation screen and vWF antigen testing will diagnose a defect. Treatment of the condition is with desmopressin, however tranexamic acid also has demonstrated efficacy. Other bleeding disorders such as thrombocytopenia and haemophilias should be considered. Involvment of a haematologist is appropriate if these diagnoses are considered or confirmed.

Ovulatory disorders

Endocrine

THYROID DEFICIENCY

Hypothyroidism may be primary in nature, originating within the thyroid, such as Hashimoto's thyroiditis; secondary, originating from the pituitary, from a deficiency in TSH due to tumour, radiation, surgery or Sheehan's syndrome; or tertiary, originating in the hypothalamus from a deficiency in TRH. Medications may also cause hypothyroidism including amiodarone, lithium and PTU.

A disruption to the hypothalamic–pituitary–ovarian (HPO) axis occurs when a deficiency in thyroid hormones promotes chronic elevations in cortisol, which in turn produces excess oestrogen which is unopposed and causes heavy and dyssynchronous endometrial shedding.

PCOS

An abnormal HPO axis results from hyperinsulinaemia, which also stimulates an increase in GnRH and therefore an imbalance between LH and FSH. This imbalance deranges the oestrogen and progesterone levels leading to immature follicles, and subsequently there is no ovulation. This anovulatory cycle leads to the AUB, with cycles that are infrequent and may occur three or more months apart. When they do occur, periods may be very heavy due to the prolonged proliferation of the endometrium under the influence of persistent oestrogen stimulation. In addition, there is an excess of androgens (more freely circulating androgens) within the woman's system that may cause virilising symptoms (acne, hair growth, central weight gain) that may accompany PCOS. This condition may be managed with lifestyle changes, with the OCP or metformin to manage the specific endocrine issues. When fertility is desired, ovulation induction and other methods of fertility assistance may be necessary. Specialist referral would be recommended in this situation.

Hepatic failure

Failure of the synthesis of clotting factors within the liver may cause unexplained bleeding. The stigmata of chronic liver disease should be apparent on physical examination and investigations to identify failure and management are dependent on the level of failure. This is a rare but important cause of AUB.

Iatrogenic

Anticoagulatory and antiplatelet medications such as warfarin, clopidogrel, dypyramidole, enoxaparin and heparin may all promote irregular or excessive uterine bleeding due to disruption of the coagulation cascade or by affecting changes to the number or function of platelets. Unopposed oestrogens may lead to AUB and eventually hyperplasia and malignancy (this effect is seen in PCOS), and should be avoided both in the premenopausal and postmenopausal woman. Progestogens should always be administered in a cyclic or continuous manner with any exogenous oestrogen in a woman who has a uterus.

Endometrium

Endometrial disorders in the absence of pelvic pathology (previously termed dysfunctional uterine bleeding) are a diagnosis of exclusion. They occur due to disruption in the normal menstrual cycling, resulting in thinning of the vascular layer and changes to the coagulation cascade. These conditions may be classified as anovulatory or ovulatory.

In the anovulatory endometrial disorders (that is, without ovulation), endometrial growth from ovarian oestrogen stimulation is no longer normally balanced by progesterone secretion from a corpus luteum postovulation. Anovulation results in a lack of progesterone to oppose the oestrogen and there is continued proliferation of the endometrium. When the endometrium becomes too thick to be adequately supported by the surrounding vasculature, focal breakdown occurs, resulting in AUB from asynchronous, incomplete shedding. The condition presents with irregular menstrual periods, often with painless, heavy bleeding, and is commonly found in PCOS, adolescents, endocrine disorders, and stress conditions.

There are few abnormalities on physical examination and no structural abnormalities with imaging. If anovulation is suspected, empirical medical treatment in the form of progestogens with or without oestrogens will restore normal hormonal cycling to initiate endometrial growth and demise.

In the ovulatory situation, the pathophysiology is less clear. Where no structural or specific cause for the bleeding is identified (and the woman has heavy, regular menstrual cycles), it is hypothesised that local defects in the endometrium may affect haemostasis through imbalances in prostaglandin synthesis to cause the heavy and variable bleeding. Investigations show no abnormality and treatment options are considered below.

HISTORY

When presented with a woman who has AUB, the cornerstone of identifying the cause begins with a detailed menstrual history. The patient's age is important to consider the beginning and end of reproductive age.

Menstrual history should include:

- menarche
- cycle regularity and length of intermenstrual intervals
- volume of flow, e.g. number and type of sanitary products used and changes in the flow during menses
- flow, e.g. clots, flooding (the symptom of blood loss onto clothing despite the use of sanitary products)
- contraception
- signs of ovulation, e.g. pain, cervical mucus changes, breast tenderness, mittelschmerz pain
- intermenstrual bleeding
- parity, e.g. the risk of adenomyosis increases with number of pregnancies.

In addition:

- sexual and obstetric history including Pap smear results
- STIs
- pregnancies
- symptoms of anaemia, e.g. shortness of breath, palpitations, fatigue, dizziness
- symptoms of thyroid dysfunction, e.g. weight gain, skin and hair changes, intolerance to cold
- symptoms of bleeding disorders, e.g. easy bruising, mucosal bleeding, prolonged bleeding from wounds, and family history
- symptoms of malignancy, e.g. unexplained weight loss
- medication history, e.g. anticoagulations, tamoxifen use, hormone therapy, herbal preparations, e.g. soya
- other medical history
- family history.

It is worthwhile considering how to quantify 'heavy' menstrual bleeding, since assessment of the volume of loss has been demonstrated to be variable. Heaviness that affects a woman's quality of life, represents a change from her usual menstrual pattern, with a history of clots and flooding and the necessity to change sanitary protection more than 2-hourly are all good indicators of blood loss that may lead to anaemia. Specifically asking about these issues will help with the history-taking and assessment of heavy menstrual bleeding.

The examination for this condition should follow the outline specified in chapter 3, The fundamentals of gynaecology.

INVESTIGATIONS

There are a limited number of investigations that are required for most causes of AUB. It is always important to exclude pregnancy with a βhCG and pregnancy should be considered in women who could be pregnant.

Biochemical investigations may include:

- serum quantitative βhCG to exclude pregnancy, ectopic and trophoblastic disease
- Full blood count for anaemia, platelet disorders
- Coagulation profile for bleeding diatheses
- TSH and thyroid hormone levels if suspecting thyroid dysfunction
- FSH/LH
- Progesterone (low levels in the second half of the cycle, that is day 21 of a regular 28-day cycle, may indicate anovulation)
- Others, e.g. testosterone, fasting prolactin, LFT, EUC, Pap smear.

The necessity for each of these will depend on the history and the differential diagnosis list that has been projected.

Imaging options are:

- ultrasound: grey-scale transabdominal and transvaginal ultrasonography is the mainstay of assessment of AUB and may reveal structural disorders of the uterus, cervix, ovaries and endometrium.
- sonohysterography (SHG): this requires a contrast medium — usually saline infusion into the endometrial cavity — to diagnose or better define intracavitary polyps and myomas and allow further imaging of the endometrium. It should be used as an addition to grey-scale imaging.

- hysteroscopy: allows visualisation of the uterine cavity to detect intrauterine lesions. During the procedure biopsies may be taken and lesions treated. This may be done in an outpatient setting with very fine instruments and camera equipment, with saline or other clear constrast uterine distension (including carbon dioxide).
- MRI/CT should be reserved for special situations only.

Other investigations include:
- biopsy: cervical or endometrial to diagnose underlying pathology such as carcinoma, but also to identify the histology of the endometrium (proliferative or secretory), which may assist in the selection of treatment. This may be done in the outpatient setting or as an inpatient when needed.
- dilatation and curettage: uterine curettage is not a treatment for the problem of AUB and is diagnostic only in nature. The removal of endometrial tissue by curettage may provide histopathologic examination, with a greater sample achieved than with an aspiration sampler.
- diagnostic laparoscopy: This requires general anaesthesia and is reserved for investigation and management of conditions such as endometriosis, tuboovarian abnormalities, leiomyomas, and those requiring surgical excision and removal. Laparoscopy is not commonly used for diagnosis, but is commonly considered in the management of some causes of AUB.

TREATMENTS
Conservative

When a woman is not anaemic, does not have a neoplastic or pre-neoplastic condition, and the AUB is not leading to diminished quality of life, it is reasonable to treat her conservatively with follow-up as clinically indicated.

Medical

Medical treatment may be considered even where structural and histological abnormalities have been demonstrated, pending discussion with the woman and appropriate follow-up. The choice of medical therapy is dependent on the specific aetiology and the fertility/contraceptive wishes of the patient.

Hormonal
PROGESTOGENS

These prevent proliferation of the endometrium by increasing the formation of arachidonic acid in the endometrium. This increases the ratio of $PGF2\alpha$ to PGE, contributes to glandular formation, halts endometrial growth, and eventually causes endometrial sloughing.

Oral progestogens are best given for 14–21 days and have been shown to decrease bleeding by approximately 85%. These are not licensed to be contraceptive (although they may have a contraceptive effect due to local effects on cervical mucus), and do not impact on future fertility. Side effects of progesterone may include weight gain, bloating, breast tenderness, acne and depression.

Local progestogens include the levonorgestrel intrauterine system (L-IUS, Mirena) and these may decrease bleeding by more than 90%. These are also contraceptive and are fully reversible. The most common side effect with these devices is irregular bleeding, and it may take 6 months to settle into a regular bleeding pattern. Other side effects include acne, headaches and breast tenderness. After using one of these devices for a year, 1 in 3 women will be amenorrhoeic, and it is important to counsel women that this may happen and is a normal outcome for this device.

Implanted or injected progestgens may be used. With these treatments, bleeding may be irregular or cease completely, and they also are a reversible contraceptive. The side effects are similar to those of the progestogen-containing IUS, but there may be problems with decreased bone mineral density when used for a prolonged time (>5 years) and caution is recommended in this setting.

COMBINED ORAL HORMONES

The combination of oestrogen and progesterone prevents proliferation of the endometrium and may decrease AUB by approximately 45%. It is a reversible contraceptive. Side effects are the most common issue with this medication and include mood swings, headache, nausea, fluid retention, and rarely DVT and stroke.

GONADOTROPHIN RELEASING HORMONE ANALOGUE (GnRHa)

This hormone halts production of progesterone and oestrogen from the ovary and is given by monthly injection or daily intranasal administration. It acts by preventing the usual pulsatile release of GnRH from the hypothalmus and in turn the rest of the HPO cascade. For 90% of women receiving these treatments, bleeding will cease completely, although there may be an initial 'flare' response where hormones are temporarily increased. While it is not licensed for contraceptive purposes, it prevents all ovarian function and therefore pregnancy is very unlikely. There is no impact on future fertility. While on this treatment, menopausal symptoms are very common and it may lead to bone demineralisation. The medication may only be used for a maximum of 12 months because of this effect. The drug has a limited role to play in AUB because of its temporary effect.

OTHER

Other hormonal therapies include transdermal patches and vaginal rings that release progesterone and oestrogen.

Non-hormonal

NON-STEROIDAL ANTI-INFLAMMATORIES

NSAIDs such as mefanamic acid are effective due to their ability to inhibit prostaglandin synthesis and alter the ratio between thromboxane and prostacyclin, decreasing blood loss by approximately one-third. These medications are often prescribed as first-line treatments and they are taken just at the time of menstruation, which helps with compliance. No single NSAID has a markedly greater effect than any other. They have no impact on fertility, although are not recommended at the time of implantation for women desiring pregnancy (considering they should only be used at menstruation for control of AUB, bleeding indicates pregnancy has not occurred). Side effects may include indigestion, diarrhoea, upper GI ulceration and gastric bleeding, and these side effects may limit their use.

TRANEXAMIC ACID

Tranexamic acid (trade name Cyklokapron) acts as an antifibrinolytic and decreases menstrual loss by 50%. It may be used both in the acute setting to treat severe heavy bleeding, and also in the long term for ongoing management of AUB. Studies have demonstrated a very low side effect profile. This is an excellent first-line treatment for women with many forms of AUB due to its efficacy and tolerability. Compliance is improved by the fact that it is only taken during heavy menstruation. There

is no impact on fertility. Side effects may include diarrhoea, headache and symptoms of reflux. This medication is contraindicated in women with previous thromboembolic disease.

Surgical

Localised removal

Specific localised pathologies may be best treated by surgical excision. This includes polypectomy and myomectomy for intracavitary pathology. A hysteroscopic approach requires no incisions and for small lesions is a day-surgical or even outpatient procedure using specialised equipment. Intramural or subserous myomas may be approached abdominally by laparoscopy or laparotomy, depending on the skills of the surgeon to perform these different procedures. Such localised removal allows for fertility preservation. For women who have removal of large myomas, caesarean delivery may be recommended for future pregnancies due to an increase in the risk of uterine rupture with labour. This will depend on the depth of myometrium incised to retrieve the myoma. With a deep or full-thickness myometrial incision, caesarean delivey would commonly be recommended. Figure 18.3a–d shows a laparoscopic myomectomy and full thickness myometrial repair.

Endometrial ablation

Endometrial ablation requires the surgical removal of endometrial tissue including the basal layer, aiming to prevent regeneration of this tissue and recurrence of the bleeding. It may be used as a first-line treatment or following unsuccessful medical treatments for women with AUB. It should never be recommended for women who have not completed their family or are uncertain about their future fertility. Pregnancy is possible post-procedure but is associated with significant risk, and women need to be appropriately counselled regarding contraception. Some pathologies such as polyps and myomas may also be removed with an ablation procedure.

The procedure involves a hysteroscopic approach for visual ablation using a resectoscope or rollerball electrode. The entire endometrium is excised or destroyed using an electrosurgical current. Other devices available use a mesh array with an electrosurgical current (NovaSure device) or heated fluid within a balloon that fills the cavity (Cavaterm, Thermachoice, Thermablate devices). Figure 18.4 shows the endometrial cavity before and after an

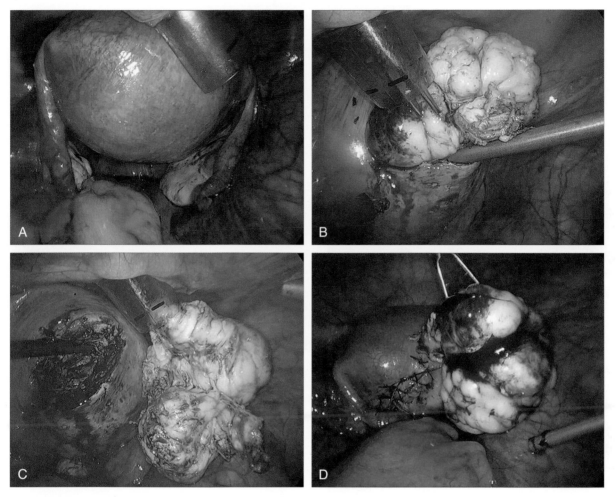

Figure 18.3

A: Enlarged uterus with a 5 cm myoma that extends intramurally to submucosally; **B**: The uterus opened and the myoma being removed. **C**: The myoma completely removed and the uterine defect seen on the left in the background. **D**: The myoma just prior to removal from the abdomen and the repaired uterus with sutures in the background. This full-thickness myomectomy will require caesarean delivery for any future pregnancy.

(Image courtesy of Jason Abbott)

endometrial ablation procedure. These devices require less surgical skill and have more consistent outcomes than first-generation endometrial ablation procedures. They are not all suitable for all pathologies or large cavities. These devices are shown in Figure 18.5.

Following endometrial ablation, which is usually performed as a day-stay surgical procedure, common effects include a watery vaginal discharge and cramping pain for 2–3 days. Risks include infection (1–2%), and rare complications include perforation of the uterus or visceral damage. Women report a decrease in bleeding of 80–90% and a decrease in dysmenorrhoea of 70–80% compared to their pre-operative levels of bleeding and pain. Approximately 30–40% of women will be amenorrhoeic following the procedure and women should be told of this in advance. The need for subsequent hysterectomy is approximately 20%.

Hysterectomy

Hysterectomy remains the definitive treatment for heavy bleeding, either as a primary option — such as when a woman wants a guarantee of freedom

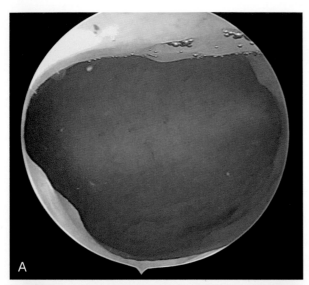

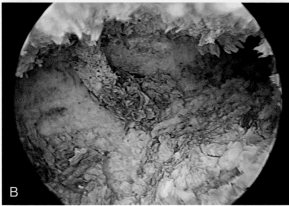

Figure 18.4
A: Normal endometrium in a women with heavy menstrual bleeding prior to endometrial ablation. The left ostium can be seen as the dark circle at the top right-hand side of the image. B: The endometrium in a woman treated by endometrial ablation. Note the absence of endometrium and the coagulated white surface of the superficial myometrium. The ostia can be seen on either side of the image.

(Image courtesy of Jason Abbott)

from bleeding — or when other treatments have failed. It is apparent that there may be no future fertility and although this is the most invasive of all treatments for AUB, it is associated with the highest satisfaction rates for women. Hysterectomy may be performed three ways:

- vaginally
- abdominally
- laparoscopically.

The choice of the surgical mode will depend on the skills of the gynaecologist to perform these different types of hysterectomy and the choice of the patient. The indication for hysterectomy, the pathology present, medical and surgical history and patient factors (such as parity, BMI) are also important considerations.

Total hysterectomy involves removal of the uterus and cervix and subtotal hysterectomy removes only the uterine corpus (body), leaving the cervix (neck) in situ. Notice that there is no reference to preservation or removal of the ovaries in hysterectomy, and ovarian removal must be discussed and the patient's informed consent obtained if this is to occur. Generally in premenopausal women where the ovaries are not affected by pathology such as in AUB, the ovaries are best retained.

Hysterectomy is a major surgical procedure and women need to be admitted to hospital, have an appropriate surgical assessment, and the procedure performed under general or regional anaesthesia. Morbidity associated with hysterectomy includes infection, haemorrhage, damage to other organs such as bowel or urinary tract, urinary dysfunction, and general complications of surgery such as thromboembolism and anaesthetic complications.

Radiological
Uterine artery embolisation

Uterine artery embolisation (UAE) is an effective treatment of heavy bleeding and large myomas as it targets the vessels to the myoma. The subsequent ischaemia reduces the size of the myoma and the AUB. The procedure is performed using a catheter fed into the femoral artery to deliver particles to the uterine vasculature under radiological guidance. The uterus has excellent collateral circulation and this prevents the uterus from necrosis.

UAE is not recommended for women who want to conserve their fertility, or when submucous myomas are present. Procedural morbidity includes vaginal discharge, severe pain, localised or systemic infection, nausea, haematoma, and ischaemia to surrounding structures, notably the endometrium, causing Ashermans syndrome or ovarian failure.

Magnetic resonance guided focused ultrasound (MRgFUS)

Magnetic resonance guided focused ultrasound (MRgFUS) is a hyperthermia therapy, using high

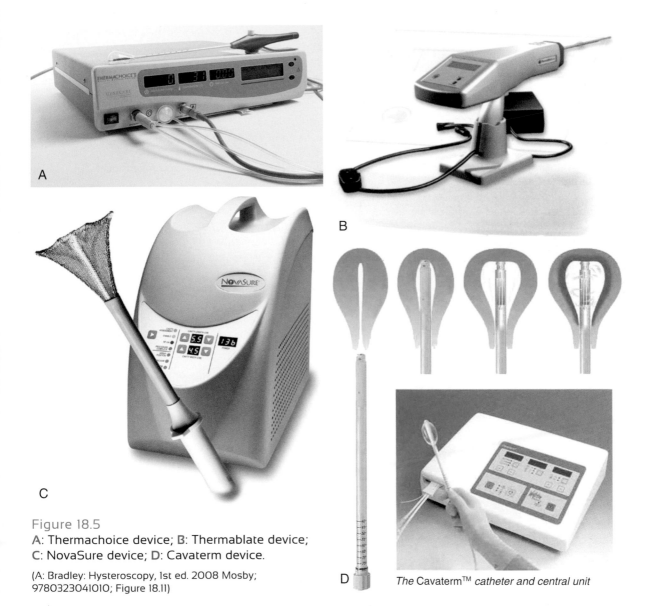

Figure 18.5
A: Thermachoice device; B: Thermablate device;
C: NovaSure device; D: Cavaterm device.

(A: Bradley: Hysteroscopy, 1st ed. 2008 Mosby;
9780323041010; Figure 18.11)

The Cavaterm™ catheter and central unit

intensity sonic energy (ultrasound) to locally heat and destroy tissue through ablation. Its main application in gynaecology is the treatment of myomas. It is currently largely a research application, although it is commercially available to patients. Under MR guidance, an ultrasound beam is focused on the myoma and the temperature is increased, causing coagulation necrosis. It is performed as an outpatient procedure, and is non-invasive. Complications include localised skin burns, visceral burns, neurological damage, and thromboembolism if patients are kept immobilised for too long during the procedure.

CONCLUSIONS

AUB is a common presentation to the medical practitioner and its causation needs to be considered in a logical manner, with exclusion of life-threatening emergency problems such as pregnancy-related complications and shock. A thorough history and examination with tailored investigations will often direct appropriate treatment. Management may be directed at specific pathology or managed empirically. A range of hormonal and non-hormonal medical treatments, as well as surgical and radiological options, are available to women, depending on the pathology present.

FURTHER READING

Munro MG, Critchley HO, Fraser IS, FIGO Menstrual Disorders Working Group. The FIGO classification of causes of abnormal uterine bleeding in the reproductive years. Fertility & Sterility 2011;95(7):2204–8. e1–3.

Salim S, Won H, Nesbitt-Hawes E, et al. Diagnosis and management of endometrial polyps: a critical review of the literature. J Minim Invasive Gynecol 2012;18(5):569–81.

Abbott J (Chairman) on behalf of the Practice Management committee of the AAGL. AAGL Practice report: Guidelines for the management of endometrial polyps. J Minim Invasive Gynecol 2012;19(1):3–9.

Burke CT, Funaki BS, Ray CE Jr, et al. ACR Appropriateness Criteria on treatment of uterine leiomyomas. J Am Coll Radiol 2011;8(4):228–34.

Huq FY. Menstrual problems and contraception in women of reproductive age receiving oral anticoagulation. Contraception 2011;84:128.

NICE. Progesterone or progesterone releasing intrauterine systems for heavy menstrual bleeding. NICE Guideline 44. Heavy menstrual bleeding. Online. Available from: www.nice.org.uk. 2013 Mar 27.

Abdel-Aleem H, d'Arcangues C, Vogelsong K, et al. Treatment of vaginal bleeding irregularities induced by progestin only contraceptives. Cochrane Database Syst Rev [Meta-Analysis Review]. 2007;2:CD003449.

Lethaby A, Irvine G, Cameron I. Cyclical progestogens for heavy menstrual bleeding. Cochrane Database Syst Rev [Meta-Analysis Review]. 2008;1:CD001016.

Lethaby A, Duckitt K, Farquhar C. Non-steroidal anti-inflammatory drugs for heavy menstrual bleeding. Cochrane Database Syst Rev [Meta-Analysis]. [Research Support, Non-US Government Review]. 2013;1:CD000400.

Cooke I, Lethaby A, Farquhar C. Antifibrinolytics for heavy menstrual bleeding. Cochrane Database Syst Rev [Review]. 2000;2:CD000249.

Marjoribanks J, Lethaby A, Farquhar C. Surgery versus medical therapy for heavy menstrual bleeding. Cochrane Database Syst Rev [Meta-Analysis Review]. 2006;2:CD003855.

Gupta JK, Sinha A, Lumsden MA, et al. Uterine artery embolization for symptomatic uterine fibroids. Cochrane Database Syst Rev [Meta-Analysis]. [Research Support, Non-US Government Review]. 2012;5:CD005073.

Hesley GK, Gorny KR, Woodrum DA. MR-guided focused ultrasound for the treatment of uterine fibroids. Cardiovasc Intervent Radiol 2013;36(1):5–13.

MCQS

Select the correct answer.

1   A 35-year-old woman has come to see you with regular heavy menstrual bleeding that is associated with minimal pain. She bleeds enough to change sanitary protection hourly and her periods last for 5 days. Which of the following series of investigations are all relevant for this woman to aid in her diagnosis?

  A   βhCG, grey-scale ultrasound, prolactin
  B   prolactin, 3D ultrasound, full blood count
  C   full blood count, βhCG, grey-scale ultrasound
  D   3D ultrasound, full blood count, thyroid-stimulating hormone
  E   thyroid-stimulating hormone, grey-scale ultrasound, prolactin

2   When considering treatment options for women who have AUB from the endometrium, which of the following statements is most correct?

  A   Mirena reduces menstrual loss by approximately 50%.
  B   Tranexamic acid reduces menstrual loss by approximately 50%.
  C   Endometrial ablation causes amenorrhoea in 90% of women.
  D   Uterine artery embolisation is safe and successful.
  E   GnRHa is effective in both the short- and long-term.

3   Sharon is a 38-year-old woman who has had AUB and a leiomyoma diagnosed by grey-scale (2D) ultrasound. Which of the following statements is the most correct regarding further investigation and management?

  A   Uterine artery embolisation should be avoided if she wants more children.
  B   Sonohysterography will better define a subserosal leiomyoma.
  C   She will need HRT if she chooses a total abdominal hysterectomy for treatment.
  D   Hysteroscopic resection is a good treatment for an intramural leiomyoma.
  E   Oestrogen-receptor profiling will indicate rate of growth of the leiomyoma.

OSCE

Erin is a 35-year-old woman who presents with heavy menstrual bleeding. What are the important features on history and examination that will direct your investigations and management? What treatment options are available to Erin for her bleeding issues?

Chapter 19

The menopause and beyond

Elizabeth Farrell

KEY POINTS

Menopause is the final menstrual period, determined after 12 months of amenorrhoea.

Premature menopause is menopause occurring before the age of 40 years and early menopause before 45 years of age. Symptoms are often more severe and are accompanied by major adjustment difficulties depending on the woman's history.

The menopause experience is unique to each woman, ranging from the cessation of menses only to severe symptoms impacting on and disturbing quality of life.

The most common symptoms of the menopause are vasomotor and urogenital symptoms.

Cardiovascular disease is the major cause of death in women and a risk assessment may be determined using Australian cardiovascular risk charts.

Osteoporosis is a consequence of loss of ovarian function with rapid bone loss within the first 5–10 years after the menopause. Up to 50% of women will experience an osteoporotic fracture in their lifetime. Fracture risk can be determined by specialised tools.

HRT is the choice in the management of osteoporosis in younger women, whereas in women over 60 years other prescriptive therapies are appropriate.

Management of the menopausal experience depends on the symptoms experienced and the woman's risk factors. Education, lifestyle advice, self-management strategies and counselling should be undertaken or offered. Available therapies include non-hormonal prescriptive medications for the vasomotor symptoms and hormone replacement therapy (HRT).

The risks and benefits of HRT should be discussed with each woman, including the benefits to symptoms, bone density and wellbeing as well as the small increase in risk of venous thromboembolism, stroke, cardiovascular disease in older women and with time the small increase in breast cancer.

The type of therapy and mode of administration of HRT will depend on whether the woman is peri- or postmenopausal. The duration of therapy will also depend on the symptom experience, requiring annual review.

Women should have a annual check with their doctor and a series of regular screening tests including Pap smear, mammography and screening blood tests, especially for lipids and glucose.

Postmenopausal bleeding is a symptom that is regarded as endometrial carcinoma until the diagnosis is excluded. Most episodes of PMB have benign causes.

INTRODUCTION

The menopause means the final menstrual period (FMP). It refers to the cessation of menstruation due to the loss of ovarian function. The average age of menopause is about 51 years, with the normal range between 45 and 57 years. Due to rapidly increasing longevity, most women will now live 30–40 years beyond the menopause. This has brought women a new way of life and a new way of death, with age-related diseases that were previously uncommon such as osteoporosis, heart disease, dementia and cancer.

The climacteric is another name for the perimenopause. It is a phase of menstrual cycle irregularity, fluctuating hormone levels and symptoms associated with ovarian senescence lasting from an average of 4–6 years before the FMP to 1 year after the menopause. About 10% of women will have symptoms that continue longer than 10 years, and the mean duration is 8 years. For some women symptoms may be long-term, and occasionally life-long.

Premature menopause is usually defined as menopause occurring under the age of 40 years. It is experienced by about 1% of women naturally (now described as premature ovarian insufficiency), with a greater percentage of women experiencing premature menopause as a result of gynaecological surgery (bilateral oophorectomy), chemotherapy and radiotherapy. With higher survival rates from cancer, the overall incidence is increasing. Oophorectomy may be necessary in conditions such as

endometriosis, chronic pelvic inflammatory disease or genital tract malignancy. In the majority of women experiencing premature menopause, the cause is unknown. Women born with gonadal dysgenesis (e.g. Turner's syndrome) are particularly at risk of the long-term consequences of oestrogen deficiency, which must be monitored regularly.

Early menopause is defined as menopause occurring before the age of 45 years. About 8% of women have spontaneously reached menopause by the age of 45 years.

Menopausal symptoms can be experienced at any time during the climacteric but are more common around late perimenopause and early postmenopause. Severe sequelae of oestrogen deficiency, such as osteoporosis and cardiovascular disease, frequently occur in later life.[1]

In the peri-and postmenopausal years women should try to optimise their quality of life by improving lifestyle, physically, psychologically and socially, as well as maintaining a healthy weight and exercising.

POTENTIAL SYMPTOMS AROUND THE MENOPAUSE

Up to 80% of women will experience some menopausal or oestrogen-deficiency-related symptoms around the menopause (Box 19.1). Each woman will have a unique experience of the menopause transition and the postmenopause, with differing intensity and frequency of symptoms. For about 20% of women menopause symptoms will impact in a significant way on quality of life so that they are unable to function normally in their daily

> ### Box 19.1 Oestrogen deficiency symptoms
>
> - Vasomotor symptoms such as hot flushes, night sweats and palpitations
> - Psychological symptoms such as anxiety, depression and feeling unloved
> - Locomotor symptoms such as joint pains, muscle pains and backache
> - Urogenital symptoms such as dry vagina, uncomfortable intercourse and urinary frequency

activities. These are the women who tend to seek help for their symptoms.

Other putative menopausal symptoms are muddled thinking and loss of memory. Women frequently complain of changes in weight and body shape, which are due to changes in fat distribution to a more android fat pattern and an increase in total body fat.

Loss of libido is not to be confused with loss of sexual function. The former includes lack of arousal and changes in orgasm, which are very complex symptoms. There are many potential influences including hormonal changes, previous sexual function, dyspareunia, ageing, general health, and psychosocial and relationship issues.

Most symptoms associated with the menopause transition, except the urogenital atrophic symptoms, will cease with time. With loss of oestrogen function the vagina loses its natural secretions, the vaginal rugae disappear, and the vaginal skin becomes thin, leading to dryness and discomfort with intercourse. There may be an increase in urinary frequency, and loss of elasticity of the pelvic tissues with an increase in the risk of prolapse and urinary incontinence.

Women from different cultural backgrounds may experience the menopause with a differing complex of symptoms. In some Asian communities, aches and pains, insomnia and lowered mood may be more prominent than vasomotor symptoms.

Women with a history of mood disorders, premature menopause or cancer are more vulnerable to depression, anxiety and other affective disorders around the menopause transition.

An example of a menopausal symptom score seen in Table 19.1 is a useful way of detecting the onset of the perimenopause and monitoring the severity of the symptoms and the response to therapy. Women without menopausal symptoms or who are being adequately treated usually score 10 or less, while women with debilitating symptoms will generally have scores varying from 20 to 50 in severity. A number of alternative menopause scoring scales, such as the Greene Climacteric Scale, are used in many menopause clinics in Australia.[2]

PREMATURE MENOPAUSE

Women undergoing premature menopause experience the symptoms, both short and long-term, that are experienced by women going through menopause at the typical age, and additionally:

- vasomotor symptoms, which are usually more severe in younger women
- severe atrophic symptoms of the genitourinary tract
- psychological distress, including depression, anger, sadness, grief, loss of femininity and body image concerns
- sexual dysfunction, including dyspareunia, loss of libido and loss of sexual function
- long-term sequelae including infertility, an increased risk of earlier onset of osteoporosis and cardiovascular disease, cognitive dysfunction, dementia and overall mortality.

Diagnosis is often delayed and should always be investigated where menstrual irregularity, oligomenorrhoea or secondary amenorrhoea occur in younger women. Hormone replacement therapy (HRT) until at least age 51 years is indicated for symptom relief and prevention of long-term complications. Usually high-dose therapy is initially prescribed, whereas low-dose therapy is initiated in women at typical age of menopause. Non-hormonal therapies may be necessary where there are contraindications to hormones, as in women with history of breast cancer. Management should include lifestyle measures for symptom control, minimising long-term risks, treatment of sexual dysfunction, infertility treatment where desired, and psychological counselling or therapy. Multidisciplinary care is recommended to manage the long-term complex needs of these women.

Causes of premature menopause include idiopathic, genetic abnormality (both X-linked and autosomal), medically induced, autoimmune and metabolic disorders, and infection. In about 60% of cases no cause is found.

OSTEOPOROSIS

Loss of bone density occurs rapidly in the first few years around menopause, with about a 15% loss in the first 5 years. Bone loss continues at a slower rate thereafter, with the risk of an osteoporotic fracture gradually increasing.

By age 65 years, one in four women has experienced an osteoporotic fracture; by age 75 years one in three women has had such fracture, and by 85 years one in two. In Australia 46% of osteoporotic fractures are vertebral, 16% are hip fractures and 16% are wrist fractures. Hip fractures may lead to increased morbidity and mortality, with up to 50%

Table 19.1 Menopause symptom score			
Oestrogen deficiency symptoms	Before therapy	3 months after starting	6 months after starting
Hot flushes			
Light-headed feelings			
Headaches			
Irritability			
Depression			
Unloved feelings			
Anxiety			
Mood changes			
Sleeplessness			
Unusual tiredness			
Backache			
Joint pains			
Muscle pains			
New facial hair			
Dry skin			
Crawling feelings under skin			
Less sexual feelings			
Dry vagina			
Uncomfortable intercourse			
Urinary frequency			
TOTAL SCORE			

Score symptoms as follows: Nil (0), Mild (1), Moderate (2) and Severe (3).

Box 19.2 Clinical risk factors for osteoporosis

- Increasing age
- Premature menopause
- Family history of osteoporosis
- Previous low trauma fracture
- Low calcium intake
- Low body mass index (<20)
- Eating disorders associated with decreased weight
- Immobilisation
- Lifestyle factors including smoking, alcoholism, lack of exercise or excessive exercise
- Medical conditions that include prolonged glucocorticoid therapy

requiring long-term care and about 15% dying within 4 months of the fracture. Once a woman has had one fracture she is at greater risk of further fractures. There is a four-fold risk of a new fracture within the first 12 months; this is termed the 'cascade effect'.

Some women are at particular risk of developing osteoporosis (Box 19.2).

Osteoporosis is best diagnosed by bone densitometry at sites such as the hip, spine and wrist (Figure 19.1). The World Health Organization defines osteoporosis as bone densities more than 2.5 standard deviations below the young normal mean (T-score <2.5).

Preventive measures should be considered in younger postmenopausal women with T-scores between −1.5 and −2.5. Treatment should be recommended for all women who have a bone mineral density (BMD) below −2.5 standard deviations and in women who have had an osteoporotic fracture.

Fracture risk can be calculated using online tools such as FRAX (www.shef.ac.uk/FRAX) or the Fracture Risk Calculator (www.garvin.org.au/promotions/bone-fracture-risk/calculator).

CARDIOVASCULAR DISEASE

Cardiovascular disease (CVD) is the main cause of death in postmenopausal women. After the menopause a woman's risk of developing CVD, including

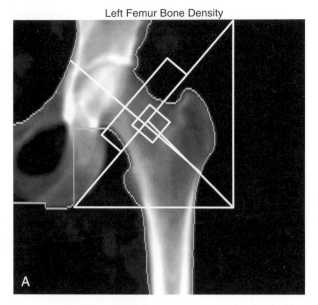

A

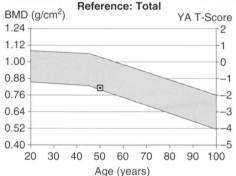

Region	BMD (g/cm²)	Young-Adult T-Score	Age-Matched Z-Score
Neck	0.893	−0.7	−0.1
Wards	0.729	−1.4	−1.3
Troch	0.592	−1.8	−1.3
Shaft	0.970	−	−
Total	0.826	−1.4	−1.8

B

Figure 19.1

Bone density (DEXA) scan of the femur of a 50-year-old woman showing early osteoporosis. The shaded zone in the graph represents the normal bone density range, which decreases from menopause. The white square represents this patient's bone density.

(Courtesy Alastair MacLennan, Department of Nuclear Medicine and Bone Densitometry, Royal Adelaide Hospital.)

coronary artery disease, hypertension, diabetes and elevated lipid levels, increases. The Australian cardiovascular risk charts and online risk assessment can be used to perform a risk assessment: www.heartfoundation.org.au/information-for-professionals/Clinical-Information/pages/absolute-risk.aspxcharts.pdf and www.cvdcheck.org.au.

NON-HORMONAL MANAGEMENT OF THE MENOPAUSE

There are many non-hormonal influences on a woman's quality of life around the age of menopause (Figure 19.2). Psychological, social and sexual issues may need to be addressed. Lifestyle factors are particularly important. Women should be encouraged to maintain their optimal weight through diet and exercise (30 minutes of weight-bearing exercise each day), avoid excessive caffeine and alcohol (less than two standard drinks per day) and stop smoking. Smoking has been associated with earlier menopause and more severe symptoms.

HRT should be avoided in women with preexisting conditions such as cardiovascular and cerebrovascular disease, history of venous thromboembolism or breast cancer. Abnormal uterine bleeding should be investigated prior to HRT being prescribed. Specialist management is advised for women with diabetes mellitus, history of endometrial cancer, abnormal liver function, active systemic lupus erythematosus (SLE) and high cardiovascular risk, where HRT may be indicated but should be used with caution.

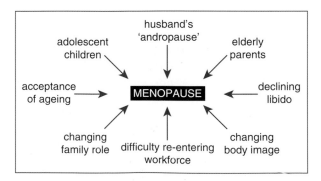

Figure 19.2
Psychological, social and sexual influences around menopause.

Vasomotor symptoms
Non-hormonal prescriptive therapies

In women with contraindications to HRT or a preference for non-hormonal preparations, vasomotor symptoms may be reduced by:
- Antidepressants, including venlafaxine, desvenlafaxine, fluoxetine, paroxetine and citalopram. Paroxetine and fluoxetine, however, should not be prescribed in women taking adjuvant tamoxifen, as the efficacy of tamoxifen may be reduced, thus increasing the risk of recurrence of breast cancer.
- Gabapentin has been shown to have equivalent efficacy to low-dose oestrogen.[3]
- Clonidine, an antihypertensive that has been used to treat hot flushes for many years.

These therapies will usually improve vasomotor symptoms by about 50–60% within about 4 weeks of therapy.

Non-prescriptive therapies

There is ongoing research into the effectiveness of vasomotor symptoms reduction by other techniques such as acupuncture, with recent evidence suggesting the effectiveness of mindfulness training and cognitive behavioural therapy.

Phytoestrogens are present in many foods such as soy, legumes and other vegetables. In large quantities, these foods may have a modest ameliorating effect on vasomotor symptoms, but in randomised placebo controlled trials to date, commercially isolated phytoestrogens such as isoflavones have not demonstrated an effect greater than placebo. Black cohosh has also not been shown to be significantly better than placebo. Most studies are short-term, and there is no long-term data on the safety and efficacy. Currently there are no significant effective alternative or complementary therapies or remedies for the menopause and its sequelae.

The effect of a placebo on hot flushes over several months is usually around 50%, and this should be remembered when assessing the many commercial claims of unregistered over-the-counter products for the menopause.

Therapies for other symptoms

Psychological symptoms can be treated with antidepressants or anxiolytics, but some women may also benefit from either short-term or long-term psychological counselling or therapy.

Locomotor symptoms may be treated with analgesics or non-steroidal anti-inflammatory agents as well as exercise and other lifestyle activities.

Vaginal products, available without prescription, include silicon-based lubricants, acidic gels, vaginal moisturisers and oils, all of which may help dryness of the vagina and uncomfortable intercourse.

Antispasmodic agents may help urinary urgency and frequency.

HORMONAL THERAPIES

The oestrogen in postmenopausal hormone replacement therapy (HRT) differs from ethinyloestradiol, a synthetic oestrogen used in most oral contraception, in that HRT usually contains biological oestrogens oestradiol, oestrone or conjugated equine oestrogens, which mostly metabolise to oestradiol and oestrone. All the progestogens available in Australia are synthetic. Biological oral progesterone is unregistered in Australia but available in New Zealand.

The average dose of oestrogens used in HRT is weaker in potency than most of the oestrogens used in oral contraception. In women with a uterus both oestrogen and a progestogen (for endometrial protection) are prescribed, but in women who have had a hysterectomy oestrogen alone is prescribed.

In the perimenopause, HRT does not inhibit ovulation and therefore is not contraceptive. In women who are non-smokers and are low risk for cardiovascular disease, combined oral contraceptives are suitable in the perimenopause for symptom control, menstrual control and contraception. When menopausal symptoms are experienced during the Pill-free week, a HRT regimen can be considered. If contraception is still required a woman may take either a low-dose oestrogen in the Pill-free week, or take the active tablets of the contraceptive continuously. Pregnancy, however, after the age of 50 years is rare. Recently two new combined oral contraceptives containing biological oestrogen (17β-oestradiol) in similar doses to HRT have become available, one of which is also approved for heavy menstrual bleeding.[4]

Tibolone is a synthetic oral hormone (a selective tissue oestrogen activity regulator), with oestrogenic, progestogenic and androgenic effects. It is effective for the management of menopause symptoms and osteoporosis.

Routes of administration

Oral therapy is generally still the first choice of route of administration. However, poor absorption or excessive metabolism of oestrogen can occur in malabsorption disorders, irritable bowel syndrome or the concurrent ingestion of H_2 antagonists for gastric reflux. If oral oestrogen is ineffective, then it is reasonable to try transdermal routes.

Some women prefer oestrogen and progestogen patches, but an oestrogen gel may be preferred when there are skin allergies or where the patches do not adhere. Skin sprays are currently unavailable in Australia. Local vaginal oestrogens can be given as tablets (oestradiol), pessaries or creams (oestriol) for vaginal symptoms with minimal systemic absorption.

Indications for hormone therapy

The two main indications for the use of HRT are relief of menopausal symptoms and the prevention and treatment of osteoporosis.

Systematic reviews of randomised controlled trials show that HRT is superior to a placebo in reducing vasomotor and urogenital symptoms (urinary frequency, atrophic vaginitis and dyspareunia).[5] Some studies also suggest that psychological symptoms and joint pains appearing around menopause may reduce with HRT.

HRT increases bone density and reduces fracture risk. It is currently the only registered therapy for the prevention of osteoporosis before the onset of an osteoporotic fracture. Its advantages are low cost, high therapy compliance, added symptom control, low numbers-needed-to-treat to prevent one fracture, and efficacy in an unscreened population. HRT should be considered as the first-line treatment for osteoporosis in young women.

Cardiovascular disease

Animal studies, laboratory studies and epidemiological studies of women taking HRT from around the age of menopause suggest that HRT may play a primary cardio-protective role through several mechanisms, including the inhibition of plaque formation in healthy arteries. However, secondary cardio-prevention studies (i.e. in women with established atherosclerosis or a past history of myocardial infarction or stroke), such as the Women's Health Initiative (WHI) study, show no benefit in initiating combined oestrogen and progesterone HRT after these events, and suggest that such HRT may be detrimental by destabilising the atheromatous plaque and increasing adverse cardiovascular outcomes by about 1% per year.[6] In the WHI oestrogen-only study, there was no increase in cardiovascular disease.[7]

Both randomised and observational WHI studies show there was no statistically significant improvement or worsening of the cardiovascular risk in the 50–59 year age group. There may be a reduction in risk of coronary artery disease in healthy women if HRT is commenced around the time of menopause or within the first 10 years. Combined hormone therapy should, however, not be prescribed in older women as it may increase their risk of cardiovascular and cardiac events.

Risk of stroke

Observational and randomised studies have revealed that both oral oestrogen and oestrogen–progestogen therapy increase the risk of stroke independent of the years since menopause. Tibolone has been shown to increase risk of stroke in women over 65. Some research suggests that transdermal oestrogen does not increase the risk of stroke.

Venous thromboembolism risk

The WHI trial has confirmed observational data that oral HRT is associated with a doubling of the risk of venous thromboembolism (VTE) and that risk increases with an increasing dose, age, smoking, body mass index, and in the first year of therapy.

Non-oral oestradiol and tibolone do not appear to increase VTE risk.

Breast cancer risk

After 5 years of use of combined HRT in the WHI trial, an increase of eight extra detected breast cancers for 10 000 women years was reported. Combined HRT increases breast density and the risk of breast cancer, especially after the age of 59 years. However, on further analysis of the trial data, the breast cancer risk was increased only in those women with prior use of HRT.

Although breast cancer was reported to increase (by 8 cases per 10 000 women years, from 30 to 38 cases per 10 000 women years), there was no overall difference in cancer rates or mortality between the placebo and combined HRT groups. This was because HRT was associated with a reduction in uterine and bowel cancers.

The WHI global index, which combined seven beneficial and adverse events, showed an increased adverse outcome for 1 per 100 patients on combined HRT. The differences in the mixed outcomes are shown in Figure 19.3. It is clear that in this population (80% being between 60 and 79 years, many with cardiovascular risk factors), long-term combined HRT cannot be recommended as a cardioprotective agent. The WHI 2004 data has been further evaluated to determine the likely risk and benefits after 5 years of combined HRT in a woman

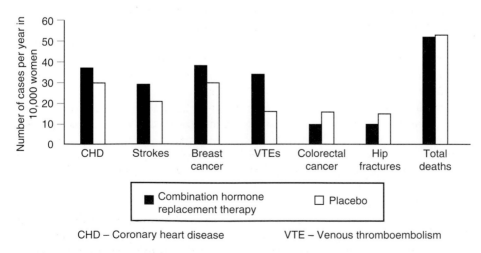

CHD – Coronary heart disease   VTE – Venous thromboembolism

Figure 19.3

WHI disease rates for women on combination hormone therapy or placebo.

(From MacLennan 2003; reproduced with permission from Australian Prescriber.)

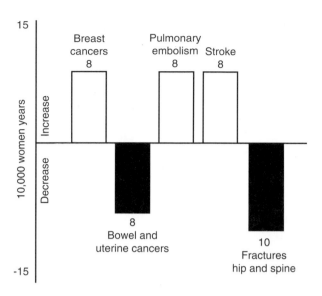

Figure 19.4
Summary of the likely significant risks and benefits after 5 years of combined HRT in a woman without cardiovascular risk factors commencing hormone therapy from early menopause.

(Based on WHI 2004.)

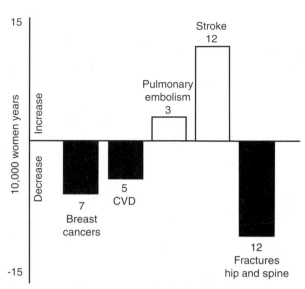

Figure 19.5
Summary of main risks and benefits of oestrogen-only HRT (CVD=cardiovascular disease).

(Based on WHI 2004.)

without cardiovascular risk factors and commencing combined hormone therapy from early menopause (Figure 19.4).

The oestrogen-only arm of the WHI trial ceased in 2004, showing no increase in breast cancer or cardiovascular disease in this study population (Figure 19.5). After 7 years of oestrogen-only therapy there was no increase in breast cancer risk. Later observational data showed an increase in risk after 15 years of use. An increase in stroke (12 per 10 000 per woman years) and a similar reduction in hip and spine fractures were observed. Thus the risk–benefit ratio is different for oestrogen-only therapy. The short duration of the WHI study prevented assessment of the long-term effects of hormone therapy.

Cognition and dementia

There is mixed evidence that HRT improves some aspects of cognitive function (e.g. verbal memory and menopausal depression), reduces the risk of dementia and improves the quality of life in symptomatic women. The hypothesis that early and prolonged HRT may give neuroprotection, that is, may slow the decline in cognitive function and reduce the risk of dementia, has yet to be tested in randomised controlled trials.

Some randomised short-term placebo-controlled trials in the early postmenopause show that oestrogen therapy improves verbal memory. In women on long-term hormone therapy (> 10 years from menopause), an observational study suggests an associated reduction in the risk of dementia (RR 0.41, CI 0.17–0.86) compared to non-users.[8] However, as with cardiovascular disease, combined hormone therapy does not appear to be neuroprotective when started in later age groups (65–79 years). Some women claim that oestrogens decrease symptoms of depression, especially if commenced around the perimenopause. Other neurological functions reportedly affected by hormone therapy include improved reaction times and postural sway compared to placebo therapy. This is relevant to the prevention of falls and may indirectly contribute to reduced fracture rates on hormone therapy.

Other effects

Short-term randomised trials show that the common early start-up side effects of oestrogen are breast tenderness and uterine breakthrough bleeding. A small number of women appear to be sensitive to the progestogen content of HRT and may complain of bloating and premenstrual-like symptoms.

Changes in the HRT regimen and in the route of administration can often reduce these problems. Transdermal preparations avoid the first pass part of metabolism and have a lower risk of VTE. Quality-of-life benefits have been described in symptomatic women on HRT but not in asymptomatic women. It may take up to 6 months to establish the most suitable HRT regimen.

Placebo-controlled trials show that weight gain is common around menopause, especially as exercise decreases, but is similar in both HRT and placebo groups. Increased gallbladder disease is a potential but as yet unproven risk associated with HRT. Potential benefits are a reduction in macular degeneration, dry eyes, tooth loss, and skin ageing.

CARE OF THE INDIVIDUAL
Assessment and counselling

It is important to allow more time for the consultation when first assessing a woman presenting with concerns about her menopause experience. A full history is necessary, including medical, surgical, menstrual, drug and other therapies, family, sexual and psychosocial issues.

It is helpful to obtain the woman's attitude to the menopause and its possible therapies, and to address any myths or common misconceptions. If HRT is being considered, there is often a fear that it may cause weight gain and other side effects including breakthrough bleeding. Details of previous side effects experienced while taking the combined oral contraceptive pill (COCP), HRT or ineffectiveness of some routes or regimens are important to allow future tailoring of possible HRT.

Examination and routine investigations

Physical examination should include breast and pelvic examination (both speculum and bimanual examination) with a cervical smear test when appropriate.

Hormone tests are rarely helpful, except as part of an assessment for premature menopause, and do not usually influence management. Serum lipids, triglyceride levels, thyroid function tests, glucose and a complete blood picture may be performed when indicated or as part of routine yearly screening. Mammography is recommended every 2 years, or yearly when there is a strong family history of breast cancer. It need not be more frequent when taking HRT. A bone density scan (e.g. dual energy X-ray absorptiometry — DEXA — of hip and spine) is appropriate when there are strong risk factors for osteoporosis or where this test will influence management. A thrombophilia screen should be performed where there has been a personal or family history of thromboembolism.

Investigations for premature menopause should include all investigations to exclude other causes of secondary amenorrhoea. Menopausal hormone levels, in particular follicle stimulating hormone (FSH) and oestradiol on two occasions at least 1–2 months apart are required for the diagnosis of premature menopause. Anti-Müllerian hormone (AMH), an ovarian hormone produced by the granulosa cells of the early developing antral follicles, may be performed as a measure of ovarian reserve.

Hormone therapy regimens

HRT consists of both an oestrogen and a progestogen and is used primarily to relieve or reduce vasomotor symptoms, aches and pains and insomnia, and promote wellbeing. The oestrogen therapy should be continuous to ameliorate symptoms without giving side effects such as breast tenderness. Around the perimenopause the progestogen therapy, in combination with the continuous oestrogen, needs to be prescribed cyclically to fit in with the endogenous ovarian cycle and to avoid breakthrough bleeding. The progestogen is usually given for 10–14 days per month. A predictable period or withdrawal bleed usually occurs after the cessation of the cyclic progestogen therapy and often the irregularity and heaviness of the perimenopausal periods are improved. Alternatively in the perimenopause the levonorgestrel-releasing intrauterine system may be used for contraception or control of heavy menstrual bleeding.

After 4 years of cyclical progestogen therapy, or if HRT is commenced more than 1–2 years after menopause, a postmenopausal regimen can be prescribed where progestogen is given continuously, usually at half the dose of the perimenopausal regimen. It is important to counsel that most women will have initial irregular breakthrough bleeding or spotting over the first 3–9 months of a continuous progestogen and oestrogen regimen before endometrial proliferation ceases and a stable atrophic endometrium is established. There is usually no need to investigate diminishing irregular bleeding in the first 12 months after the initiation of combined continuous hormone therapy regimen.

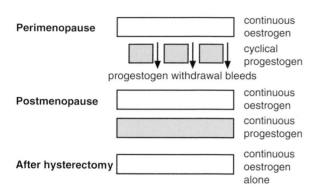

Figure 19.6
Hormone therapy regimens.

Oestrogen-only therapy

A woman who has had a hysterectomy usually does not require progestogen and receives unopposed oestrogen therapy (Figure 19.6).

Testosterone therapy

The role of testosterone in postmenopausal women is controversial. There is no correlation between serum levels of androgens and sexual dysfunction. Following bilateral oophorectomy the testosterone levels fall significantly, and it is in this group and in other women who have experienced premature menopause that testosterone therapy is considered more appropriate. Testosterone patch replacement has been shown to be beneficial in improving sexual dysfunction, especially in women following bilateral oophorectomy, but it is not available in Australia. There is insufficient data to clarify the optimal use or long-term safety of testosterone. In some women, it may help libido and anecdotally a few may experience improvement in energy and mood. Some may also experience increased feelings of aggression and in excess it can have virilising side effects. There are currently no registered preparations in Australia for women, although testosterone cream is used. Tibolone has a mild androgenic effect in postmenopausal women and can be used as an 'all in one' postmenopausal therapy, as it occupies and stimulates the oestrogen, progestogen and testosterone receptors.

Length of therapy

Women can be treated for as long as they perceive an improved quality of life from the alleviation of menopausal symptoms. This time varies greatly from woman to woman and can be from months to many years. After 4–5 years of therapy it is reasonable for women to have a trial period ceasing HRT. To avoid rebound vasomotor symptoms, the dose can be reduced over 1–2 months before cessation. Up to approximately 40% of women may experience a return of debilitating symptoms, warranting the option of a further course of therapy after counselling about the risks of longer-term therapy. Often a lower dose can be recommended with effect.

Tailoring therapy

High continuance rates can be achieved with adequate initial counselling, early follow-up, and tailoring of the regimen to minimise start-up side effects while giving effective relief of symptoms. It may take up to 6 months to establish an effective regimen. Once this regimen is established, yearly review is appropriate. About 15% of women are sensitive to progestogens and may experience premenstrual-like symptoms. They may require lower progestogen dosages or, preferably in the perimenopause, an intrauterine progestogen delivery system can be fitted that gives local endometrial protection for 5 years without adverse systemic effect in most women.

Options for the management of osteoporosis

The aim of management is the prevention of fracture, with treatment definitely prescribed when a woman has had a fragility fracture. Adequate calcium and vitamin D are necessary, with a recommended daily dose of 1000–1200 mg of elemental calcium. Daily exercise is recommended to maintain fitness and muscle mass, postural stability and improve balance, which are necessary to reduce the risk of falls as women age. In younger women with menopausal symptoms and low bone density, HRT should be considered as the first-line treatment. Early onset of osteoporosis is a risk in premature menopause, therefore regular assessment of bone density and calcium metabolism along with HRT is recommended.

HRT is not recommended for osteoporosis or prevention of fracture in women over 60 years, either as continuing therapy or to be initiated at this time. In an older woman with cardiovascular risk factors and a recent low-trauma fracture but few menopausal symptoms, other therapies need to be discussed.

- Bisphosphonates are antiresorptives that are effective in treating osteoporosis with or without fracture, but do accumulate in bone. There are side effects of oesophageal symptoms, including ulceration, if the therapy is not taken strictly according to the instructions. Potential but very rare risks of osteonecrosis of the jaw and atypical subtrochanteric fractures may occur. Recently it has been recommended that the therapy be ceased after 5 years for a variable period of time depending on the individual's fracture risks. The bisphosphonates available are alendronate, risedronate, etidronate or zolendronic acid, and are prescribed as a daily, weekly, monthly or yearly dose.
- Raloxifene, a selective oestrogen-receptor modulator (SERM), reduces the risk of vertebral fracture. It has also been shown to significantly reduce breast cancer risk and is anti-oestrogenic on the endometrium, but has an increased risk of VTE similar to HRT.
- Strontium ranaleate, which stimulates bone formation and inhibits absorption, reduces both spine and hip fracture risk. It is given in a daily dose and is often prescribed where bisphosphonates are not tolerated or have been discontinued.
- Parathyroid hormone, which stimulates bone formation, can be given by a subcutaneous injection daily for a maximum of 18 months but is very expensive.
- Denosumab is a monoclonal antibody to the receptor activator RANK ligand, a protein that acts as the primary signal to promote bone removal, and reduces vertebral, non-vertebral and hip fractures. It is given by a subcutaneous injection 6-monthly.

The most appropriate form of therapy will depend on the risk of osteoporosis fracture, the woman's age, her medical risks, previous fracture and menopausal status. Referral to an endocrinologist may be necessary.

LONG-TERM GOALS FOR HEALTHY AGEING

Menopause is a significant life transition in most women's lives and optimising health is necessary for healthier ageing.

In the women with premature menopause their long-term health management is vital to avoid premature onset of major medical conditions. These women have special needs and should be managed by a caring and competent health practitioner or team of practitioners. A caring team of health professionals has been demonstrated to improve therapy adherence and long-term wellbeing.

Increasing longevity has brought with it an increased number of disability years. Disability years are defined as those when an individual is in the care of others for assistance with day-to-day living. Women now have an average of 9 disability years before death. The most common reasons for disability are cardiovascular disease, locomotor disorders such as arthritis and osteoporosis, and incontinence and dementia. The menopause and its subsequent management may influence all these. There is a need for more research into improving the quality of life after menopause and reducing the disability years.

Annual screening with health checks is appropriate, including 2-yearly Pap smears until the recommended age of 70 and 2-yearly mammography until age 70. The BreastScreen Australia program provides free 2-yearly mammography for all women between 50 and 70 years, and will screen women between 40 to 50 years and over 70 years on request.

POSTMENOPAUSAL BLEEDING

Postmenopausal bleeding (PMB) is a symptom, not a diagnosis, but cancer must be excluded.

It refers to any bleeding (including very light bleeding, spotting or staining) that occurs 12 months or more after the final menstrual period. The true incidence of postmenopausal bleeding is unknown. In Australia in 2000–01, there were over 46 000 hospital admissions for diseases of the pelvic organs and genital tract in women over 50 years of age. Many of these admissions would have been for evaluation of postmenopausal bleeding. Proper steps must be taken to exclude gynaecological cancer, including referral to a specialist gynaecologist. A careful explanation, including the likelihood that cancer will not be found, will greatly reduce the woman's anxiety. Blood loss is usually not heavy but will influence decisions regarding management, including:

- Urgency of referral to a specialist for evaluation
- Prescription of continuous oral progestogens to manage bleeding
- Emergency transfer to hospital for blood transfusion, vaginal packing or emergency

radiological or surgical intervention (all rarely required).

Clinical evaluation

An appropriate history, examination and investigations are required. Take a careful history of the bleeding, its quality including amount, duration and whether associated with other symptoms such as pain and change in medications, including lack of adherence.

Speculum examination of the vagina and cervix, a Pap smear, bimanual examination of the pelvic organs and an abdominal examination must be performed. If hysterectomy and/or oophorectomy have been performed, the histology and details of possible remaining ovarian, uterine or cervical tissue must be established. The contribution of transvaginal ultrasound to evaluation of postmenopausal bleeding lies in the high negative predictive value of a thin endometrium for cancer, thus reliably identifying such women, who may avoid endometrial sampling. In a multicentre trial, visualisation of an endometrial echo 5 mm or less had a 99% negative predictive value for a diagnosis of cancer. The positive predictive value for disease of an endometrial echo greater than 5 mm was 9%, and if restricted to serious disease (cancer or atypical hyperplasia) was only 4%.[9]

Transvaginal ultrasound assessment of endometrial thickness may suggest the presence of a malignancy but is not diagnostic. The diagnosis of endometrial cancer is made on endometrial tissue obtained by endometrial biopsy, with or without hysteroscopy. Biopsy without hysteroscopy may, however, miss some benign causes of postmenopausal bleeding including intrauterine polyps or submucosal fibroids. Hysteroscopy with dilatation and curettage may also be performed.

Over the last 20 years, rates of obesity and unhealthy weight have increased in people aged 25–64 years with the proportion of overweight women increasing from 27% to 47%. Excess body weight predisposes women to endometrial as well as other cancers.

Risk of endometrial cancer is increased in women with a body mass index (BMI) greater than 30 kg/m^2 and the risk increases linearly with increasing BMI. In the United Kingdom, approximately 50% of endometrial cancers are attributable to obesity, with the incidence of endometrial cancer rising in postmenopausal women but with improved

5-year survival rates. The incidence peak is in the postmenopausal years, mainly between 60–79 years.[10]

Benign causes of PMB

Recent cessation or current use of hormones may be a simple explanation for the bleeding. Breakthrough bleeding in the first year of continuous oestrogen and progestogen hormone replacement therapy does not need investigation, but endometrial biopsy and hysteroscopy could be considered after this time. Sometimes PMB in the initial 2–3 years after the FMP is due to some persistent hormonal fluctuation. Other causes of PMB include the following:

- Urogenital atrophy with thinning of the vagina and cervical epithelium and the endometrium may cause bleeding because of fragility of the epithelium. After exclusion of malignancy vaginal oestrogen therapy is the treatment of choice.[11]
- Endometrial polyps or submucosal fibroids may cause bleeding in the postmenopause and may be diagnosed on transvaginal ultrasound. At hysteroscopy, once identified they can be treated by polypectomy and resection respectively. The risk of endometrial cancer in endometrial polyps is only about 1%.
- Endometrial hyperplasia when simple is not premalignant, but if it has progressed to atypical hyperplasia it will progress to carcinoma in about 40%. Treatment may be by high-dose progestogen but definitively with simple hysterectomy.[12]
- Other tumours, rarely, such as uterine sarcomas, ovarian granulosa cell tumours, vaginal or vulval cancers, may present as PMB.

While not diagnostic, transvaginal ultrasound may demonstrate this range of benign to malignant pathology (Figure 19.7). Most episodes of PMB are due to benign causes, however a thorough evaluation is necessary to exclude malignancy.

Endometrial cancer

Endometrial cancer spreads locally to lower uterus, cervix, ovaries and pelvic lymph nodes. The recommended treatment is total abdominal hysterectomy, bilateral salpingo-oophorectomy, and pelvic node sampling. Postoperative radiotherapy is often recommended to prevent local vaginal vault recurrence. Pelvic radiotherapy may be the primary

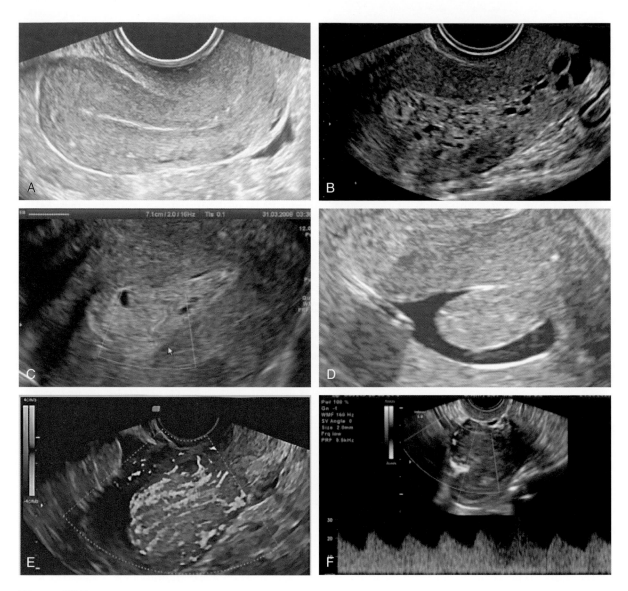

Figure 19.7

Ultrasound images in women with postmenopausal bleeding. A: Thin regular endometrium 2.2 mm; B: Thickened cystic endometrium suggestive of endometrial hyperplasia; C: Thickened endometrium suggestive of polyp with associated feeder vessel; D: Saline hysterography outlines the polyp in the fluid filled cavity; E: Markedly thickened highly vascular endometrium, histology confirmed carcinoma (sagittal section of uterus); F: Pulsed Doppler pattern of high velocity low resistance flow in an aggressive endometrial carcinoma, which occupies most of the body of the uterus (transverse section of uterus). Ultrasound is not diagnostic for endometrial hyperplasia or carcinoma.

(Images courtesy of S Atkinson, D Sutton and S Meagher, Monash Ultrasound for Women.)

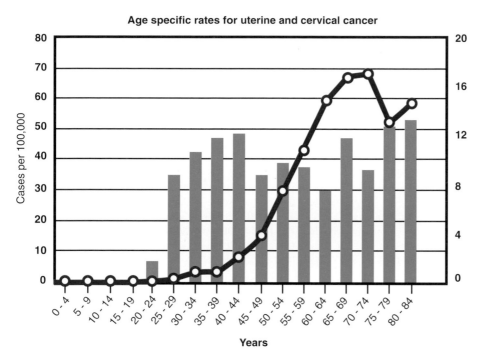

Figure 19.8

Age-adjusted rate of cancers of the endometrium and cervix in Australian women. Blue line diagram represents endometrial (uterine cancer) (range 0–68 cases per 100 000). Green bar chart represents cervical cancer (range 0–13 cases per 100 000).

treatment when the cancer is diagnosed too advanced for therapy. In Australia the 5-year relative survival rate for women diagnosed with endometrial cancer in 1998–2004 is 82%.

Cervical cancer

Cervical cancer has a bimodal age distribution. Cervical cancer in the postmenopausal period is often in the absence of a previous Pap smear. The diagnosis may be evident on a Pap smear but a histological diagnosis is required for confirmation. Cervical cancers are about 70% squamous cell origin due to human papillomavirus (HPV), with the other 30% being adenosquamous, adenocarcinoma and other forms. Unfortunately, a Pap smear does not as readily detect adenocarcinoma of the cervix.

Studies have shown that the 5-year relative survival rate for the earliest stages of invasive cervical cancer is 92%, however combining all stages the 5-year survival rate is about 73%.[13] Cervical cancer

spreads locally (lower uterus, cervix, vagina and adjacent structures) and to the pelvic lymph nodes. The preferred management is an extended total abdominal hysterectomy and pelvic node sampling or pelvic radiotherapy, depending on available expertise. Sometimes the tumour is reduced by radiotherapy before surgery. In appropriate cases, postoperative radiotherapy is offered to prevent local recurrence. If the disease is too advanced for surgery or the patient unfit for surgery, pelvic radiotherapy is offered. Local recurrence may be managed surgically, with radiotherapy or chemotherapy.

Figure 19.8 shows the age-adjusted rate of cancers of the endometrium and cervix in Australian women.

Non-gynaecological causes

Non-gynaecological causes of PMB are rare and include blood dyscrasias, but may also be from the urinary tract, especially from the urethra in older women, or from the rectum.

REFERENCES

1. Sturdee DW, Pines A, for the International Menopause Society Writing Group. Updated IMS recommendations on postmenopausal hormone therapy and preventative strategies for midlife health. Climacteric 2011;14:302–20.

2. Greene JG. Constructing a standard climacteric scale. Maturitas 1998;29:25–31.

3. Aquirre W, Chedraui P, Mendoza J, et al. Gabapentin vs. low-dose transdermal estradiol for treating post-menopausal women with moderate to very severe hot flushes. Gynecol Endocrinol 2010;26:333–7.

4. Kiley JW, Shulman LP. Estradiol valerate and dienogest: a new approach to oral contraception. Int J Womens Health 2011;3:281–6.

5. MacLennan AH, Lester S, Moore V. Oral oestrogen replacement therapy versus placebo for hot flushes. Cochrane Database Syst Rev 2001;1. Online. Available: www.update-software.com/cochrane.

6. WHI (Writing Group for the Women's Health Initiative Investigators) Risks and benefits of estrogen plus progestin in healthy postmenopausal women. Principal results from the Women's Health Initiative Randomised Controlled Trial. JAMA 2002;288:321–33.

7. WHI (Women's Health Initiative Steering Committee) Effects of conjugated estrogen in postmenopausal women with hysterectomy. The Women's Health Initiative Randomized Controlled Trial. JAMA 2004;291:1701–12.

8. Zandi PP, Carlson MC, Plassman BL, et al. for the Cache County Memory Study Investigators. Hormone therapy and incidence of Alzheimer's disease in older women: the Cache County Study. JAMA 2002;288:2123.

9. Langer RD, Pierce JJ, O'Hanlan KA, et al: Transvaginal ultrasonongraphy compared with endometrial biopsy for the detection of endometrial disease. N Engl J Med 1997;337:1792.

10. Reeves GK, Pirie K, Beral V, et al. Cancer incidence and mortality in relation to body mass index in the Million Women Study: cohort study. BMJ. 2007;335(7630):1134.

11. Tan O, Bradshaw K, Carr BR. Management of vulvovaginal atrophy-related sexual dysfunction in postmenopausal women: an up-to-date review. Menopause 2012;19:109–17.

12. Lethaby A, Farquhar C, Sarkis A, et al 2003 Hormone replacement therapy in postmenopausal women: endometrial hyperplasia and irregular bleeding. Cochrane Database Syst Rev 2003;2. Online. Available from: www.update-software.com/cochrane.

13. Australian Institute of Health and Welfare & Australasian Association of Cancer Registries. Cancer in Australia: an overview, 2010. Cancer series no. 60. Cat. no. CAN 56. Canberra: AIHW; 2010.

FURTHER READING AND USEFUL WEBSITES

The Australian Institute of Health and Welfare www.aihw.gov.au

The Australasian Menopause Society www.menopause.org.au, with links to the International Menopause Society, the North American Menopause Society and the Jean Hailes Foundation

ALGORITHMS

Menopause — A management algorithm. www.jeanhailes.org.au/health-professionals/menopause-algorithm

Vaginal bleeding in post-menopausal women. A diagnostic guide for general practitioners and gynaecologists. www.canceraustralia.gov.au

MCQS

Select the correct answer.

1   Which is the most appropriate hormonal regimen for a 56-year-old postmenopausal woman with a uterus who has many menopausal symptoms?

   A   combined cyclical oestrogen and cyclical progestogen
   B   combined continuous oestrogen and continuous progestogen
   C   combined continuous oestrogen and cyclical progestogen
   D   combined cyclical oestrogen and continuous progestogen
   E   cyclical or continuous oestrogen alone, depending on her wish for periods

2   A well 55-year-old woman whose last menstrual period was 4 years ago and who has never used HRT presents with vaginal bleeding. Which of the following is correct?

   A   Evaluation is not required if she has had a hysterectomy.
   B   An ultrasound scan to measure endometrial thickness is mandatory.
   C   This is likely to be endometrial cancer.
   D   This is likely to be cervical cancer.
   E   The woman should be referred to a specialist for evaluation.

3   Which one of the following therapies is **not** an evidence-based therapy for the reduction of osteoporotic fractures?

   A   raloxifene
   B   bisphosphonates
   C   phytoestrogens
   D   vitamin D
   E   hormone therapy

OSCE

Mary is a 56-year-old woman who presents with postmenopausal bleeding two months ago. What are the important points that you need to assess on history and examination? What investigations and management options are important for a woman with this presentation?

Chapter 20

Incontinence

Paul Duggan

KEY POINTS

Urinary and faecal incontinence are prevalent conditions in women.

Incontinence is costly and has a significant adverse effect on quality of life and mental function.

Incontinence is caused by sphincter failure and/or dysfunction of the neural control of the bladder and bowel.

Related symptoms of urgency and frequency are also significant health problems.

There are few effective preventive strategies.

Diagnosis is usually clinical but complex cases may require complex investigations.

Treatment often requires a multidisciplinary approach.

INTRODUCTION

All babies are incontinent and for many adults regression to incontinence will occur in the later years. This chapter will predominantly consider urinary incontinence and related dysfunction of the lower urinary tract in women. If you have ever wondered 'Why do babies wet their nappies?', 'How do toddlers become dry?', 'Why do previously healthy women start wetting themselves years after their children were born?' and 'How can this be treated, and, better still, prevented?' then this is the chapter for you.

URINARY INCONTINENCE

Urinary incontinence is the unintentional loss of urine. Most children achieve daytime continence between 3 and 5 years of age.[1] Nocturnal enuresis is, however, relatively common, even in later childhood. There appears to be a familial relationship between enuresis and daytime incontinence for parents and children of both sexes. Urinary incontinence is reported in approximately 13% of Australian women aged 18–23 years, increasing to more than 35% in those over 45.[2] Women who are incontinent have a poorer quality of life and are more likely to be anxious or depressed than women who are continent.[3] Incontinence is not by itself a reason for admission of elderly people to residential care facilities, but it may be a factor in the decision to place an elderly person in residential care. Inappropriate management of incontinence (e.g. use of nappies) in acute-care settings in the elderly may contribute to regression. Rates of incontinence in men are generally much lower than in women, but elderly men exhibit a catch-up phenomenon, partly as a result of prostatic disease and its treatment, and partly as a consequence of senescence.

Urinary incontinence is often associated with other urinary symptoms (particularly overactive bladder and voiding dysfunction), faecal incontinence, and genital and rectal prolapse. There are many mechanisms involved in continence and thus many types of incontinence. High-quality evidence supporting current investigation and treatment modalities is often lacking. Management generally requires a multidisciplinary approach.

APPLIED ANATOMY AND PHYSIOLOGY

The key anatomical structures controlling micturition are the brain, spinal cord, autonomic and somatic nerves, bladder and urethra. Simplistically, the bladder is a storage vessel and the urethra a valve. The bladder is a muscular organ predominantly lined by transitional epithelium (squamous metaplasia at the trigone is commonly observed). The detrusor muscle is comprised entirely of smooth muscle. Neural pathways controlling micturition are complex, widely distributed in the central and peripheral nervous system, and involve many different neurotransmitters.[1]

There is rich autonomic innervation of the submucosa of the bladder, the detrusor and the urethra. Sympathetic innervation arises in the thoracolumbar part of the spinal cord. Sympathetic nerves release noradrenaline, which binds to β-adrenergic receptors in the detrusor, causing relaxation, and to α-adrenergic receptors in the urethra and bladder neck, causing contraction. Thus, sympathetic activity promotes storage of urine.

Parasympathetic and somatic innervation originates in the S2–S4 segments of the spinal cord. Acetylcholine is the best known postganglionic neurotransmitter but there are many others. There are a number of different types of muscarinic receptor. In the detrusor the binding of acetylcholine to M3 receptors initiates a contraction. Conversely, activation of M1 or M4 receptors in nerve terminals can enhance or suppress the release of acetylcholine to the detrusor. The pudendal nerve supplies the striated muscle of the external urethral sphincter and carries the sensory nerves from the bladder neck and urethra. Pelvic and hypogastric nerves convey sensory information from the bladder to the spinal cord. Cell bodies of these sensory fibres are located in dorsal root ganglia in the T11–T12 and S2–S4 segments of the spinal cord. These cell bodies synapse with neurons involved in spinal reflexes and with spinal tract neurons that communicate with higher centres in the brain.

It has only recently been appreciated that the urinary epithelium and its submucosal layer respond to chemical and mechanical stimuli and communicate via many transmitters with nerves in the bladder wall. It is possible that many of the clinical effects attributed to anticholinergic therapies are in fact mediated not through relaxation of the detrusor but through direct effects on the sensory components of the urinary epithelium and submucosa.

Dysfunction in the brain, spinal cord or periphery are all potential causes of urinary incontinence and other abnormalities of bladder function. Problems in these sites are not mutually exclusive.

The urethra in women is 4 cm long and lined by transitional epithelium near the bladder and stratified squamous epithelium distally. The urethral sphincter comprises striated muscle that surrounds the mid-urethra. In premenopausal women there are many mucosal folds observed in cross-sections of the urethra. The female urethra has oestrogen receptors, and the degree of mucosal folding and 'bulk' of the submucosal tissue is responsive to (increased by) oestrogen. This helps explain the improvement in lower urinary tract symptoms seen in postmenopausal women following oestrogen supplementation.

Control of micturition is a complex process. In the baby (and some adults with spinal injuries), micturition is a reflex process involving afferent and efferent autonomic and somatic pathways. As the bladder fills, stretch receptors send signals of increasing amplitude, which ultimately overwhelm spinal inhibitory signals and result in a reflex contraction of the detrusor muscle coordinated with relaxation of the urethral sphincter. Result = wet nappy. As the central nervous system matures the toddler is able to centrally augment spinal inhibitory signals and delay voiding. Result = dry nappy. Earlier, during pregnancy, the baby's mother may have had her first encounter as an adult with urinary incontinence.

There are a number of factors that may account for urinary incontinence in pregnancy. There is relative polyuria, increased intraabdominal pressure, hormonally mediated relaxation of connective tissue supports (e.g. by relaxin) and smooth muscle (e.g. by progesterone), and, in late pregnancy, the possibility of ischaemic injury (e.g. by pressure effects on the vasa nervorum) or trauma (birth-related) affecting pelvic nerves. Pelvic neuropathy is significantly correlated with dysfunction of the lower urinary tract.[7] However, for the majority of women, despite evidence of pelvic neuropathy persisting for at least 6 months postpartum, urinary function eventually returns to normal without treatment following normal childbirth.[4]

To properly evaluate lower urinary tract symptoms it is necessary to know what is normal. For the healthy adult female:

- the bladder should comfortably retain 400–500 mL of urine
- voiding up to seven times per day is normal
- awaking to void once if under 60 years old and twice if over 60 is normal
- voiding is usually a quick and efficient process — there should be no straining, and the bladder should be almost completely emptied (<25 mL residual volume)
- urine is sterile but often contaminated with vaginal flora — an infected sample should have a pure growth of a pathogen ($>10^5$ colony counts) and ≥ 10 white blood cells per high power field.

Causes

Urinary incontinence may occur as a result of injury to or dysfunction of the central or peripheral nervous system, striated muscles, connective tissue and ligaments of the pelvic floor, or the smooth muscle and mucosa of the bladder and urethra. Direct injury to these structures usually results from pregnancy and delivery. Trauma, ischaemia or malignancy may injure the spinal cord or central nervous system. Pelvic radiotherapy may damage blood supply to soft tissue and nerves.

Many drugs may affect urinary function; for example alpha blockers may cause urinary incontinence by sphincter relaxation, anticholinergic medications may cause urinary retention by detrusor relaxation, diuretics may cause urinary frequency. Duloxetine hydrochloride is a balanced selective serotonin and noradrenaline reuptake inhibitor that activates efferent neurons in the sacral segment of the spinal cord, contributing to contraction of the urethral sphincter and relaxation of the detrusor. It has been used overseas in the management of stress incontinence but is not currently licensed for use in Australia.

Many medical conditions are associated with lower urinary tract dysfunction. Dysuria and frequency caused by urinary tract infections (UTI) are well recognised, but incontinence may be the only symptom of a UTI in the elderly. In diabetes mellitus urinary frequency may be a sign of poor glycaemic control or UTI. Neuropathy related to disease (e.g. diabetes, multiple sclerosis) or pelvic surgery may present with complex urinary symptoms including incontinence and retention. Autoantibodies to M3 receptors in women with Sjögren's syndrome have been implicated as a cause of lower urinary tract dysfunction. These women are notoriously difficult to treat as they already have a very dry mouth and eyes — drugs with anticholinergic properties do not suit them. Women with joint hypermobility disorders (including Marfan and Ehlers-Danlos syndromes) have higher rates of urinary incontinence and genital prolapse than expected in the general population. Reduction in mobility (e.g. arthritis, stroke) may make the difference between getting to the toilet in time or not. Nocturia may be a sign of congestive heart failure or, particularly in the elderly, failure of diurnal secretion of vasopressin (antidiuretic hormone) from the posterior pituitary.

Behavioural and psychological factors also need to be considered. For some children, or adults with intellectual impairment, urinary incontinence may be a means of gaining attention. Habitual excessive fluid intake may present as urinary urgency, frequency and nocturia. It is a widely held view that drinks containing caffeine affect the bladder. The diuretic effect of caffeine is not sustained beyond the first few days after first starting to drink tea or coffee regularly. It is uncertain to what extent drinks containing caffeine stimulate the detrusor via activation of cAMP. It is possible that volume rather than contents of a drink is a more important contributor to sensations of frequency and urgency.

Types of urinary incontinence

Urinary incontinence and related conditions may be defined by any or all of subjective symptoms, clinical observation or urodynamic diagnoses (Table 20.1). More than one type of incontinence may be present. The coexistence of incontinence and voiding dysfunction is particularly challenging (Table 20.1).

EFFECT OF URINARY INCONTINENCE

Surprisingly, many women regard incontinence as a normal burden to endure and treatment is not sought. This may be because of a belief that incontinence is incurable, because the needs of dependants may be given a higher priority than personal health, because of embarrassment, or because of

Table 20.1 Common or important types of incontinence and related bladder dysfunction

Type of urinary dysfunction	Definition	Symptoms	Signs	Urodynamic diagnosis	Causes
Stress incontinence	A loss of urine associated with activities that cause an increase in pressure within the abdominal cavity	Leaking reported with coughing, sneezing, lifting or exercise	Leaking observed with coughing, sneezing, Crede's or Valsalva manoeuvres	Leaking observed during a urodynamic study resulting from an increase in intraabdominal pressure and in the absence of a detrusor contraction	Congenital or acquired defects in function of the urethral sphincter; chronic cough; obesity; iatrogenic (e.g. medications that cause sphincter relaxation or chronic cough; some surgical procedures)
Urge incontinence (now called 'urgency incontinence')	A loss of urine associated with an uncontrollable desire to void	Leaking associated with urgency; may be precipitated by cues such as running water, turning the house key in the lock	Usually not observed as a clinical sign	Not applicable	Poorly understood, may result from a breakdown in neurological control, may be seen in women with sphincter weakness, possible psychological and behavioural elements in some cases
Detrusor overactivity	A urodynamic diagnosis made when an observed detrusor contraction is associated with the strong desire to void in a person who is trying to inhibit micturition. This may occur with or without associated leakage. In idiopathic detrusor overactivity there is no identifiable cause. In neurogenic detrusor overactivity there is an identifiable neurological cause.	Symptoms are not a reliable guide. Many but not all women will report overactive bladder and/or urge incontinence. Neurogenic patients often have urinary retention in addition to urinary incontinence.	As per definition	As per definition	A breakdown in neural control of urinary storage at some point(s) in the highly complex pathways. By definition, idiopathic is unexplained and neuropathic is associated with a recognised neurological condition.

Mixed incontinence	A combination of stress and urgency incontinence or stress incontinence and detrusor overactivity	A combination of stress and urgency incontinence	As for stress and urgency incontinence	A combination of stress incontinence and detrusor overactivity	As for stress and urgency incontinence and detrusor overactivity
Insensible incontinence	Loss of urine that is not associated with urgency or 'stress' as defined above	Unexplained wetness	Frequently damp pad. Sometimes difficult to distinguish between urine loss and 'watery' vaginal discharge and/or perspiration. A 'vitamin B test' may be useful – urine is coloured bright yellow following ingestion of vitamin B supplements. Bright yellow staining on pad indicative of urine loss.	No consistent urodynamic findings. Any of the above or a normal study are possible.	Some women have marked sphincter weakness. Sometimes no cause is established. Rarely, may be caused by *vesicovaginal fistula* – an abnormal connection between the epithelium of the bladder and the vagina, which may result from trauma, malignancy, infection or radiotherapy.
Overactive bladder	Urinary frequency and urgency, plus or minus urgency incontinence. Often associated with nocturia.	As per definition	Not applicable	Record of voids and episodes of incontinence in a frequency volume chart (bladder diary) recorded by the woman in her normal environment is an important adjunct to testing in the urodynamic clinic.	Usually unexplained. Urinary tract infection must be excluded. If haematuria present also consider tumour. May be iatrogenic – diuretics and other medications (always look up – too many medications to list), or related to urogynaecological surgery.

Continued

Table 20.1 Continued

Type of urinary dysfunction	Definition	Symptoms	Signs	Urodynamic diagnosis	Causes
Nocturia	Interruption of sleep to micturate. It is normal for women under 60 years to get up once at night and twice at night aged over 60 years	As per definition	Not applicable	Not applicable	Habituation of night-time voiding related to poor sleep is not strictly nocturia but may present as such, 'overactive bladder', excessive drinking, iatrogenic (diuretics, medications that cause dry mouth), congestive cardiac failure, age-related loss of diurnal vasopressin secretion
Voiding dysfunction	Abnormal voiding as defined by symptoms and/or urodynamic parameters	Straining to void, intermittent stream, weak stream, prolonged emptying time, feeling of incomplete emptying, may be associated with recurrent urinary tract infections. Complete urinary retention in severe cases.	Rarely, loin tenderness secondary to hydronephrosis following vesicoureteric reflux	Maximal or average flow rates below 5th centile for age, high post-void residuals (which may be measured by ultrasound or in–out catheterisation). Common to see artifactual 'obstructive voiding' in urodynamic clinics due to inhibition. Repeat measurements required if an abnormality suspected.	Often unexplained. Sometimes seen with high stage vaginal prolapse. Iatrogenic (medication, urogynaecological surgery). Urinary retention often seen in patients with neurogenic detrusor overactivity. Acute urinary retention related to surgery, herpetic infection relatively common, beware serious neurological causes (e.g. cauda equina syndrome)

other barriers to health care (e.g. living in a remote community). Incontinence may affect quality of life and self-esteem in many ways. Women may become socially isolated due to the fear of embarrassing leakage in public, urgency and frequency that is difficult to control, and the fear of a urine smell. Stress incontinence may affect participation in sport and exercise. Leakage during intercourse may affect sexual relationships. Regular use of pads to keep clothing dry is a significant financial cost. Significant leakage may also require frequent laundering of clothes and/or bedding. Urine or chafing from pads may irritate vulval skin and cause chronic dermatitis. Painful symptoms of cystitis and nocturia may affect sleep, leading to chronic fatigue and depression.

CAN URINARY INCONTINENCE BE PREVENTED?

Studies of prevention of urinary incontinence in women have considered the role of elective caesarean delivery and antenatal and postnatal pelvic floor exercises.

Elective caesarean delivery appears to produce a short-term clinical benefit in the postnatal period compared with vaginal delivery. However, this benefit appears to have dissipated within 2 years. Similarly, caesarean delivery appears to offer no benefit in terms of subsequent sexual function once an episiotomy or vaginal tear has healed.[5] Decisions regarding elective caesarean versus vaginal delivery are complex, but given the higher morbidity of the former there is little to recommend abdominal delivery other than on obstetric grounds.

Antenatal and postnatal pelvic floor exercises have been shown to provide short-term benefit with statistically significant reductions in episodes of incontinence in women undergoing treatment compared with controls.[6] Unfortunately, data have seldom been collected beyond 3 months postpartum. It is uncertain if the short-term benefit from pelvic floor exercises is sustained in the long term.

INVESTIGATION AND MANAGEMENT
History

Key features in the history include the woman's age, the nature of the problem, the effect that the problem is having on her life, the type and outcomes of treatments that have been tried (if any), in addition to medical, drug, surgical and social history. Look for contributing factors (chronic cough, neurological dysfunction, obesity, reduced mobility or pelvic floor injury associated with pregnancy or previous surgery) and patient-specific risks of possible treatments. Note antibiotic allergies, as UTI may require treatment. You should establish what a woman means by 'her problem', and specifically inquire about other abnormal urinary or bowel symptoms, symptoms of prolapse, sexual dysfunction, oestrogen deficiency, emotional and psychiatric symptoms.

Examination and investigation

Perform an abdominal, vaginal and pelvic examination to assess oestrogenisation, perineal excoriation, prolapse, pelvic masses and strength (by squeezing against the examiner's fingers) of pelvic floor muscles. Ask the woman to cough, and record whether or not leakage was observed (Figure 20.1). A urine sample should be tested to exclude haematuria and infection.

Some experts advise asking the woman to keep a bladder diary, usually a record of times and volumes voided, fluid intake and leakage episodes, for 2 or more consecutive days (Figure 20.2). Excessive and reduced fluid intake can be assessed this way. This type of record gives additional insight into the woman's bladder function and habits, and the diary can be compared with a new record after treatment. Completion of the bladder diary also gives an indication of the woman's motivation.

Management

Management of urinary incontinence depends on the type of incontinence, the individual's preferences, and the range of treatment options available to her.

Short-term data support the role of pelvic floor exercises in stress and mixed incontinence.[7] Results may be better if an appropriately trained physiotherapist, continence nurse adviser or medical practitioner with a special interest gives the instruction. These professionals can provide education and additional motivation to the woman, assess adequacy of her technique, and provide supplementary methods such as vaginal cones and biofeedback techniques for women who are having difficulty learning to contract their pelvic floor muscles. Pelvic floor exercises may also assist women experiencing urinary frequency, urgency and faecal incontinence. These exercises should probably be performed lifelong.

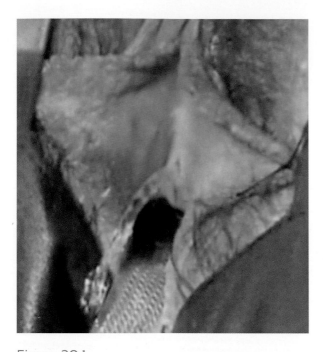

Figure 20.1

Screen snapshot of intraoperative video image showing a substantial stream of clear fluid expressed per urethra by Crede's manoeuvre (suprapubic pressure) with 300 mL normal saline in the bladder in a woman undergoing a tension-free vaginal tape procedure for severe stress incontinence (uninserted tape seen in lower section of picture). Elimination of incontinence following insertion of the tape can be demonstrated by repeating the Crede's manoeuvre (not shown).

(Image courtesy of author.)

Using current best evidence, Imamura and colleagues[8] concluded pelvic floor exercise is a cost-effective first-line approach to management of stress incontinence. However, in their conclusions the authors acknowledged that absence of long-term data was a significant limitation. In an 8-year follow-up of 230 women randomised antenatally to physiotherapist-supervised or pamphlet-based instruction in pelvic floor exercises, the substantially lower rate of stress incontinence reported in the supervised group at 3 months postpartum (19% versus 33%, $p=0.02$) was no longer evident at 8 years (35% versus 39%, $p=0.7$).[4] Poor long-term compliance with pelvic floor exercises was noted as a factor. Success rates for surgical management of stress incontinence also diminish over time. It remains appropriate to reserve surgery for women who have not responded to pelvic floor exercises.

Oestrogen supplementation, often given intravaginally, is used as an adjunctive therapy in postmenopausal women and may reduce symptoms of overactive bladder. To date no clinical benefit for stress incontinence has been observed in randomised controlled trials comparing oestrogen with placebo.

If surgery is being considered for stress incontinence, some authorities recommend that urodynamic investigations be undertaken first. The purpose of preoperative urodynamic testing is to confirm the diagnosis and to exclude other significant functional problems of the lower urinary tract. Urodynamic testing has three components: voiding studies, cystometry (Figure 20.3a) and imaging (Figure 20.3b). Confirming the diagnosis by urodynamics is important if the history is not clearcut and stress incontinence has not been confirmed by clinical examination. If a preexisting voiding problem is uncovered that may affect the decision to operate. Australian gynaecologists tend to utilise preoperative urodynamic tests less frequently than their UK counterparts partly because of less access to the technology and partly because of differences between countries in the models of standards of care.[9]

Many operations for stress incontinence have been described. Midurethral sling procedures such as the 'tension-free' vaginal tape (TVT) are the most commonly performed operations at the present time. Complications include short-term or long-term urinary retention, urinary, wound and chest infections, haemorrhage, bladder perforation, very occasionally ureteric injury, de novo detrusor overactivity, deep venous thrombosis and, rarely, bowel perforation and death. Surgery is expensive, requiring day or overnight admission and 2–4 weeks off normal activities for simple procedures and 2–7 days in hospital and 6–12 weeks off normal activities for complex procedures that combine surgery for incontinence and genital prolapse.

Women presenting in the primary care setting with overactive bladder are typically managed in a multimodal manner. Attention is paid to normalising fluid intake (1.5 L a day is a reasonable baseline) and to avoiding constipation. Bladder drill, requiring a conscious effort to delay voiding, may be recommended in conjunction with pelvic floor exercises. Anticholinergic medication is more effective than placebo[10] and typically results in improvement,

The Bladder Diary

Start at 7 or 8 am, when you get up in the morning.

Day 1

Time	Fluid Intake (mL)	Urine Output (mL)	Incontinence	Wet bed
6am	50ml	130		
7am				
8am				
9am		150		
10am	150		15mls	
11am	150		20MIs	
12pm				
1pm				
2pm	150	170		
3pm				
4pm	150	70	10mls	
5pm	150	120		
6pm	160	70		
7pm	200	130	10mls	
8pm	250			
9pm		70		
10pm	50			
BED				
11pm		150		
12am				
1am				
2am				
3am				
4am		160		
5am				

Day 2

Time	Fluid Intake (mL)	Urine Output (mL)	Incontinence	Wet bed
6am				
7am				
8am	50	150		
9am			5mls	
10am	200			
11am				
12pm	100	150	5mls	
1pm	200	100	5mls	
2pm		170		
3pm	200	100		
4pm				
5pm				
6pm	200	60	5mls	
7pm		60		
8pm				
9pm	250	100		
10pm				
BED		40		
11pm	50			
12am				
1am				
2am				
3am				
4am				
5am		250		

Figure 20.2

A 2-day bladder diary recorded by a 64-year-old woman presenting with symptoms of overactive bladder. There appears to be some restriction in fluid intake, which is a common and usually ineffective management strategy. Eight episodes of urinary incontinence are recorded (the woman has estimated the volume of urine lost) and the apparent bladder capacity of 170 mL is well below normal for her age. This could be explained either by a true reduction in bladder capacity or incomplete bladder emptying. In this case the incontinence is urge incontinence, however very similar charts can be seen in women with severe stress incontinence. The woman is voiding up to nine times during the day (abnormal) and up to twice at night (age-dependent, normal for this patient).

(Image courtesy of author.)

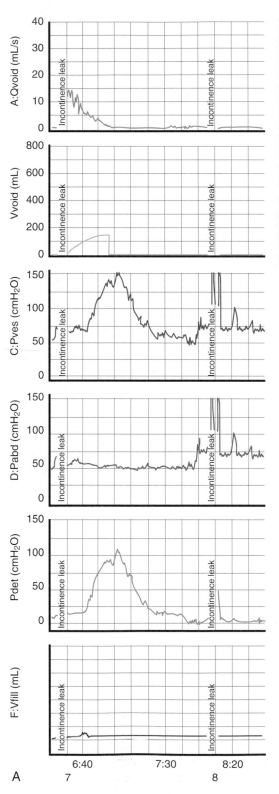

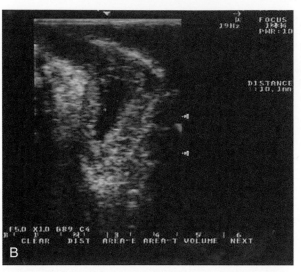

Figure 20.3

A: Section of cystometric recording and **B**: ultrasound imaging of bladder, in a woman with mixed urinary incontinence that had failed to respond to pelvic floor exercises and anticholinergic medication. Figure 20.3A shows that retrograde filling of the bladder has stopped at 150 mL (the woman was reporting marked urgency). Soon after cessation of filling most of the content of the bladder has been lost as result of a spontaneous detrusor contraction. This is recorded as the first incontinence leak — diagnosis severe idiopathic detrusor overactivity. There is an offset between the recorded leakage and the detrusor contraction due to latency in transmission of pressure in the very long fluid-filled lines and the pressure transducers. The patient was then asked to cough and a small volume of fluid was lost and in the absence of a detrusor contraction — diagnosis urodynamic stress incontinence. This is recorded as the second incontinence leak. The transvaginal image of the bladder was taken using a specialised probe and shows an almost empty bladder with a measured detrusor thickness of 10.1 mm, which is significantly increased and suggestive of a chronic problem with hypercontractility of the detrusor.

(Images courtesy of author.)

not cure. Anticholinergic side effects are common and may be a reason for cessation of therapy. In Australia, oral oxybutynin hydrochloride is first-line drug therapy. It is often necessary to prescribe more expensive alternatives due to side effects and/or lack of efficacy. If there have been multiple failures of therapy the diagnosis needs to be reconsidered and urodynamic testing undertaken.

Stress incontinence and mixed incontinence are the most common diagnoses made in general urodynamic clinics.[11,12] These women are a selected group and most will be referred for surgery. The small proportion (15–20%) with pure detrusor overactivity can be very difficult to manage as they have often been through the range of readily available therapies for overactive bladder. There is no explanation for the condition, and it is assumed that there is a breakdown in the neurological pathways that inhibit the detrusor muscle and/or dysfunction of the sensory pathways. Operations devised for stress incontinence or prolapse are inappropriate when detrusor overactivity is the sole cause of the woman's incontinence. The approach in these cases is to review and optimise what has been done before (e.g. consider referral for review of pelvic floor exercise technique to an appropriately trained physiotherapist or continence nurse adviser, to use different dose regimens of medications previously tried) and prescribe alternative anticholinergic and antispasmodic medications and oestrogen replacement in appropriate cases. In refractory cases, sacral neuromodulation may be considered. Sacral neuromodulation is an expensive procedure that involves the subcutaneous implantation of electrodes usually into the S2 or S3 sacral foramina and attached to an implanted battery-powered pulse generator. Electrical pulses are set at an amplitude and frequency to maximise response for the individual. Overall, a substantial reduction in episodes of urge incontinence and reduced frequency and nocturia can be expected.[13] The substantial cost of sacral neuromodulation and potential complications related to the implanted leads and pulse generator are major limitations. Intradetrusor injection of dilute botulinum A toxin is a promising alternative with similar efficacy in the short term. Botulinum toxin is currently not licensed for this purpose. Other limitations of botulinum toxin include a small but significant risk of prolonged urinary retention, requirement for repeat reinjection (perhaps annually), variability in dose regimens

employed to date, and absence of long-term data on efficacy and cost effectiveness.

If there is an identified neurological cause to incontinence, the diagnosis is neuropathic detrusor overactivity. Spinal cord injuries, stroke, diabetes and demyelinating disorders may result in this diagnosis. These patients are typically managed in specialised, multidisciplinary clinics.

Immobility can be an important contributor to urge incontinence, simply as a result of the woman's inability to get to the toilet in time. Assistance may be required with household aids and appliances, in addition to other therapy. Often, a multidisciplinary approach is required under these circumstances.

There is a wide variety of continence aids, including various pads, nappies and permanent catheters. Pads come in a variety of sizes. They are expensive, and may cause chafing and contribute to excoriation. Permanent catheters are the last resort (due to discomfort and ever-present risk of infection) but will improve quality of life in women with severe incontinence when other therapies have failed or are unsuitable.

Outflow obstruction in women that is not the result of surgery is mainly due to detrusor failure. The reason for detrusor failure is seldom identified. Intermittent clean self-catheterisation is the first-line treatment for these cases, although some women may benefit from sacral neuromodulation. If obstruction has resulted from surgery, reoperation to relieve the obstruction may be effective.

FAECAL INCONTINENCE

Faecal incontinence can lead to social isolation and reduced quality of life. Up to 7% of healthy people over 65 years and up to a quarter of women attending urogynaecological clinics report faecal incontinence.

Structure and function of the anal canal

In the adult the anal canal is about 5 cm long. The anal sphincter is cylindrical and comprises internal (smooth muscle) and external (striated muscle) layers. The internal layer is a continuation of the muscularis of the rectum and ends about 1 cm above the end of the external sphincter. The external layer in its upper part is a sling-like structure comprising fibres of the puborectalis muscle and its lower part completely encircles the anal canal. In women, the external sphincter is about 2.5 cm long posteriorly and 1.5 cm long anteriorly; the anterior part of the sphincter is at risk from birth trauma. The upper part of the anal canal is innervated by autonomic fibres and the lower part (demarcated by the dentate line) is innervated by somatic fibres in the inferior rectal branch of the pudendal nerve and perineal branch of the fourth sacral nerve. In common with the urinary tract, motor and sensory control is complex and involves many levels in the central and peripheral nervous system.

Causes of faecal incontinence

The causes of faecal incontinence are numerous but obstetric trauma is one of the most common factors identified. Here the causes appear to be nerve damage and/or direct trauma to the anal sphincter complex. Trauma to the sphincter complex is associated with forceps delivery, high birth weight, median episiotomies and occipital posterior positions.

Investigation and management

Anterior external anal sphincter defects may be obvious at delivery. Third and fourth degree tears (involving the external anal sphincter only and sphincter plus anal mucosa respectively) occur in 0.5–1.0% of vaginal deliveries and are highly associated with midline episiotomies.

Sphincter trauma is more often occult and, with anal endosonography, up to 35% of primiparous women can be shown to have evidence of sphincter complex disruption. The mainstay of treatment for occult sphincter defects is pelvic floor exercises. For childbirth-related disruption of the sphincter complex, the treatment is usually surgical. It is unclear whether an overlapping external sphincter repair (which is technically more challenging) or end-to-end repair is the better technique.[14] Patients with lesser disability from incontinence, who decline operative treatment, are unfit for surgery or who do not respond to surgery may, in conjunction with pelvic floor exercises, try dietary manipulation, the use of constipating agents (loperamide, codeine phosphate), or biofeedback. Management is usually multidisciplinary.

It has been routine clinical practice, supported by expert opinion, to advise elective caesarean delivery in any future pregnancies in women who have experienced birth-related trauma to the anal sphincter and have undergone surgical repair (secondary prevention). A recent meta-analysis has showed no benefit of elective caesarean delivery in the primary prevention of anal sphincter injury.[15]

Sacral neuromodulation has recently become available in Australia in the treatment of faecal incontinence. This technique appears to significantly reduce the number of episodes of faecal incontinence. Results have been mixed in patients who report both faecal and urinary incontinence.

CONCLUSION

In adult women, bladder dysfunction increases with age. The problems are multifactorial, with genetics, parity, lifestyle and behavioural factors making a significant contribution. Quality of life and mental health are adversely affected. Complete prevention of incontinence is unattainable, but risk reduction by attention to lifestyle factors such as maintaining a normal weight, not smoking, and performing pelvic floor exercises regularly appears sensible. Treatment strategies are tailored to the individual and may need to take into account related problems of genital prolapse and faecal incontinence. There is a wide range of treatment options and a multidisciplinary approach to treatment is recommended.

REFERENCES

1. Fowler CJ, Griffiths D, de Groat WC. The neural control of micturition. Nat Rev Neurosci 2008;9(6):453–66.
2. Chiarelli P, Brown W, McElduff P. Leaking urine: prevalence and associated factors in Australian women. Neurourol Urodynam 1999;18:567–77.
3. Coyne KS, Kvasz M, Ireland AM, et al. Urinary incontinence and its relationship to mental health and health-related quality of life in men and women in Sweden, the United Kingdom, and the United States. Eur Urol 2012;1:88–95.
4. Agur W, Steggles P, Waterfield M Freeman R. The long-term effectiveness of antenatal pelvic floor muscle training: eight-year follow up of a randomised controlled trial. BJOG 2008;115:985–90. doi: 10.1111/j.1471-0528.2008.01742.x.
5. Dean N, Wilson D, Herbison P, et al. Sexual function, delivery mode history, pelvic floor muscle exercises and incontinence: a cross-sectional study six years post-partum. Aust N Z J Obstet Gynaecol. 2008;48(3):302–11.
6. Hay-Smith J, Mørkved S, Fairbrother KA, et al. Pelvic floor muscle training for prevention and treatment of urinary and faecal incontinence in antenatal and postnatal women. Cochrane Database Syst Rev 2008;4:CD007471. doi: 10.1002/14651858. CD007471.

7. Dumoulin C, Hay-Smith J. Pelvic floor muscle training versus no treatment, or inactive control treatments, for urinary incontinence in women. Cochrane Database Syst Rev 2010;1:CD005654. doi: 10.1002/14651858.CD005654.pub2.

8. Imamura M, Abrams P, Bain C, et al. Systematic review and economic modelling of the effectiveness and cost-effectiveness of non-surgical treatments for women with stress urinary incontinence. Health Technol Assess 2010;14(40):1–188, iii–iv.

9. Duggan PM, Wilson PD, Norton P, et al: Utilization of preoperative urodynamic investigations by gynecologists who frequently operate for female urinary incontinence. Int J Urogyn Pelvic Floor Dys October 2003;14(4):282–7.

10. Nabi G, Cody JD, Ellis G, et al. Anticholinergic drugs versus placebo for overactive bladder syndrome in adults. Cochrane Database Syst Rev 2006;4:CD003781. doi: 10.1002/14651858.CD003781.pub2.

11. Duggan P. Urodynamics or history? Clinical decision-making in women presenting with urinary incontinence. Aust N Z J Obstet Gynecol 2010;50:556–61.

12. Duggan P. Urodynamic diagnoses and quality of life in women presenting for evaluation of urinary incontinence. Aust N Z J Obstet Gynecol 2011;51(5):416–20.

13. Herbison GP, Arnold EP. Sacral neuromodulation with implanted devices for urinary storage and voiding dysfunction in adults. Cochrane Database Syst Rev 2009;2:CD004202. doi: 10.1002/14651858.CD004202.pub2.

14. Fernando RJ, Sultan AHH, Kettle C, et al. Methods of repair for obstetric anal sphincter injury. Cochrane Database of Systematic Reviews 2006;3:CD002866. doi: 10.1002/14651858.CD002866.pub2.

15. Nelson RL, Furner SE, Westercamp M, et al. Cesarean delivery for the prevention of anal incontinence. Cochrane Database Syst Rev 2010;17(2):CD006756. doi: 10.1002/14651858.CD006756.pub2.

MCQS

Select the correct answer.

1 Which of the following is most characteristic of urinary stress incontinence?

   A Considerable quantities of urine are lost.
   B Bed wetting occurs at night.
   C There is a desire to empty the bladder again immediately after micturition.
   D It occurs with a sudden and unexpected increase in intraabdominal pressure.
   E It is most commonly found in teenagers.

2 Mary, aged 58 years, has been having difficulty with the control of her blood pressure. She had been taking an antihypertensive for 2 years in increasing doses and her GP added a second antihypertensive medication 6 weeks ago to control her blood pressure. Her only other medication is amitryptiline 25 mg which she says she takes at night to help her sleep. Since she started the second antihypertensive she has been using a panty liner to manage urinary stress incontinence. Which one of the following is most likely to be responsible for her stress incontinence?

   A amitryptiline
   B irbesartan+hydrochlorthiazide
   C prazosin hydrochloride
   D atenolol
   E nifedipine

3 Angela, age 36 years, presents to her GP for management of stress incontinence. She has children aged 5 and 7 years, and is unable to bounce on the trampoline with them without wetting herself. She denies any other symptoms. Angela was taught pelvic floor exercises antenatally during her second pregnancy but they have not helped. On examination, there is a minor degree of prolapse of the anterior vagina and a spurt of urine was observed when she was asked to cough. Which one of the following is the most appropriate next step in management?

   A insert a ring pessary
   B confirm the diagnosis by urodynamic studies
   C refer to a gynaecologist for surgical management
   D prescribe duloxetine hydrochloride
   E refer to a physiotherapist for pelvic floor exercises

4 Maria is a 75-year-old woman presenting with a 6-month history of isolated nocturia that is now affecting her sleep and daytime functioning. She lives with her husband and is fully independent. She is otherwise well, walks regularly in 'the hills', is a non-smoker, doesn't drink alcohol and is on no medication. She drinks 1.4 L (mixture of water and coffee) a day evenly spaced between breakfast and 9 p.m. Cardiovascular and respiratory examination are normal. She has no vaginal prolapse though there is a small urethral caruncle visible. Urinalysis and ultrasound of the lower urinary tract are normal. Which one of the following is the best option to manage her nocturia?

A intravaginal oestrogen supplementation
B desmopressin nasal spray nocte
C spironolactone taken at midday
D oxybutynin hydrochloride nocte
E fluid restriction after 7 p.m.

5 Audrey is a 45-year-old nulliparous woman who has presented to her GP complaining of urinary frequency, urgency and urge incontinence. This has been a problem for years and has been particularly bad in the last 12 months. Voiding is normal. She has previously used oxybutynin hydrochloride tablets, prescribed last year by another GP, but did not tolerate this (very dry mouth). Examination and urinalysis are normal. The GP asks Audrey to complete a bladder diary (figure 20.2) and refers her to a physiotherapist. Which one of the following additional options available to the GP would currently be most appropriate in the management of this condition?

A oxybutynin hydrochloride patch
B M3-selective anticholinergic tablet
C intravaginal oestrogen supplementation
D bladder scan
E advise fluid restriction

6 Petunia, age 27, is presenting for antenatal counselling at 12W gestation in her second pregnancy. She experienced a fourth degree anal tear in her first pregnancy following a difficult ventouse extraction of a 3600 g baby girl. The tear was repaired in operating theatre soon after delivery and Petunia was subsequently managed by the hospital's obstetrics and continence nursing services. She reported some minor flatus incontinence in the first few weeks but has had completely normal bowel control since. She continues to do pelvic floor exercises regularly. In relation to prevention of anal sphincter injury in this pregnancy, which one of the following is the most appropriate advice to give Petunia?

A It is appropriate to plan for a normal vaginal birth at this point.
B The decision regarding mode of delivery should be deferred until estimation of fetal weight by ultrasound at 36W.
C Elective caesarean section should be planned for 39W gestation.
D Pelvic floor exercises are protective.
E Perform regular perineal stretching with the Epi No inflatable device from 37W.

OSCE

Tracey is a 36-year-old woman presenting in a primary care setting with urinary incontinence.

Take a history and list the important features on examination for Tracey and consider investigations and management options for her.

Chapter 21

Genital prolapse

Paul Duggan

KEY POINTS

Uterovaginal prolapse is a herniation of some or all of the genital tract — a prevalent condition in women aged 50+ years.

Parity, birth weight of babies, increasing age, chronic cough and obesity are the most significant risk factors.

Symptomatic prolapse causes pelvic and vaginal discomfort and is often associated with bladder, bowel and sexual dysfunction.

Prolapse is usually caused by direct trauma to the connective tissue and muscular supports of the pelvic floor, or, indirectly, by pelvic neuropathy.

There are no effective preventive strategies.

Diagnosis is clinical.

Failure of conservative and surgical treatment is common, reflecting poor anatomical design, and vulnerability of structures of the pelvic floor to injury and re-injury.

INTRODUCTION

Genital prolapse refers to abnormal descent of the uterus and/or vagina. This chapter will focus on symptomatic genital prolapse. However, genital prolapse may be asymptomatic and detected only by vaginal examination, usually when a health professional is undertaking a routine Pap smear. Although it is commonly believed that prolapse is a result of childbirth, this is an oversimplification. Symptomatic prolapse in parous women may present well after the last delivery and also occurs in nulliparous women.

PREVALENCE AND INCIDENCE

A Scandinavian survey of randomly selected women aged 40–60 years reported symptoms of pelvic heaviness in 15%, the presence of a genital bulge in 4%, and use of fingers in the vagina or on the perineum to assist defecation in 12%.[1] A survey of randomly selected women in South Australia found that 9% aged 50 years and older had had at least one prolapse repair and 9% had current symptoms of prolapse.[2] Over 10% reported difficulties with defecation and 5% vaginal laxity. A Western Australian study has estimated the lifetime risk for women of undergoing surgery for pelvic organ prolapse to be 19%.[3]

APPLIED ANATOMY AND PHYSIOLOGY

The uterus and vagina are mobile and distensible, with connective tissue supports predominantly comprised of smooth muscle and collagenous matrix. The cord-like round ligament, the relatively dense infundibulopelvic ligament and the thin broad ligament attach the uterus to the pelvic side wall. The relatively strong uterosacral ligament and loose paracervical tissue attach the cervix to the sacrum and to the pelvic side wall. These attachments comprise peritoneal folds, connective tissue,

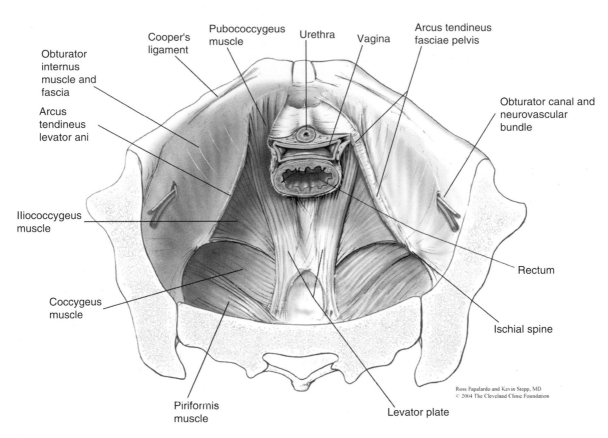

Cooper's ligament

Pubococcygeus muscle

Urethra

Vagina

Arcus tendineus fasciae pelvis

Obturator internus muscle and fascia

Arcus tendineus levator ani

Obturator canal and neurovascular bundle

Iliococcygeus muscle

Coccygeus muscle

Rectum

Ischial spine

Piriformis muscle

Levator plate

Ross Papalardo and Kevin Stepp, MD
© 2004 The Cleveland Clinic Foundation

Figure 21.1
The relationships of the muscles of the pelvic floor and sidewalls and their attachments from an abdominal view. The arcus tendineus fasciae pelvis has been removed on the left, showing the origins of the levator ani muscles. On the right, the arcus tendineus fasciae pelvis remains intact showing the attachment of the lateral vagina via the endopelvic fascia (cut away).

(Walters: Urogynecology and Reconstructive Pelvic Surgery, 3rd ed. 2006 Mosby. Figure 2.7; 9780323029025)

nerves, lymphatics and blood vessels. The uterosacral and infundibulopelvic ligaments may be surgically attached to the vaginal vault to aid support of the upper vagina following hysterectomy.

The connective tissue and levator ani striated muscle group provide the principal support of the pelvic floor.

Integrity of connective tissue is very important in the maintenance of normal anatomy and function of the pelvic floor. The arcus tendineus fascia pelvis (ATFP) is the name given to the connective tissue that attaches anteriorly the vagina to the obturator internus muscle (Figure 21.1). The ATFP, also called the 'white line', describes an arc between the ischial spine and posterior symphysis pubis. This curvilinear attachment is responsible for the normal

appearance of the sulci of the anterior vagina. Disruption of the ATFP results in loss of these sulci and is an important cause of anterior vaginal prolapse. The sulci are sited laterally. Anterior prolapse may also occur with the ATFP intact through the mechanism of disruption of central connective tissue of the anterior vagina. The relative importance of these two mechanisms is debated. Similar principles are at play in relation to posterior vaginal prolapse.

There is some controversy regarding whether it is the pudendal nerve (originating in S2–S4 nerve roots) or the levator ani nerve (originating in S3–S5 nerve roots) that innervates the levator ani in humans.[4] It is plausible that there may be individual variation. Both nerves are closely related at the ischial spine, and thus pudendal nerve blocks may affect both nerves as may surgical dissection or injudicious suture placement. Fibres carried in either nerve are also at risk of injury in pregnancy and childbirth. Strengthening of the levator ani muscles by pelvic floor exercises has been shown to improve symptoms of prolapse, overactive bladder and incontinence.

Hydronephrosis resulting from ureteric kinking may occur in more severe forms of genital prolapse. Urinary retention due to descent of the bladder base below the urethra may also occur (note that many women with such a degree of prolapse do not have urinary retention, suggesting that detrusor function is also important). Rectal prolapse, haemorrhoids and faecal incontinence are sometimes seen in association with genital prolapse. Not infrequently, a multidisciplinary approach may be required to optimally manage complex cases. This may involve some of the following groups: gynaecologists or urogynaecologists, physiotherapists, continence nurse advisers, urologists, colorectal or general surgeons, geriatricians.

RISK FACTORS

Parity and birth weight have been consistently reported as independent risk factors for prolapse.[5] Incidence increases with age, postmenopausal status, smoking, chronic lung disease and obesity.

PREVENTION OF PROLAPSE

There are few data addressing the role of primary or secondary prevention and currently an effective strategy has not been identified. Addressing lifestyle and behavioural factors is appropriate (e.g. not smoking, maintaining a healthy body weight). The place of elective caesarean delivery and pelvic floor exercises is unclear. In the short term, benefit may be observed with either approach.[6] However, there are significant concerns that these short-term benefits are not durable.

CLINICAL EVALUATION

The typical symptoms of prolapse include a dragging or bearing down sensation in the vagina and the appearance of a lump or bulge at the vaginal entrance (Figures 21.2, 21.3). Often there are associated difficulties with bladder- or bowel-emptying and/or urinary and faecal incontinence. Rectal prolapse or haemorrhoids may also be present. Menstruating women may report difficulties with insertion of tampons. Many women report low back

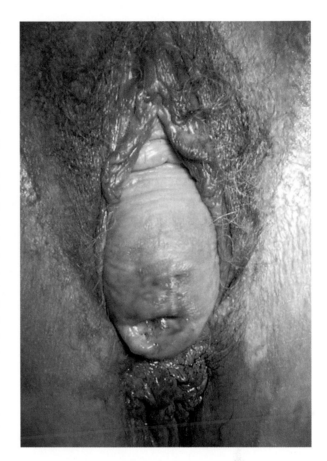

Figure 21.2
Complete genital eversion. The anterior lip of the cervix (POPQ point C) is clearly visible. Points Aa and Ba are also visible but more difficult to identify because the external urethral meatus is hidden and because it is not clear to novices where the cervix ends and anterior vagina begins. In practice, once identified, the distance between the points and the hymenal ring are measured with a tape. With that caveat, a reasonable estimate from this two dimensional image is that point C is between +8 cm and +10 cm, Ba is about +8 cm (note where the concentric lines that identify the vagina end) and Aa is about +2 cm.

(Photo courtesy of author.)

pain, which may also be due to other causes. Although dyspareunia is not consistently a problem in women who are sexually active and have a prolapse, the presence of prolapse may affect a woman's confidence to continue a normal sex life. Ulceration of prolapsed epithelium may occur and result in discharge or bleeding. Other causes of vaginal

Table 21.1 Definitions of POPQ points used in the description of genital prolapse*[7]

Compartment	Point	Definition
anterior	Aa	anterior vaginal wall 3 cm from hymenal ring
	Ba	most distal point of the anterior vaginal wall between points Aa and C. By definition point Ba = point Aa if point Aa is the most distal part of the prolapse.
apical	C	most distal part of anterior lip of cervix or leading edge of hysterectomy scar
	D	location of posterior vaginal fornix. This is omitted if there is no cervix.
posterior	Ap	posterior vaginal wall 3 cm from hymenal ring
	Bp	most distal point of the posterior vaginal wall between points Bp and D or C. By definition point Bp = point Ap if point Ap is the most distal part of the prolapse.

*The POPQ system describes the maximal observed descent in each compartment when the woman strains (Valsalva manoeuvre).

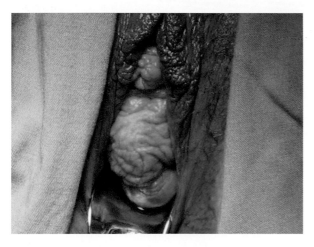

Figure 21.3
Anterior and apical compartment prolapse (previous hysterectomy). The posterior compartment is retracted by the Sims speculum.

(Photo courtesy of author.)

discharge and postmenopausal bleeding need to be excluded. Prolapse in young nulliparous women raises the possibility of connective tissue disorders.

Genital prolapse is best identified using a Sims' speculum and sponge forceps, either by examining the woman in the left lateral position or in dorsal lithotomy.

Staging of prolapse

The Pelvic Organ Prolapse Quantification (POPQ) system is now widely accepted internationally as the default system for staging genital prolapse. In this system the genital tract is divided into three compartments: anterior, apical, and posterior (Table 21.1). Each compartment is staged separately (Table 21.2).

For the anterior compartment, two POPQ points are described (Figure 21.4). Point Aa is a fixed point in the midline on the anterior vaginal wall exactly 3 cm from the external urethral meatus. Aa has a possible range of values from −3 to +3 cm relative to the hymen. Point Ba is a floating point that describes the distance in cm of the furthest point of the anterior compartment prolapse in relation to the hymenal ring. Point Ba has no fixed range of values, but could reasonably be expected to be any value between −8 and +8 cm.

Two POPQ points are described for both the apical and posterior compartments. For the posterior compartment these are called Ap and Bp and they mimic points Aa and Ba on the anterior wall. For the apical compartment the points are called C and D. Point C describes the position at maximal straining of the anterior lip of the cervix and point D the position of the posterior vaginal fornix. The difference between C and D is the length of

Table 21.2 POPQ staging of pelvic organ prolapse[7]

Stage	Definition
Stage 0	No prolapse demonstrated. Points Aa, Ap, Ba, Bp ≤ −3 cm, C or D ≤ −[TVL−2] cm.
Stage I	The most distal portion of the prolapse is < −1 cm
Stage II	The most distal portion of the prolapse is between −1 cm and +1 cm
Stage III	The most distal portion of the prolapse is > +1 cm but < +[TVL−2] cm
Stage IV	Essentially, complete eversion of the genital tract. The most distal portion is ≥ +[TVL−2] cm

TVL = total vaginal length. The hymenal ring is the reference point and is given a value of zero. If the prolapse extends beyond the hymenal ring the POPQ score is positive; the POPQ score is negative if the prolapse is above the hymenal ring. Note that the POPQ system describes the maximal observed descent in each compartment when the woman strains (Valsalva manoeuvre) except for TVL, which is measured at rest.

the visible, intravaginal part of the cervix. If the woman has had a hysterectomy point C becomes the scar line at the vaginal apex and there is no point D.

Points Aa, Ba and C should be readily identifiable on Figure 21.1.

The POPQ system was devised to improve communication between gynaecologists in relation to the anatomical description of prolapse and is an essential component in clinical research. However, for women presenting with symptomatic prolapse there is not a good correlation between POPQ stage and severity of symptoms.[8] Evaluation of symptoms to make a diagnosis and assess the outcome of treatments is a critical component of clinical practice and is undertaken by a detailed history. In research (and increasingly in clinical practice) the evaluation of symptoms includes disease-specific quality of life questionnaires, discussed later.

It takes some practice to get used to the POPQ system and medical students are not expected to be experts in it. However, they will inevitably encounter POPQ terminology in correspondence and publications so should have a basic understanding of it. POPQ staging is arbitrary and its value is debated, so Table 21.2 can be used for reference. However, students should become conversant with describing prolapse in three compartments and at least be able

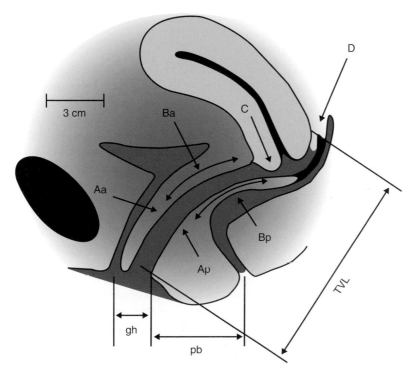

Figure 21.4
Schematic line drawing identifying POPQ points Aa, Ba, C, D, Ap and Bp. TVL = total vaginal length, gh = width of genital hiatus, pb = width of perineal body.

(Katz, Comprehensive Gynecology 5th edition Mosby 2007.)

to estimate the maximal point of descent for each compartment.

Older terminology

The terms urethro-cystocele, rectocele and enterocele describe prolapse of the anterior vaginal compartment, posterior vaginal compartment and vaginal apex (or vaginal vault) respectively. These older terms are still widely used.

Quality of life

There are a number of validated, prolapse-specific quality of life (QoL) questionnaires.[9,10] In common, QoL questionnaires provide a score for 'domains' that evaluate the severity of the prolapse and the impact of the prolapse on function. Scores are calculated from the Likert scale responses to questions. An example is provided by the short form 7 version of the Pelvic Floor Impact Questionnaire (Figure 21.5). The scoring system allows quantification of the effect of prolapse within each domain and statistical testing of response to treatment.

MANAGEMENT

Management options are tailored to the individual woman. These options include strengthening exercises for the pelvic floor, intravaginal oestrogen supplementation, vaginal packing, vaginal pessaries, and corrective surgery. Reassurance is appropriate in all cases, particularly as prolapse is not a life-threatening condition. Potentially reversible risk factors should be identified and managed (e.g. obesity, constipation, oestrogen deficiency, chronic cough related to medication, smoking or asthma).

Pelvic floor exercises

These have been shown to be effective in the short term for POPQ stage I and stage II prolapse[11] but exercises are far less likely to reduce higher stages of prolapse. Vaginal oestrogen supplementation may enhance the effect of pelvic floor exercises in postmenopausal women.[12] Involvement of a physiotherapist or continence nurse adviser is often helpful and essential if the woman is having difficulty with pelvic floor exercises. Long-term compliance with pelvic floor exercises may be poor.[13]

Vaginal packing

Chafing and ulceration of externalised epithelium occurs in neglected cases and may be managed by vaginal packing with cotton gauze liberally smeared with oestrogen cream. The prolapse is reduced by the pack, which should be liberally covered in oestrogen cream and replaced daily. Ulceration managed in this way will respond in 2–3 weeks, when definitive treatment (pessary or surgery) may then be undertaken. These women are usually elderly with limited mobility. If admitted, prophylaxis for venous thromboembolism is advisable.

Vaginal pessaries

An appropriately selected and fitted pessary (Figure 21.6) should reduce the prolapse, and if the woman is sexually active should not affect either partner's enjoyment of intercourse. Pessaries need to be removed, washed and reinserted periodically to minimise ulceration of vaginal epithelium and prevent incarceration. Every 3–6 months is sufficient for ring pessaries but pessaries with a large surface area in contact with vaginal epithelium may require more frequent changing. Pessaries may increase physiological vaginal discharge and rates of anaerobic vaginal infection. Supplemental vaginal oestrogen therapy for postmenopausal women may minimise these problems. However, for vaginal pessaries the long-term continuation rate may be low, due to complications including excessive vaginal discharge, bleeding, pain, constipation and expulsion.[14] About 50% of women elect surgery due to dissatisfaction with a pessary.

Surgery

The principles of surgery for genital prolapse are to correct the anatomical defect, to maintain sexual function and to treat associated urinary and bowel dysfunction. Traditional surgical repair involves all or some of vaginal hysterectomy, midline suturing of vaginal connective tissue ('fascia') and excision of redundant vaginal epithelium — an operation that has changed little in the last 100 years. Many newer operations have been described that utilise vaginal, abdominal or laparoscopic techniques. Repair may involve suturing of native tissue, and/or implantation of biological grafts or synthetic mesh. Non-absorbable synthetic materials may provide a more durable repair but are associated with complications, including erosion of material through the vaginal epithelium or, rarely, the bladder. Procedures that obliterate the vaginal cavity (e.g. Le Fort) can be performed under local anaesthesia and may be appropriate in selected cases. Long-term

Instructions: Some women find that bladder, bowel or vaginal symptoms affect their activities, relationships, and feelings. For each question, place an X in the box next to the response that best describes how much your activities, relationships, or feelings have been affected by your bladder, bowel, or vaginal symptoms or conditions over the past 3 months. Please be sure to mark an answer in all 3 columns for each question. Thank you for your cooperation.

How do your symptoms or conditions usually affect your:	Bladder or urine	Bowel or rectum	Vagina or pelvis
1. Ability to do house chores (cooking, housecleaning, laundry)?	☐ Not at all ☐ Somewhat ☐ Moderately ☐ Quite a bit	☐ Not at all ☐ Somewhat ☐ Moderately ☐ Quite a bit	☐ Not at all ☐ Somewhat ☐ Moderately ☐ Quite a bit
2. Ability to do physical activities such as walking, swimming, or other exercise?	☐ Not at all ☐ Somewhat ☐ Moderately ☐ Quite a bit	☐ Not at all ☐ Somewhat ☐ Moderately ☐ Quite a bit	☐ Not at all ☐ Somewhat ☐ Moderately ☐ Quite a bit
3. Entertainment activities such as going to a movie or concert?	☐ Not at all ☐ Somewhat ☐ Moderately ☐ Quite a bit	☐ Not at all ☐ Somewhat ☐ Moderately ☐ Quite a bit	☐ Not at all ☐ Somewhat ☐ Moderately ☐ Quite a bit
4. Ability to travel by car or bus for a distance greater than 30 minutes away from home?	☐ Not at all ☐ Somewhat ☐ Moderately ☐ Quite a bit	☐ Not at all ☐ Somewhat ☐ Moderately ☐ Quite a bit	☐ Not at all ☐ Somewhat ☐ Moderately ☐ Quite a bit
5. Participating in social activities outside your home?	☐ Not at all ☐ Somewhat ☐ Moderately ☐ Quite a bit	☐ Not at all ☐ Somewhat ☐ Moderately ☐ Quite a bit	☐ Not at all ☐ Somewhat ☐ Moderately ☐ Quite a bit
6. Emotional health (nervousness, depression, etc.)?	☐ Not at all ☐ Somewhat ☐ Moderately ☐ Quite a bit	☐ Not at all ☐ Somewhat ☐ Moderately ☐ Quite a bit	☐ Not at all ☐ Somewhat ☐ Moderately ☐ Quite a bit
7. Feeling frustrated?	☐ Not at all ☐ Somewhat ☐ Moderately ☐ Quite a bit	☐ Not at all ☐ Somewhat ☐ Moderately ☐ Quite a bit	☐ Not at all ☐ Somewhat ☐ Moderately ☐ Quite a bit

Figure 21.5
Pelvic Floor Impact Questionnaire short form 7.

(From Barber MD, Walters MD, Bump RC. Short forms of two condition-specific quality-of-life questionnaires for women with pelvic floor disorders (PFDI-20 and PFIQ-7). 2005). Am J Obstet Gynecol 2005 Jul;193(I):I03–I3. Reproduced by permission.)

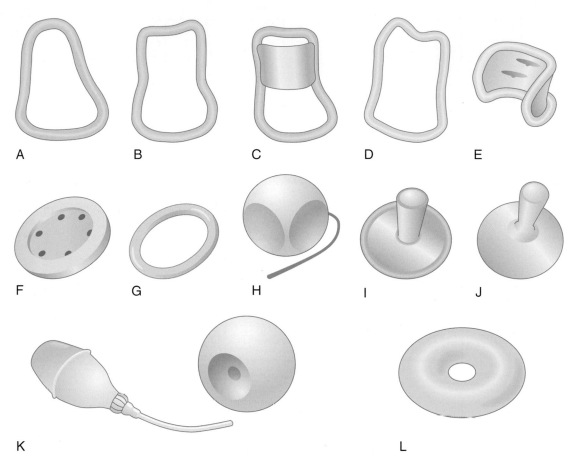

Figure 21.6
Types of vaginal pessary. **A**: Smith's, **B**: Hodge's, **C**: Hodge's with web support, **D**: Risser, **E**: Gehrung, **F**: ring with web support, **G**: ring, **H**: cube, **I**: Gelhorn, rigid, **J**: Gelhorn, flexible, **K**: Inflatoball, **L**: doughnut. In Australia, the most commonly used are the ring and Gelhorn pessaries.

(From Duthie: Practice of Geriatrics, 4th ed. 2007 Saunders. 9781416022619, Figure 42.1)

randomised data are required to properly evaluate newer mesh techniques.[15]

Re-operation for prolapse is common (expected in 10% and 30% of cases following traditional posterior and traditional anterior repair, respectively), and the time intervals between repeat procedures generally decrease with each successive repair.[16] Repeat prolapse operations are associated with progressive scarring, loss of vaginal length and calibre, and deterioration in sexual, bladder and bowel function. The latter may be due to progressive pelvic neuropathy from the underlying defect that caused the prolapse. However, surgery may also exacerbate pelvic neuropathy by direct trauma to autonomic and peripheral nerves. Surgical procedures on the posterior vaginal wall and perineal body may cause dyspareunia.

Women contemplating prolapse repair must be made aware that the results of pelvic floor reconstructive surgery may be adversely affected by subsequent pregnancy. Treatment of prolapse may improve a woman's confidence to resume intercourse but may not result in increased sexual enjoyment if this was a problem before treatment. Other contributors to sexual dysfunction, including low libido, relationship problems, inflammatory conditions of the vulva and vagina, and psychological influences, must be considered.

SUMMARY

Genital prolapse is a common condition that increases in prevalence with age. Pregnancy and childbirth are important risk factors. Management is tailored to the individual woman, should include reassurance, and may include pelvic floor exercises, oestrogen supplementation, vaginal packing, pessaries or surgery. A multidisciplinary approach is usually worthwhile.

REFERENCES

1 Eva UF, Gun W, Preben K. Prevalence of urinary and fecal incontinence and symptoms of genital prolapse in women. Acta Obstetricia et Gynecologica Scandinavica 2003;82(3):280–6.

2 MacLennan AH, Taylor AW, Wilson DH, et al. The prevalence of pelvic floor disorders and their relationship to gender, age, parity and mode of delivery. BJOG 2000;107(12):1460–70.

3 Smith FJ, Holman CD, Moorin RE, et al. Lifetime risk of undergoing surgery for pelvic organ prolapse. Obstet Gynecol 2010;116(5):1096–100.

4 Thor KB, de Groat WC. Neural control of the female urethral and anal rhabdosphincters and pelvic floor muscles. Am J Physiol Regul Integr Comp Physiol 2010;299:R416–38. doi: 10.1152/ajpregu.00111.2010.

5 Jelovsek JE, Maher C, Barber MD. Pelvic organ prolapse. Lancet 2007;369(9566):1027–38.

6 Braekken IH, Majida M, Engh ME, et al. Can pelvic floor muscle training reverse pelvic organ prolapse and reduce prolapse symptoms? An assessor-blinded, randomized, controlled trial. Am J Obstet Gynecol 2010;203(2):170.e1–7.

7 Bump RC, Mattiasson A, Bø K, et al. The standardization of terminology of female pelvic organ prolapse and pelvic floor dysfunction. Am J Obstet Gynecol 1996;175(1):10–17.

8 Duggan P. Preoperative staging of prolapse does not correlate with symptoms and quality of life. Pelviperineology 2011;30:27–30.

9 Barber MD, Walters MD, Bump RC. Short forms of two condition-specific quality-of-life questionnaires for women with pelvic floor disorders (PFDI-20 and PFIQ-7). Am J Obstet Gynecol 2005;193(1):103–13.

10 Digesu GA, Khullar V, Cardozo L, et al. P-QOL: a validated questionnaire to assess the symptoms and quality of life of women with urogenital prolapse. Int Urogynecol J 2005;16:176–81. doi: 10.1007/s00192-004-1225-x.

11 Hagen S, Stark D, Glazener C, et al. A randomized controlled trial of pelvic floor muscle training for stages I and II pelvic organ prolapse. Int Urogynecol J Pelvic Floor Dysfunct 2009;20(1):45–51.

12 Sartori MG, Feldner PC, Jarmy-Di Bella ZI, et al. Sexual steroids in urogynecology. Climacteric 2011;14(1):5–14.

13 Agur W, Steggles P, Waterfield M, et al. The long-term effectiveness of antenatal pelvic floor muscle training: eight-year follow up of a randomised controlled trial. BJOG 2008;115:985–90. doi: 10.1111/j.1471-0528.2008.01742.x.

14 Sarma S, Ying T, Moore KH. Long-term vaginal ring pessary use: discontinuation rates and adverse events. BJOG 2009;116(13):1715–21.

15 Maher C, Feiner B, Baessler K, et al. Surgical management of pelvic organ prolapse in women. Cochrane Database of Systematic Reviews 2010;4:CD004014. doi: 10.1002/14651858.CD004014.pub4.

16 Olsen AL, Smith VJ, Bergstrom JO, et al. Epidemiology of surgically managed pelvic organ prolapse and urinary incontinence. Obstetrics and Gynecology 1997;89(4):501–6.

MCQS

1   A 55-year-old parous woman presents with symptoms of a vaginal bulge. On examination, there is a prolapse of the anterior vaginal wall (cystocele), which on straining descends almost as far as the vaginal entrance (Points Aa and Ba=−1 cm). Her cervix descends to within 4 cm of the vaginal entrance. There is no posterior prolapse. Her BMI is 25, she is a non-smoker, she has no significant medical history and takes no medications. She is now 2 years postmenopause, is divorced and has not had sex for 3 years. She has recently met a man and has put off sexual intimacy because she is embarrassed and concerned that he will be put off by the prolapse. Which one of the following is the most appropriate first step in management?

   A   Refer for surgical management.
   B   Refer for pelvic floor physiotherapy.
   C   Prescribe intravaginal oestrogen cream.
   D   Offer reassurance.
   E   Insert a vaginal ring pessary.

2   A 55-year-old parous woman presents with prolapse of the anterior vaginal wall (cystocele). Her primary symptom is a feeling of pelvic discomfort that gets worse throughout the day and improves when she rests. She reports normal sexual function. Her BMI is 25, she is a non-smoker, she has no significant medical history and takes no medications. On examination, Points Aa and Ba=−1 cm. Which one of the following indicates that surgery for the prolapse should now be considered?

   A   She has been under the management of a pelvic floor physiotherapist for 6 months.
   B   On examination, the vaginal epithelium appears pink and with prominent rugae.
   C   She reports occasional stress urinary incontinence.
   D   On examination, point C=−6 cm and point D=−8 cm.
   E   She works full time as a cleaner.

3   A 62-year-old woman presents with a symptomatic vaginal bulge and difficulties in defecation. She notices a vaginal lump the size of a table-tennis ball and now has to press on this lump to empty her bowel. She is otherwise well and there is no other relevant history. On examination, points Ap and Bp=+2 cm, points C and D=−8 and −10 cm, points Aa and Ba=−3 cm. Which one of the following management options is most appropriate?

   A   pelvic floor exercises
   B   vaginal ring pessary
   C   posterior vaginal repair
   D   intravaginal oestrogen
   E   oral loperamide

4   A 35-year-old woman, married with two children, presents to her GP for a routine Pap smear. She is completely well, takes no medication, and there is no other relevant history. The vaginal walls are patulous and fold inwards between the blades of the speculum and the GP is initially unable to locate the woman's cervix. The doctor removes the speculum, sheaths it in a condom, cuts the end of the condom, and tries again. After successfully taking the smear, to better delineate any prolapse the doctor re-examines the woman with a single blade from the speculum. What additional component is essential for the doctor to be able to complete the assessment?

    A   assistance (a second pair of hands)
    B   an accessible sponge forceps
    C   knowledge of the birthweights of the two children
    D   evaluation of the oestrogenisation of the vaginal epithelium
    E   positioning with stirrups in dorsal lithotomy

OSCE

Mary is a 47-year-old woman who is presenting in a primary care setting for evaluation of a vaginal bulge. What are the important features at history and on examination to determine appropriate investigations and management for this presentation?

Chapter 22

Germ cell tumours of the ovary

Naven Chetty

KEY POINTS

Benign germ cell tumours (ovarian dermoids) are among the most common ovarian cysts.

Benign ovarian dermoids may be monitored clinically (by ultrasound) and if intervention is considered, surgical removal is appropriate.

Malignant germ cell tumours are rare.

Malignant germ cell tumours may often be diagnosed clinically by their tumour marker profile.

Malignant germ cell tumours are most usually treated by combination surgery and chemotherapy.

INTRODUCTION

All medical practitioners will come across an ovarian germ cell tumour during a reasonable course of practice. The vast majority of these tumours are benign, and only a small number are malignant. Similar tumours can arise from the testis in males, extragonadal cells retroperitoneally in the midline or mediastinum, and rarely in the CNS, including in the pineal gland and pituitary. Unlike epithelial ovarian cancers, malignant germ cell tumours occur in younger women, present at an earlier stage, are extremely chemosensitive, and fertility preservation is possible. Malignant germ cell tumours are unique, as they can often be diagnosed preoperatively from their tumour marker profile.

EPIDEMIOLOGY

Germ cell tumours are common, accounting for approximately 30% of primary ovarian tumours, of which 95% are benign, mature, cystic teratomas. The peak incidence for ovarian germ cell tumours is in young women and adolescent girls, where they account for 58% of ovarian tumours, one-third of which are malignant. Malignant germ cell tumours comprise 3% of all ovarian malignancies in Western countries, with a higher incidence reported in Asian, Pacific Islander and Hispanic populations, compared with Caucasians. More than 83% of malignant germ cell tumours of the ovary are diagnosed in women younger than 40 years of age. A review of 1262 malignant germ cell tumours reported that 32.8% were dysgerminomas; 35.6% were immature teratomas with malignant differentiation; and 28.7% had mixed histological features. Other malignant germ cell tumours are extremely rare. Differentiating the benign from the malignant is clearly important, and there is a variety of factors that can assist with this diagnosis.

CLASSIFICATION OF GERM CELL TUMOURS

Germ cell tumours are classified according to the World Health Organization (WHO) Classification of Tumours. There are three broad categories:

1 primitive germ cell tumours
2 biphasic or triphasic teratomas
3 monodermal teratomas and somatic-type tumours associated with dermoid cysts.

Primitive germ cell tumours

Primitive germ cell tumours contain malignant germ cell elements other than teratoma. There are six recognised subtypes:

1 Dysgerminoma: this is the only malignant germ cell tumour that has significant bilaterality, with 10% of diagnoses made in both ovaries concurrently. Macroscopically, they are encapsulated, solid, lobular and light tan in colour, while microscopically there are large cells with clear cytoplasm and a centrally placed nucleus, giving a 'fried egg' appearance. The macroscopic and microscopic features are seen in Figures 22.1 and 22.2.

2 Yolk sac tumour: these tumours show differentiation into multiple endodermal structures. Typically they produce alpha-fetoprotein (AFP) that may be used for both diagnosis and post-treatment surveillance. Macroscopically, these tumours are soft, grey-yellow, with areas of necrosis and liquefaction giving a honeycomb appearance. Microscopically, Schiller-Duval bodies (papillary fibrovascular projections lined by epithelium) are found in 13–20% of these lesions and are characteristic of this type of tumour.

3 Embryonal carcinoma: these are rare tumours, composed of epithelial cells resembling those of the embryonic disc.

4 Polyembryoma: these are rare tumours composed of embryoid bodies resembling the early embryo.

5 Non-gestational choriocarcinoma: this is another rare germ cell tumour composed of cytotrophoblast, syncytiotrophoblast and extravillous trophoblast. Clinically, these are large haemorrhagic tumours with associated luteinised ovarian cysts in the contralateral ovary due to beta human chorionic gonadotropin (β hCG) secretion. As with other hormone producing tumours, β hCG can be used to track response to treatment. These tumours have a worse prognosis than does gestational choriocarcinoma (see chapter 23), so distinction is important to allow for more tailored treatment.

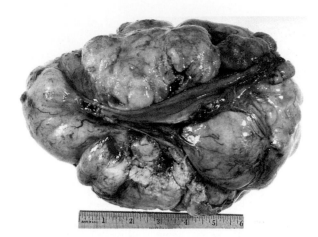

Figure 22.1

Macroscopic image of a dysgerminoma. The tumour has a cerebriform architecture. The fallopian tube is attenuated along the surface.

(Crum: Diagnostic Gynecologic and Obsetric Pathology, 2nd ed. 9781437707649; Figure 29.31, Copyright © 2011 Saunders, An Imprint of Elsevier)

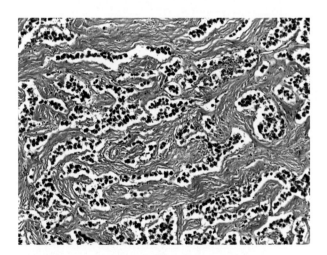

Figure 22.2

Photomicrograph of a dysgerminoma. This tumour has linear arrays of neoplastic cells in a fibrous stroma.

(Crum: Diagnostic Gynecologic and Obsetric Pathology, 2nd ed, 9781437707649; Figure 29.34. Copyright © 2011 Saunders, An Imprint of Elsevier)

6 Mixed germ cell tumour: as their name suggests, these tumours are composed of at least two different germ cell elements, and as a result their tumour marker profile will vary.

Biphasic or triphasic teratomas

Biphasic and triphasic teratomas are the most common of the ovarian germ cell tumours and are composed of derivatives or two or three primary germ layers; that is, ectoderm, mesoderm or endoderm. Accordingly, these tumours can give rise to any tissue that may be seen in the body. They are divided into immature and mature subtypes, which also correlates with malignant or benign nature.

1 Immature teratomas are tumours that contain a varying amount of immature tissue, which is usually immature neuroectoderm. They make up 20–35% of malignant germ cell tumours of the ovary. Immature teratomas tend to be unilateral, solid, have a fleshy consistency, and are tan in colour. Immature teratomas are the only malignant germ cell tumour that is histologically graded, from well differentiated (grade 1) to poorly differentiated (grade 3), with the grade used to guide adjuvant treatment.

2 Mature teratoma or ovarian dermoid cysts are benign cysts composed of mature tissues, most frequently sebaceous material, hair and bone. They may present at any age from 2 to 80 years, with a mean age of 32 years. Approximately 5% of tumours present postmenopausally. Mature teratomas are common and comprise up to 58% of all benign ovarian tumours. Ovarian torsion is a common cause for presentation and is reported in 10–16% of cases, secondary to the fat content within the cyst that causes the cyst to float on peritoneal fluid and render it more easily twisted, particularly as the cyst enlarges. Spontaneous cyst rupture is rare and is reported in only 1% of cases, however rupture may result in a chemical peritonitis that presents as an acute abdomen. Dermoid cysts are bilateral in 8–15% of cases. Macroscopically they have a smooth, reflective surface and a cyst wall of variable thickness. Microscopically, they may take on any mature tissue structure, and nodules composed of fat and bone that project into the cyst may be present; these are called Rokitansky protuberances. The macroscopic and microscopic appearances of a dermoid cyst are demonstrated in Figures 22.3 and 22.4.

Monodermal teratomas and somatic-type tumours associated with dermoid cysts

Monodermal teratomas are a rare group of tumours made up of teratomas composed of a single tissue type, derived from one embryonic layer. They include struma ovarii — mature teratomas containing thyroid tissue that may be benign or malignant.

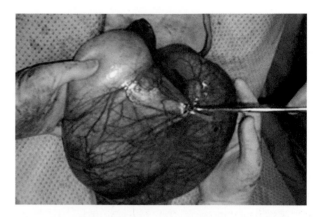

Figure 22.3
Large mature teratoma removed at laparotomy.

(DiSaia: Clinical Gynecologic Oncology, 7th ed. 9780323074193 Figure 10.6A. Copyright © 2007 Mosby, An Imprint of Elsevier)

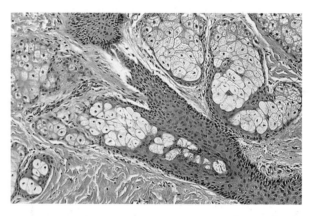

Figure 22.4
Photomicrograph of a mature teratoma (dermoid) of the ovary with the multiple types of cells demonstrated.

(DiSaia: Clinical Gynecologic Oncology, 7th ed. 9780323074193 Fig 10.6B. Copyright © 2007 Mosby, An Imprint of Elsevier)

Also included in this group are carcinoid tumours composed of neuroendocrine cells resembling those of the gastrointestinal tract. Carcinoid syndrome secondary to production of serotonin occurs in 33% of these tumours. Presentation of carcinoid syndrome may include flushing and diarrhoea, and in some cases tricuspid valve injury secondary to effects of serotonin that bypasses the liver and remains in an activated form. These tumours have an excellent prognosis, with most presenting as stage I disease.

This group also includes neuroectodermal tumours, sarcomas, carcinomas arising in a dermoid, sebaceous tumours and melanocytic tumours, but all are extremely rare and will not be discussed further.

STAGING

Malignant germ cell tumours are staged according to the International Federation of Gynecology and Obstetrics (FIGO) system. All ovarian malignancies (epithelial and germ cell tumours) are staged surgically, requiring cytology and biopsies for histological assessment. Table 27.2 in the chapter on cancer of the ovary reports the FIGO staging of both ovarian germ cell and epithelial tumours.

PRESENTATION

Presentation of a germ cell tumour is variable, and may be non-specific with abdominal distension or the finding of a mass with associated bladder or bowel symptoms. It may also cause severe abdominal pain, particularly when associated with an ovarian torsion or cyst rupture. Tumours that release hCG may present with menstrual irregularities or symptoms of pregnancy such as nausea and breast tenderness. Fortunately, more than two-thirds of malignant germ cell tumours are stage I at the time of diagnosis, involving the ovary only. These tumours metastasise via direct peritoneal spread or the lymphatic system, and rarely patients may present with symptoms secondary to metastatic disease.

INVESTIGATIONS

The history and examination of a suspected germ cell tumour is as for ovarian malignancy (see chapter 27), taking into consideration the age of the patient, since many patients with germ cell tumours may be young and specific attention should be placed on secondary sexual characteristics and menstrual history. As malignant germ cell tumours tend to produce characteristic tumour marker profiles, tumour markers will allow for an accurate diagnosis of an ovarian mass. Routine tumour markers that should be requested include:

1. CA 125
2. CA 19.9
3. Alpha fetoprotein (AFP)
4. β hCG (non pregnancy)
5. Lactate dehydrogenase (LDH)

While CA 125 and CA 19.9 are unhelpful in the diagnosis of malignant germ cell tumours, when faced with an ovarian mass, these may aid

Table 22.1 Tumour marker profile for malignant germ cell tumours

Germ cell tumour type	Tumour marker		
	AFP	β hCG	LDH
Dysgerminoma	–	–	+
Yolk sac tumour	+	–	–
Embryonal carcinoma	+	+	–
Non-gestational choriocarcinoma	–	+	–
Immature teratoma	–/+	–	–
Mixed germ cell tumour	–/+	–/+	–/+

differential diagnosis from an epithelial ovarian cancer. Table 22.1 summarises the tumour marker profile for the more common malignant germ cell tumours.

The initial imaging should be a pelvic ultrasound, transvaginal where appropriate, because it offers superior image quality. An ovarian dermoid cyst may be accurately diagnosed sonographically due to its fat content, calcification and Rokitansky protuberance. These cysts are usually negative for hCG, AFP and LDH, but may have mild elevations in CA 125 and CA 19.9 depending on peritoneal irritation or the presence of gastrointestinal type tissue in the cystic mass. The remaining germ cell tumours cannot be differentiated sonographically and the presence of a complex adnexal mass in conjunction with elevated tumour markers will support the diagnosis of a malignant germ cell tumour. Once a malignant germ cell tumour is suspected then a CT scan of the abdomen and pelvis and either chest X-ray or CT is required. The presence of ascites, extra-ovarian lesions and lymphadenopathy will support the diagnosis of a metastatic process. Figure 22.5 demonstrates an ultrasound image of a typical ovarian dermoid cyst.

MANAGEMENT

Management of ovarian germ cell tumours is often surgical as histological assessment is required.

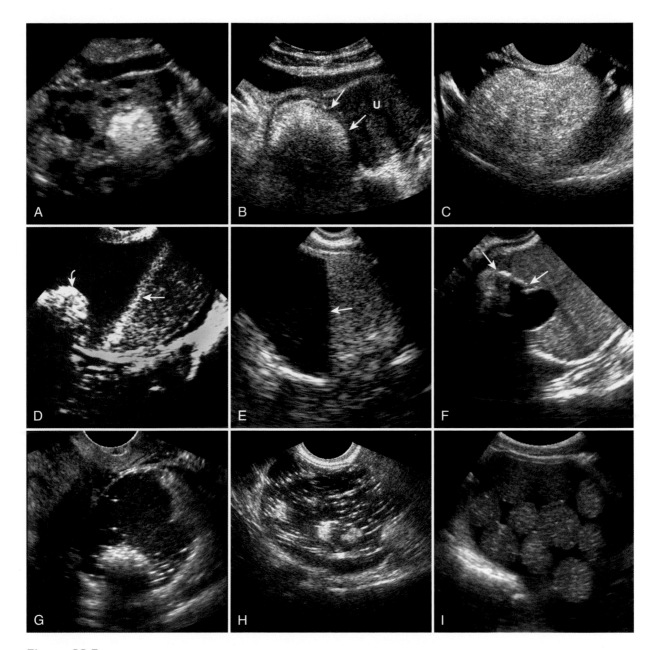

Figure 22.5
Ultrasound images of ovarian dermoids.

(Rumack: Diagnostic Ultrasound, 4th ed. Copyright © 2010 Mosby, An Imprint of Elsevier; 9780323053976; Figure 15.42.)

Simple cystectomy, conserving the ipsilateral ovary, is appropriate for suspected dermoid cysts. This is frequently undertaken by laparoscopy but laparotomy may also be performed. For suspected malignant germ cell tumours, surgery should involve peritoneal washings for cytology, unilateral salpingo-oopherectomy, omental and peritoneal biopsies, and biopsies of any suspicious lesions that may be seen or palpated in the abdomen and pelvis, including lymph nodes. Since malignant germ cell tumours are chemosensitive fertility may be preserved during reproductive years, with no change in prognosis when macroscopic disease is confined to the ovary.

All malignant ovarian germ cell tumours will require adjuvant chemotherapy using bleomycin, etoposide and cisplatin, except stage Ia dysgerminomas and well-differentiated stage Ia, immature teratomas. Administration of the oral contraceptive pill during chemotherapy does not appear to help protect ovarian function. There is no role for radiotherapy in managing germ cell tumours.

Following diagnosis and treatment, patients should be reviewed every 2–4 months for the first 2 years and yearly thereafter, until 10 years post treatment. Follow-up should include history, examination and evaluation of all tumour markers, since tumour recurrence may be in a different cell type. Sonographic or radiological imaging may be deferred until a suspicion of recurrent disease is raised via tumour markers, symptoms or examination. Persistent disease following chemotherapy requires second-line chemotherapy rather than surgery.

Overall 5-year survival for malignant germ cell tumours is high at 91.0%, and 10-year survival is 90%. With the vast majority of this type of cyst being stage I at presentation, these have a higher survival rate of 98% and 96% respectively.

FURTHER READING

International Federation of Gynecology and Obstetrics. www.figo.org/files/figo-corp/docs/staging_booklet.pdf.

Kumar S, Shah JP, Bryant CS, et al. The prevalence and prognostic impact of lymph node metastasis in malignant germ cell tumors of the ovary. Gynecol.Oncol 2008;110(2):125–32.

Lai CH, Chang TC, Hsueh S, et al. Outcome and prognostic factors in ovarian germ cell malignancies. Gynecol Oncol 2005;96(3):784–91.

Low JJ, Perrin LC, Crandon AJ, et al. Conservative surgery to preserve ovarian function in patients with malignant ovarian germ cell tumors. A review of 74 cases. Cancer 2000;89(2):391–8.

Murugaesu N, Schmid P, Dancey G, et al. Malignant ovarian germ cell tumors: identification of novel prognostic markers and long-term outcome after multimodality treatment. J Clin Oncol 2006;24(30):4862–6.

National Cancer Institute. Surveillance, Epidemiology and End Results (SEER) database 1988–2001. US National Institutes of Health. Online. http://seer.cancer.gov.

Nawa A, Obata N, Kikkawa F, et al. Prognostic factors of patients with yolk sac tumors of the ovary. Am J Obstet Gynecol 2001;184(6):1182–8.

Nichols CR, Catalano PJ, Crawford ED, et al. Randomized comparison of cisplatin and etoposide and either bleomycin or ifosfamide in treatment of advanced disseminated germ cell tumors: an Eastern Cooperative Oncology Group, Southwest Oncology Group, and Cancer and Leukemia Group B Study. J Clin Oncol 1998;16(4):1287–93.

Nurman RJ, Norris HJ. Malignant germ cell tumors of the ovary. Hum Pathol 1977;8(5):551–64.

Pectasides D, Pectasides E, Kassanos D. Germ cell tumors of the ovary. Cancer Treat Rev 2008;34(5):427–41.

Salani R, Backes FJ, Fung MF, et al. Posttreatment surveillance and diagnosis of recurrence in women with gynecologic malignancies: Society of Gynecologic Oncologists recommendations. Am J Obstet Gynecol 2011;204(6):466–78.

Smith HO, Berwick M, Verschraegen CF, et al. Incidence and survival rates for female malignant germ cell tumors. Obstet Gynecol 2006;107(5):1075–85.

Tavassoli FA, Devilee P, editors. World Health Organization Classification of Tumours of the Breast and Female Genital Organs. Lyon: IARC Press; 2003.

MCQS

Select the correct answer.

1   A 28 year old presents for ultrasound investigating a right adnexal mass. The report states: 'there is a 6 cm complex ovarian mass with mixed echogenicity and areas that are suggestive of fat within the ovary. The other ovary and the uterus are normal and there is no ascites or free fluid in the pouch of Douglas.' Which of the following statements is correct?

   A   Ultrasound should be repeated in 8 weeks to see if the cyst resolves.
   B   Ultrasound should be complemented with CT in this situation.
   C   Ultrasound is diagnostic in this setting.
   D   Ultrasound is helpful but further investigations are required.
   E   Ultrasound is not helpful in this situation.

2   A 28-year-old woman presents with the finding of a left-sided asymptomatic mass found at routine Pap smear. She is menstruating regularly and is not currently sexually active. A transvaginal ultrasound shows a 6 cm complex mass in the left ovary. Her β hCG is negative, her AFP is negative and her LDH is 4000. Which of the following is the most likely diagnosis?

   A   dermoid
   B   dysgerminoma
   C   yolk sac tumour
   D   corpus luteal cyst
   E   embryonal carcinoma

3   A 28-year-old nulligravid woman is diagnosed with a yolk sac tumour confined to the right ovary on macroscopic examination at laparotomy. Which of the following statements is correct?

   A   She should have the ovary removed and proceed to chemotherapy.
   B   She should have the ovary removed and proceed to radiotherapy.
   C   She should have the ovary removed and commence the OCP.
   D   She should have both ovaries removed and commence the OCP.
   E   She should have both ovaries removed and proceed to chemotherapy.

OSCE

Justine, a 23-year-old nulligravid woman, presents with generalised abdominal distension. Describe the features in the history and examination that you wish to explore with her regarding her presentation.

Chapter 23

Gestational trophoblastic disease

Rhonda Farrell

KEY POINTS

Gestational trophoblastic disease (GTD) is uncommon–rare.

Hydatidiform mole is a benign GTD that may be partial or complete.

There are typical pathological and cytogenetic differences in complete and partial molar pregnancies.

Follow-up is essential.

Malignant GTD is rare and requires referral and expert oncological care.

INTRODUCTION

Gestational trophoblastic disease (GTD) describes a group of tumours that arise from the fetal trophoblast. It is an essential characteristic of normal human trophoblast to invade the endometrium and maternal blood vessels. Usually this invasive behaviour is limited, but in trophoblastic tumours there are abnormally proliferating trophoblasts capable of unlimited growth, invasion and, in some cases, metastatic spread.

Trophoblastic tumours may be benign (hydatidiform mole) or, more rarely, malignant (gestational trophoblastic neoplasia). The malignant tumours include invasive mole, placental site trophoblastic tumour, and choriocarcinoma. Both the benign and malignant tumours have the following characteristics:

- They occur in association with a pregnancy, ranging from early pregnancy loss to a full-term normal pregnancy.
- The tumour DNA always differs from that of the patient's own DNA.
- Human chorionic gonadotrophin (hCG) produced by the trophoblast is an excellent tumour marker, allowing reliable diagnosis and management.
- They are so sensitive to chemotherapy as to permit a nearly 100% cure rate, often without loss of reproductive function.

These are rare tumours, but they are so specific to gynaecology that it is essential for all junior doctors to be aware of them. The key to diagnosis is to know that they exist, think about the possibility, and perform serial β hCG when concerned that your patient has GTD.

BENIGN TROPHOBLASTIC TUMOUR: HYDATIDIFORM MOLE

Macroscopically, the products of conception in a molar pregnancy consist largely of numerous clear vesicles that vary in size from a few millimetres to more than 1 cm and are said to resemble a bunch of grapes. Microscopically, they resemble chorionic trophoblast, characterised by stromal oedema, loss of capillary formation, and profound trophoblast proliferation at the surface of the vesicles (see Figures 23.1 and 23.2).

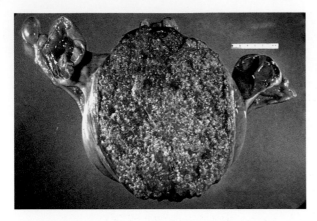

Figure 23.1
Complete molar pregnancy.

(Kumar: Robbins and Cotran Pathologic Basis of Disease, Professional Edition, 8th ed. 9781437707922; Figure 22.58. Copyright © 2009 Saunders, An Imprint of Elsevier)

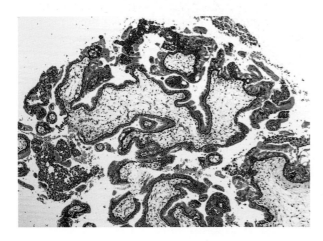

Figure 23.2
Photomicrograph of molar pregnancy.

(Kumar: Robbins and Cotran Pathologic Basis of Disease, Professional Edition, 8th ed. 9781437707922; Figure 22.59. Copyright © 2009 Saunders, An Imprint of Elsevier)

Hydatidiform mole can be classified as partial or complete. The differences between these two presentations are summarised in Table 23.1.

With a complete hydatidiform mole, early pregnancy may be complicated by early or recurrent hyperemesis (a factor related to the abnormally high β hCG), and rarely the early onset of preeclampsia or hyperthyroidism. Later, the uterus is unusually large for dates and feels very soft. Imaging by ultrasound provides a classical picture due to the many vesicular structures present (Figure 23.3) and may also indicate the presence of large ovarian cysts (these luteal cysts arise from the high hCG levels). Fetal

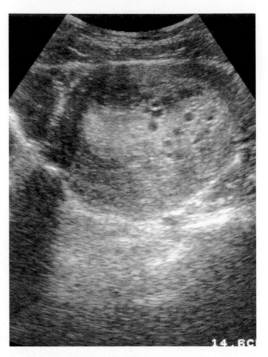

Figure 23.3
Ultrasound image of hydatidiform mole, showing vesicle-like echolucent areas.

(Photo courtesy Peter Farkas/Royal Darwin Hospital.)

structures and heart motion are absent at ultrasound. Vaginal blood loss, sometimes containing a few of the characteristic vesicular structures, may be the first sign of a complete molar pregnancy.

With a partial mole, embryonic death usually occurs first, followed later by miscarriage, often after the end of the first trimester (13–16 weeks), or it may present as a silent (missed) miscarriage. It is often diagnosed only after histological examination of evacuated products of conception, which partly accounts for the wide prevalence reported in the literature. Pathological examination of the products of conception is mandatory to differentiate the clinical diagnosis from hydropic degeneration of the placenta, which may occur after fetal death or in anembryonic pregnancies, but which never leads to persistent trophoblastic disease. Figures 23.4A–C show macroscopic and microscopic features of a partial molar pregnancy.

Treatment for a molar pregnancy consists of suction curettage. Preferably, this is performed with concomitant ultrasound examination, oxytocic support and careful cervical dilatation to avoid perforation of the very soft uterus. Haemorrhage at the time of curettage is an important risk and must

Table 23.1 Comparison of partial and complete mole

Characteristics	Complete mole	Partial mole
Frequency*	1 in 2000 pregnancies	1 in 1000 pregnancies
Usual origin	• Paternal only • Fertilisation of an oocyte without genetic material by one spermatozoon that subsequently doubles its chromosomes	• Maternal and paternal • Fertilisation of a normal egg cell by two spermatozoa (dispermy)
Karyotype	Diploid — mostly 46XX	Triploid — mostly 69XXY
Pathology	• Hydropic oedema of all villi • Substantial hyperplasia • No embryonic structures • No fetal erythrocytes	• Hydropic oedema of part of the villi • Moderate hyperplasia • Embryonic structures present • Fetal erythrocytes may be present
Clinically	• Uterine size frequently large for dates • Usually presents as abnormal vaginal bleeding in early pregnancy (often with passage of vesicular tissue), unless diagnosed by ultrasound earlier	• Uterine size usually normal or smaller than expected • Mostly presents as a silent (missed) or incomplete miscarriage (embryonic death usually occurs before 10 weeks) • Often recognised only on histological examination of evacuated products
hCG levels	Usually high	May be high
Progression to gestational trophoblastic neoplasia	15–20%	2–4%

*Reported frequencies range widely and are 3–4 times higher in Japan and Asia than in Australia, Europe and the United States.

be managed promptly. Anti-D immunoglobulin should be administered to Rhesus-negative women. Additional management consists of careful follow-up by hCG tracking to detect gestational trophoblastic neoplasia that may be noted by an elevation in the hCG level. This involves weekly hCG assays until two consecutive negative results have been obtained, followed by monthly assays for 6 months in the case of complete molar pregnancy. Reliable contraception should be used during this time to ensure that follow-up is not complicated by a new pregnancy. Combined oral contraception and progestogen based contraceptives (see chapter 4) are safe for that purpose.

MALIGNANT TROPHOBLASTIC DISEASE: GESTATIONAL TROPHOBLASTIC NEOPLASIA

Should hCG levels fail to decrease consistently following treatment for a molar pregnancy, this may signify persistent abnormal trophoblastic tissue, a condition now classed as malignant and called gestational trophoblastic neoplasia. Irregular vaginal bleeding or subjective symptoms of pregnancy may

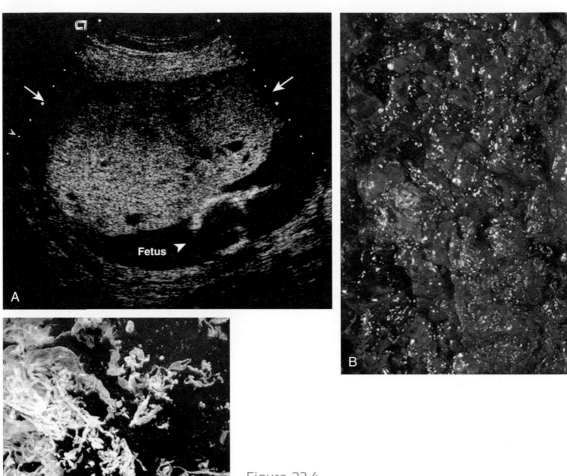

Figure 23.4

Partial molar pregnancy. **A**: Sonographic image of a 13-week gestation with triploidy demonstrating the placenta (arrows) to be markedly thickened, containing scattered small cystic areas consistent with villous swelling. The fetus (fetus, arrowhead) is seen within the amniotic cavity. **B**: Immature placenta with focal villous enlargement. **C**: Early partial mole with scattered swollen villi (upper centre) seen in the dissecting microscope.

(Crum: Diagnostic Gynecologic and Obstetric Pathology, 2nd ed. 9781437707649; Figure 33.48. Copyright © 2011 Saunders, An Imprint of Elsevier)

accompany this clinical finding. The risk for gestational trophoblastic neoplasia is higher in complete than in partial mole.

Gestational trophoblastic neoplasia is diagnosed by any one of the following that occurs after evacuation of a molar pregnancy:

- hCG levels that do not decrease by at least 10% 3 weeks after evacuation of a molar pregnancy, or an increase of more than 10% over a 2-week interval

- Persistence of detectable levels of hCG more than 6 months after molar evacuation
- Histological evidence of choriocarcinoma in the products.

Any of the above findings in the absence of a new pregnancy warrants further investigation and treatment. While gestational trophoblastic neoplasia is potentially lethal, its sensitivity to chemotherapeutic agents means that the disease is usually curable, provided it is recognised and treated in a timely manner. It requires careful gynaecological and general examination and thorough investigation of the many areas to which the trophoblast may have spread. Spread of the disease most frequently occurs locally in the pelvis and by haematogenous spread, notably affecting the liver, lungs and brain. Investigations should therefore include:

- detailed gynaecological examination (including examination for vaginal metastases)
- chest X-ray
- CT scan of the abdomen and pelvis
- consideration of CNS imaging by MRI or testing the spinal fluid for hCG in the presence of neurological symptoms or signs.

There are three possible types of gestational trophoblastic neoplasia:

1 Invasive mole, defined as persistent trophoblast that invades deeply into the myometrium following a molar pregnancy. There may be metastases, usually in the lungs and vagina. Microscopically, it is characterised by oedematous chorionic villi with trophoblast proliferation, as seen with a non-invasive mole.

2 Choriocarcinoma — this may occur after any form of pregnancy, including a normal full-term pregnancy. Histological assessment does not demonstrate the usual chorionic villi, but reveals large fields of invasive hyperplastic and anaplastic trophoblastic tissue. Metastasis is by the haematogenous route, usually to the lungs, liver and brain. During the monitoring phase of a molar pregnancy, a continuing rise in hCG to well above normal levels of pregnancy, associated with evidence of metastatic disease on imaging, is sufficient to make a clinical diagnosis of choriocarcinoma and commence treatment with chemotherapy without the need for a histological diagnosis. Figure 23.5 shows the macroscopic image of a hysterectomy specimen affected by choriocarcinoma.

3 Placental-site trophoblastic tumour — this consists of placental-bed trophoblast invading the myometrium from the site of placental implantation. This differs from choriocarcinoma in that the hCG level is usually much lower and the diagnosis is made only histologically. The condition is rare, accounting for only 0.1–0.2% of trophoblastic tumours.

Treatment of gestational trophoblastic neoplasia is usually with chemotherapy. For low-risk disease, single-drug regimens (methotrexate/folinic acid) are adequate, but multidrug regimens are recommended

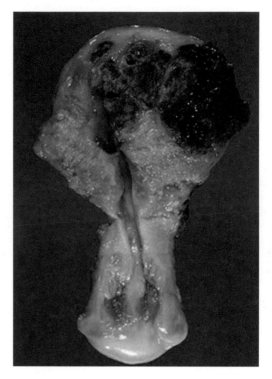

Figure 23.5
Choriocarcinoma.

(Nucci & Oliva: Gynecologic Pathology, 1st ed. 9780443069208; Figure 16.19. Copyright © 2009 Churchill Livingstone, An Imprint of Elsevier)

for high-risk disease. An international scoring system has been adapted by FIGO to predict women at low-risk or high-risk disease (see Table 23.2).

Surgery has a limited place in the treatment of trophoblastic disease. Hysterectomy is the recommended treatment for the few cases of placental site trophoblastic tumour, and may be the solution for a woman with an invasive molar pregnancy who has no further desire for pregnancy. Follow-up with hCG levels after hysterectomy are mandatory to detect any metastatic disease. In isolated cases, surgical excision of localised metastatic lesions that are relatively resistant to chemotherapy (e.g. in the lung or an easily accessible part of the brain) may be warranted to reduce tumour load.

Most cases of gestational trophoblastic neoplasia can be cured by chemotherapy without losing subsequent reproductive function. In the absence of metastases outside the pelvis, 99% of patients with invasive mole can be cured, with 95% maintaining reproductive function if they so desire. However, 5-year survival rates are markedly reduced when brain or liver metastases are present.

Table 23.2 FIGO adapted modified WHO prognostic scoring system for gestational trophoblastic neoplasia

FIGO scoring	0	1	2	4
Age	<40	>40	–	–
Antecedent pregnancy	Mole	Miscarriage/termination	Term pregnancy	–
Interval months from index pregnancy	<4	4–<7	7–<13	≥13
Pre-treatment serum hCG (IU/L)	$<10^3$	$<10^3$–$<10^4$	$<10^4$–$<10^5$	$>10^5$
Largest tumour size (in cm)	<3	3–<5	≥5	–
Site of metastases	Lung	Spleen	Gastrointestinal	Liver, brain
Number of metastases	–	1–4	5–8	>8
Previous failed chemotherapy			Single drug	2 or more drugs

Low risk: Score 0–6
High risk: Score 7 or greater

RECURRENCE

Molar pregnancies carry a risk of recurrence in a subsequent pregnancy that ranges from 1% after a single molar pregnancy to around 20% after two or more molar pregnancies. Therefore, ultrasound (at 10–12 weeks) is recommended for early diagnosis in any subsequent pregnancy after a diagnosis of molar pregnancy.

FURTHER READING

FIGO Committee on Gynecologic Oncology. Current FIGO staging for cancer of the vagina, fallopian tube, ovary, and gestational trophoblastic neoplasia. Int J Gynaecol Obstet 2009;105:3–4.

Hoffner L, Surti U. The genetics of gestational trophoblastic disease: a rare complication of pregnancy. Cancer Genetics 2012;205(3):63–77.

Goldstein DP, Berkowitz RS. Current management of gestational trophoblastic neoplasia. Hematology–Oncology Clinics of North America 2012;26(1):111–31.

Milenkovic V, Jeremic K, Lazovic B, et al. Fertility sparing therapy for metastatic gestational trophoblastic disease in young patients. Int J Gynaecol Obstet 2012;116(2):170–1.

Kani KK, Lee JH, Dighe M, et al. Gestational trophoblastic disease: multimodality imaging assessment with special emphasis on spectrum of abnormalities and value of imaging in staging and management of disease. Current Problems in Diagnostic Radiology 2012;41(1):1–10.

Osborne RJ, Filiaci V, Schink JC, et al. Phase III trial of weekly methotrexate or pulsed dactinomycin for low-risk gestational trophoblastic neoplasia: a gynecologic oncology group study. Journal of Clinical Oncology 2011;29(7):825–31.

Lurain JR. Gestational trophoblastic disease II: classification and management of gestational trophoblastic neoplasia. American Journal of Obstetrics & Gynecology 2011;204(1):11–18.

Seckl MJ, Sebire NJ, Berkowitz RS. Gestational trophoblastic disease. Lancet 2010;376(9742):717–29.

You B, Pollet-Villard M, Fronton L, et al. Predictive values of hCG clearance for risk of methotrexate resistance in low-risk gestational trophoblastic neoplasias. Annals of Oncology 2010;21(8):1643–50.

MCQS

Select the correct answer.

1 Gestational trophoblastic neoplasia receives the highest score for prognostic purposes if it develops after:

   A complete mole.
   B partial mole.
   C spontaneous abortion.
   D ectopic pregnancy.
   E full-term delivery.

2 Which of the following combinations denotes a complete molar pregnancy?

   A diploid karyotype, maternal and paternal transmission, up to 50% progression to gestational trophoblastic neoplasia, no fetal parts present
   B diploid karyotype, paternal transmission, up to 20% progression to gestational trophoblastic neoplasia, fetal parts present
   C diploid karyotype, paternal transmission, up to 20% progression to gestational trophoblastic neoplasia, no fetal parts present
   D triploid karyotype, paternal transmission, up to 20% progression to gestational trophoblastic neoplasia, no fetal parts present
   E triploid karyotype, maternal and paternal transmission, up to 50% progression to gestational trophoblastic neoplasia, no fetal parts present

3 When a diagnosis of complete molar pregnancy is made, which of the following is the optimal management plan?

   A suction curettage with ultrasound control, prevention of haemorrhage with oxytocics, follow-up β hCG for 2 years
   B suction curettage with ultrasound control, prevention of haemorrhage by oxytocics, follow-up β hCG for a minimum of 6 months after treatment
   C suction curettage with ultrasound control, prevention of haemorrhage by bimanual compression, follow-up β hCG for 2 years
   D hysterectomy with ovarian conservation, follow-up β hCG for 6 months
   E hysterectomy with ovarian conservation, follow-up β hCG for 2 years

OSCE

Janelle is a 22-year-old woman who presents to the Early Pregnancy Assessment Service at 10 weeks with nausea and vomiting that is uncontrolled with anti-nausea agents. She has had bright red and painless bleeding.

What are the important features on history and examination that are important for this presentation? What investigations would you recommend?

Chapter 24

Cervical cancer screening

Jonathan Carter

KEY POINTS

Worldwide, cervical cancer is a leading cause of death in women.

Cervical screening programs aid in preventing progression of pre-invasive cervical disease to invasive disease.

The link between HPV and cervical pre-invasive and invasive disease is well established.

HPV vaccinations are available. Their effect on the need to screen and prevalence of disease is not known at this time.

All medical practitioners should have a knowledge of the limitations of screening methodologies.

Counselling women who have an abnormal smear is a very common requirement for medical practitioners.

INTRODUCTION

The worldwide burden of cervical disease is enormous, with over 300 million new cases of HPV infection, 30 million new cases of low-grade squamous intraepithelial lesions (LGSIL) and 10 million new cases of high-grade squamous intraepithelial lesions (HGSIL) diagnosed annually. While perhaps somewhat under-appreciated in developed countries, the worldwide burden of cervical cancer is immense, with over 500 000 new cases of cervical cancer diagnosed each year, resulting in 250 000 deaths. The prevalence of cervical cancer is highest in underdeveloped and Third World countries, particularly sub-Saharan Africa, Central and Southern America, Eastern Europe and Asia.

Cervical screening is presented as a separate chapter in this text as it is a vital part of women's health and needs to be understood at every level of medical contact. Screening for cervical cancer is both possible and highly effective, and is one of the most effective medical screening programs in the world.

ANATOMY AND HISTOLOGY OF THE CERVIX

The uterine cervix is the lower part of the uterus, measuring approximately 3 cm in length and protruding into the upper vagina. On its outside or ectocervix it is covered by a non-keratinising stratified squamous epithelium. The inside or endocervix is covered by columnar, mucus-secreting epithelium. The junction where these two epithelia meet is referred to as the squamo-columnar junction (SCJ) or, more correctly, the 'new' SCJ. Before puberty the original junction is located on either the vagina or the ectocervix. The area or region between the original and new SJC is referred to as the transformation zone. It is an area of active cellular change, where the exposed columnar epithelium undergoes a process of squamous metaplasia. This process commonly occurs at three phases in a woman's life:

1 during fetal development
2 at puberty
3 during the first pregnancy.

The process is enhanced by an acid pH environment and greatly influenced by oestrogen. It is in this region of the transformation zone that HPV-infected metaplastic cells undergo dysplastic change.

WHAT CAUSES CERVICAL CANCER?

To develop cervical cancer, it is necessary (although not sufficient) to have persistent infection of the cervix with high-risk or oncogenic HPV (hrHPV). It has been shown that virtually all cervical cancers test positive for HPV DNA, and that the attributable risk of HPV for cervical cancer is higher than smoking is for lung cancer and hepatitis B virus is for liver cancer. While HPV infection is necessary, other associated cofactors are required that may include smoking, long-term oral contraceptive pill (OCP) use, human immunodeficiency virus (HIV) coinfection, high parity, herpes simplex virus (HSV), and *Chlamydia trachomatis* (CT) infection, an uncircumcised male parter(s), immune suppression, and nutritional and dietary factors.

Natural history

The natural history of HPV-related disease is initiated by an acute infection resulting in viral replication, leading to the development of either a subclinical, or a clinically evident, infection. Subclinical infections may be self-limiting with viral clearance, with clinically evident disease occasionally

producing external genital lesions (warts), LGSIL or HGSIL, the latter being a consequence of persistent infection with hrHPV.

Previously, it was thought that there was a natural and orderly progression of cervical intraepithelial neoplasia (CIN) from CIN I to CIN II to CIN III and finally invasive cervical cancer. We now understand that the majority of low-grade lesions will regress without treatment (and this has led to the rationale for not treating), while most high-grade lesions (HGSIL or CIN III) will progress to invasive cancer if left untreated; this is why treatment for these lesions is recommended (see Figure 24.1).

Generally it takes 7–10 years to develop an invasive cervical cancer from CIN III, with a mean transition time of about 4.5 years. Some patients may progress more rapidly (see Table 24.1). Variables associated with progression of HGSIL to

Table 24.1 Transition time of cervical intraepithelial neoplasia

Stages	Mean transition time (years)
Normal to CIN I	1.62
Normal to CIN II	2.20
Normal to CIN III	4.51

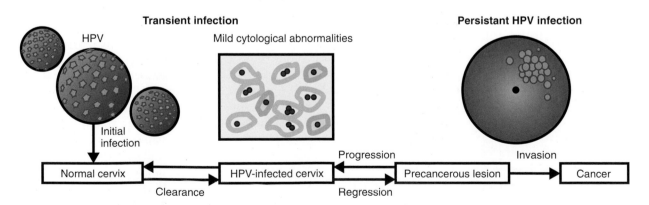

Figure 24.1

Natural history of HPV infection and CIN.

(From Xian Wen Jin. Cervical screening and prevention, p. 1212, Figure 1. Adapted from Wright TC, Schiffman M. Adding a test for human Papillomavirus DNA to cervical cytology. N Eng J Med 2003;348:489–490.)

cancer include increasing age, large lesion sizes and a higher degree of cellular abnormality.

What is HPV?

HPV has been discussed in chapter 5 on STIs. Here, it is important to note that 15 types of HPV cause cervical cancer, with types 16 and 18 the most common in cervical lesions and accounting for 60–80% of all cervical cancer. The typical HPV structure is demonstrated in Figure 24.2. There is wide variation in the prevalence of HPV types throughout Africa, Asia and other parts of the world. HPV is generally transmitted through sexual contact, with penetrative heterosexual intercourse the most common mode of transmission. HPV infection is very common in sexually active young women, with a point prevalence of about 25% and a cumulative prevalence of greater than 80%. As such, and as a descriptor to patients, it is often referred to as a marker of normal sexual maturity. After the age of 30 the prevalence of HPV infection declines dramatically to about 5%, and the key determinants of infection remain age of coitarche (the time of first intercourse), number of sexual

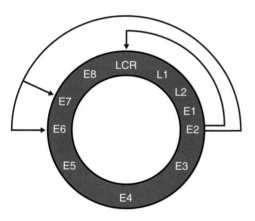

Figure 24.2

Structure of the HPV virus. Most HPV exists in episomal (circular) DNA. The important genomic sites are called open reading frames (ORFs). In the episomal state, E2 regulates both the long control region (LCR), which is responsible for regulation of viral transcription, and E6 and E7, the two sites most often responsible for malignant transformation.

(From Cox JT: Clinical Proceedings, Association of Reproductive Health Professionals, September 2003, p 5, with permission. Adapted from: Lawson HW. Cervical Cancer Screening. chapter 11, page 124, figure 11-5.)

partners (high risk determined by the number of new sexual partners per month), and male partners' sexual behaviour.

Most HPV infections are transient with viral clearance by cell-mediated immune mechanisms usually within 6 months. Some HPV infections, particularly those of high-risk genotypes, may take between 12–24 months to clear. Factors modulating cervical disease progression include ongoing HPV exposure, HPV genotype and its molecular variant and the HPV viral load, as well as the immune status of the host.

Immune response

The HPV life cycle takes place entirely within the cervical squamous epithelial cell, and thus is effectively 'hidden' from the host immune system. Unlike other infections, there is no systemic response, no viraemia, and no blood-borne phase. The infected epithelial cells:

- undergo 'non-lytic cell death'
- are not destroyed
- are able to release newly synthesised virus
- do not evoke an inflammatory reaction
- block the release of inflammatory cytokines that normally occurs in response to an invader.

If or when an immune response can be generated after natural infection, then there is exudation of L1-neutralising antibodies at the basement membrane, preventing viral binding. Additionally, transudation of IgG and IgA antibodies through the epithelium binds the HPV before it is able to infect cells.

HPV vaccines

With the development of recombinant DNA technology, HPV vaccines have been produced with L1 proteins assembled into virus-like particles (VLP) and added to aluminum salts to improve the immune response to the vaccine. VLPs are very similar in external appearances to native HPV viral particles. As the VLP contains no viral DNA it is not infectious, but it is able to elicit a significant neutralising antibody response.

Currently there are two vaccines available. Gardasil is quadrivalent and Cervarix is a bivalent vaccine. Both are very efficient in reducing HPV 16 and HPV 18 disease of the lower genital tract; in addition Gardasil is also effective against lesions related to HPV 6 and HPV 11 infections.

Table 24.2 Features of commercially available HPV vaccines[1]

	Gardasil	Cervarix
Manufacturer	MSD	GlaxoSmithKline
Ages	9–45 (females) 9–15 (males)	10–45
HPV types	6, 11, 16, 18	16, 18
Expression system	Yeast *Saccharomyces cerevisiae*	Baculovirus in insect cells
Adjuvant	Aluminium hydroxy phosphate sulfate	ASO4 (Adjuvant System 04): $Al(OH)_3$+MPL
Cross reactivity	Demonstrated	Demonstrated
Program	0, 2 and 6 months (IMI)	0, 1 and 6 months (IMI)
Recommended in pregnancy	No	No
Volume per dose	0.5 mL	0.5 mL
Efficacy in preventing incident/transient infections	91%	92%
Efficacy in preventing persistent infections	100%	100%

Franco E, Harper D. Vaccination against human Papillomavirus infection: a new paradigm in cervical cancer control. Vaccine 2005;23:2388–94.

Vaccine-induced protection appears to last for a number of years, and while HPV antibodies are primarily type-specific, both vaccines have shown some cross-protection against other HPV types, including types 31, 33 and 45. Generally the vaccines are well tolerated following administration but may produce local discomfort or pain, redness, fatigue, headache and myalgia. While a number of potential vaccine adverse effects have been demonstrated, overall many of these adverse effects are not specifically related to the vaccine and it remains safe without significant adverse effects. Table 24.2 compares a variety of characteristics and findings of two proof-of-principle randomised controlled trials that assessed the efficacy of these commercially available prophylactic vaccines to prevent HPV infection and cervical abnormalities.

SCREENING

All women aged 18–70 who have ever had sexual intercourse should have a Pap test performed every 2 years. The Australian National Cervical Screening Program (NCSP), one of the most successful cervical cancer screening programs in the world, screens just over 2 million women annually. In 2007, 28 188 abnormalities were detected by histology, of which 13 709 were low-grade and 14 479 were high-grade lesions.

The financial impost on countries for cervical disease prevention is huge. In the United States, it has been estimated that the cost of screening, follow-up and treatment of cervical cancer approximates US$6 billion/year; while in Australia the screening program costs $138 million dollars annually.

Pap test

The Pap test performed today is largely unchanged since its first description by Georgios Papanikolaou in the 1940s. However, rather than obtaining an aspirate from the posterior vaginal fornix as described by Papanikolaou, in the modern Pap test

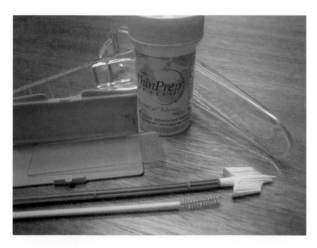

Figure 24.3
Tools used to perform a Pap test.

(Image courtesy of author.)

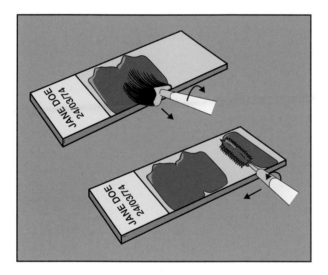

Figure 24.4
Preparation of the conventional Pap smear slide.

(Adapted from: Lawson HW. Cervical Cancer Screening. Chapter 11, page 126, figure 11-8.)

the cervix is brushed to obtain cells that are then transferred to a glass slide (Figures 24.3 and 24.4).

The Pap test does have limitations, and in a meta-analysis of 62 studies, the mean sensitivity of the Pap test is 58% and mean specificity is 69%. It is less accurate for glandular lesions, with a 40% false negative rate. Not collecting cells properly; not transferring them to the slide; and poor cellular preservation account for two-thirds of the errors in the test. In the remaining third, problems arise from screening or interpretation errors, where abnormal cells are missed or incorrectly interpreted. Inter-observer variability also accounts for errors in interpretation, with a recent study reporting that in Pap tests originally interpreted as high grade, 53% were reinterpreted as LGSIL, atypical squamous cells of unknown significance (ASCUS), or negative.

Improving the system

In an attempt to improve the accuracy of the Pap test, a number of strategies have been employed including liquid-based cytology and HPV testing.

Liquid-based cytology

ThinPrep and SurePath are liquid-based cytology (LBC) technologies that produce a uniform, thin-layer slide that minimises obscuring artifacts such as red blood cells and mucus. With the ThinPrep Pap test, the cervix is brushed with a sampling device, which is rinsed in transport media where the sample is dispersed, randomised, filtered and a representative sample is transferred to the slide. With the SurePath Pap test the cervix is brushed using a sampling device with a detachable head, which is placed in the transport medium, capturing the entire sample. The test uses a sedimentation process where samples are enriched to remove debris, followed by centrifuging to generate a pellet, a portion of which is than applied for slide analysis.

The advantages of LBC are that more artifacts are removed, a greater number of cells are collected and transferred, and cell morphology is better preserved, resulting in an overall better smear. It is unclear as to how much benefit LBC provides in detecting high-grade lesions compared to conventional cytology, with a recent meta-analysis showing no difference in their ability to diagnose high-grade disease.

Human papilloma virus testing

Using a commercial RNA probe-ELISA kit, the Hybrid Capture2 assay is an accurate and reproducible method of detecting the presence of HPV DNA. HPV testing is more sensitive but less specific than cytology, and as sensitive as immediate colposcopy for detecting high-grade disease. Using HPV testing as a primary screening tool would spare those women who were HPV-negative the need to undergo colposcopic evaluation. It offers a 99% negative predictive value when the Pap report determines atypical squamous cells of undetermined significance (ASCUS), with a sensitivity of 92.5% to

Table 24.3 Risk of CIN III on follow-up

HPV status	Pap test	Risk (%)
Negative	Normal	1
	Any other Pap	<5
Positive	Normal	7
	ASCUS/LGSIL	11
	HGSIL	45
	HGSIL + HG colposcopy	67

Box 24.1 Epithelial cell abnormalities used to describe cervical cytology specimens

Squamous abnormalities

- Atypical squamous cells of undetermined significance (ASCUS)
- Possible low-grade squamous intraepithelial lesion
- Low-grade squamous intraepithelial lesion (LGSIL)
- Possible high-grade squamous intraepithelial lesion
- High-grade squamous intraepithelial lesion (HGSIL)
- Squamous cell carcinoma

Glandular abnormalities

- Atypical endocervical cells of undetermined significance
- Atypical glandular cells of undetermined significance
- Possible high-grade glandular lesion
- Endocervical adenocarcinoma in situ
- Adenocarcinoma

detect CIN II or worse and 95.6% to detect CIN III or worse. In patients who are HPV-negative, it is a good predictor of the absence of disease. HPV negativity is associated with a very low risk of cervical cancer, while even among women who have a normal cervical cytology, persistent detection of HPV greatly increases their risk of progression to CIN III and cervical cancer (see Table 24.3).

Potential advantages for incorporating HPV testing include the reduction of many repeat Pap tests and subsequent referral for colposcopy and biopsy. Additional benefits for the patient include reduced time off work, reduced need to re-attend for results, and reduced anxiety. Currently in Australia, testing for HPV DNA is only indicated for post-treatment surveillance as recommended by the Medical Services Advisory Committee (MSAC).

CERVICAL SCREENING TERMINOLOGY

The terminology used in cervical screening has been varied, with a number of systems used internationally. In 2006 in Australia, the 'Australian Modified Bethesda System 2004' (AMBS 2004) was implemented to replace the previous nomenclature and bring our terminology in line with international standards. The change occurred due to a greater understanding of the natural history of both HPV and CIN and the realisation that progression of CIN I to high grade CIN II and CIN III was not inevitable.

The significant changes with the AMBS 2004 include:

1 use of the terms outlined in Box 24.1 to describe squamous abnormalities and glandular abnormalities on cervical screening tests
2 conservative management for low-grade Pap smear changes
3 when low-grade change confirmed, a 'no treatment' recommendation for CIN I
4 formal HPV DNA testing was used as a 'test of cure' after treatment.

The benefits of a cervical cancer screening program in part come from diagnosing and treating women with high-grade disease, while most of the harm comes from over-investigating and treating women with low-grade disease.

LGSIL

Most low-grade Pap smears represent an acute HPV infection, the majority of which will resolve spontaneously. However, as discussed above, the Pap test

Table 24.4 Outcome			
Outcome	Mean	6 months	12 months
Regression (LGSIL to ASCUS or normal)	10.5	51%	78%
Progression (LGSIL to HGSIL)	86.4	1.7%	3.6%

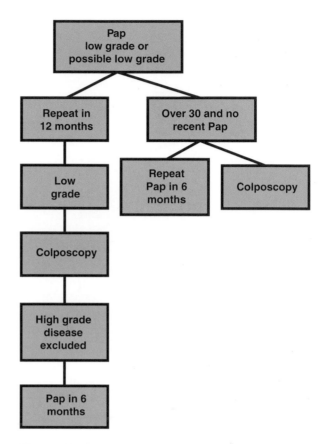

Figure 24.5
Management algorithm for possible LGSIL or LGSIL.
(Image courtesy of author.)

is imperfect, and overall 11% of smears that report low-grade disease indeed have an underlying high-grade abnormality and 20% of all CIN III comes from the low-grade reported group. This is more likely in women over age 30 and is the rationale for either immediate colposcopy or repeat smear in 6 months in this age group. A contributor to this discrepancy in reporting is that the mean lesion size of CIN III is very small in patients with a low grade smear (0.6 mm) compared to those with a high grade smear (9.5 mm) and this may represent a sampling issue. The majority of LGSIL will regress to ASCUS or normal within a mean time of 10.5 months. By 6 months 51% and by 12 months 78% of LGSIL have regressed (Table 24.4).

Rarely will LGSIL progress to HGSIL. The mean time to progression is 86.4 months with only 1.7% progressing by 6 months and 3.6% progressing at 12 months. The risk of an invasive cancer after a low-grade smear is 0.1%.

The AMBS 2004 guidelines indicate that biopsy-proven low-grade lesions do not require treatment, because these lesions will nearly always resolve spontaneously. Instead, the recommendation is to repeat the smear at 12 and 24 months. If these two Pap smears are negative, the woman can return to normal screening. If either Pap smear shows low-grade change, repeat annually until at least two negative smears, then return to normal screening. If any repeat Pap smear shows high-grade change, refer for colposcopy (see the flow diagram for managing a LGSIL, Figure 24.5).

HGSIL

All patients with a possible or high-grade lesion (squamous or glandular) should be referred for colposcopy (Figures 24.6 and 24.7).

SPECIAL CIRCUMSTANCES
Pregnancy

Generally, pregnancy should not cause deviation from either performing a Pap test or the evaluation of a smear-detected abnormality. The only provisos would be in a patient with a known low-lying placenta. Due to increased pelvic vascularity and lax vaginal walls, colposcopic evaluation during pregnancy may be difficult and ideally should be performed by an expert colposcopist.

Immune-suppressed

It is recommended that immune-suppressed patients have annual Pap tests with colposcopy reserved for any detected abnormality.

Post-hysterectomy

Where a subtotal hysterectomy has been performed (i.e. cervix retained), patients should continue with routine biennial screening. For patients having had

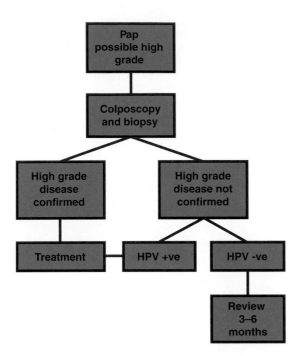

Figure 24.6
Management algorithm for possible HGSIL.

(Image courtesy of author.)

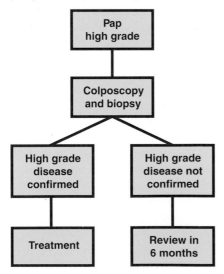

Figure 24.7
Management algorithm for HGSIL.

(Image courtesy of author.)

a total hysterectomy for benign conditions that have a normal prior smear history, no further screening is required. For patients with a prior history of lower genital tract dysplasia including CIN, continued screening is recommended with biennial vaginal vault Pap tests.

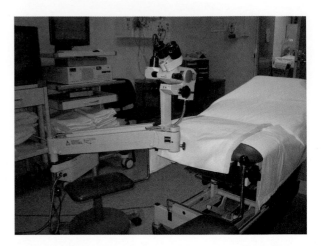

Figure 24.8
Colposcopic equipment used for examination of cervix.

(Image courtesy of author.)

Adolescents

In the management of abnormalities in adolescents it is important to avoid over-treatment. Young and adolescent patients have a high rate of regression of disease and in appropriate patients a period of conservative observation with Pap test and colposcopy should be undertaken at 6 monthly intervals for 1–2 years with the expectation of complete or partial regression in a large majority of patients.

COLPOSCOPY

Colposcopy is an examination of the cervix and lower genital tract with a low power, stereoscopic microscope with an attached light source (Figure 24.8). The cervix and vagina are cleaned of any blood and debris with normal saline, and, after inspecting the cervix and vagina, a dilute 3–5% solution of acetic acid is applied to the cervix. Acetic acid dehydrates the cells and causes a reversible coagulation of the nuclear proteins. Characteristic acetowhite epithelial changes will occur in cells rich in proteins such as dysplastic cells. Significant acetowhite features include intensity or colour tone, margins and surface contour, and vascular changes. A solution of Lugol's iodine may be applied, being taken up by glycogen-rich cells and leaving dysplastic and immature cells as iodine negative.

A number of colposcopic scoring systems have been proposed. The most commonly used and widely reported of these, the Reid Colposcopic

Table 24.5 Modified Reid colposcopy

	Score			
	0	1	2	3
Colour	Low intensity semitransparent, indistinct	Shiny, grey-white intermediate	Dull, oyster-white, grey	Yellow, necrotic, friable
Margins	Microcondylomatous, feathered, flocculated, angular, jagged	Regular, symmetrical, smooth	Rolled, peeling edges, internal borders	Exophytic, nodular, ulcerated
Mosaic, punctation	Fine	None	Coarse	

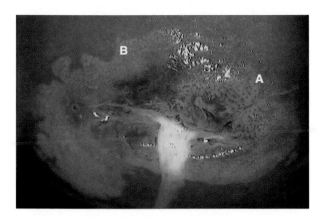

Figure 24.9
Colpo-photograph of a high grade lesion with punctation (A) and mosaicism (B).

(Image courtesy of author.)

Index, is shown in Table 24.5. Characteristic vascular patterns include the presence of punctuation and mosaicism. Punctuation is the presence of looped capillaries viewed end-on, whereas vessels running parallel to the surface are seen as cobbled areas of mosaicism (Figure 24.9).

Colposcopy is a subjective assessment tool, and results are variable, based on the training and experience of the colposcopist. The main aim of colposcopy is the identification of the worst appearing microscopic region to allow for a directed biopsy. The ability to differentiate normal cells from high-grade lesions by colposcopy has a sensitivity of 54–85% and specificity of 69%.

TREATMENT MODALITIES

When there is an abnormality determined by the combination of cervical cytology, colposcopy and cervical biopsy, treatment can either be conservative (ablation or excisional) or definitive, that is, hysterectomy. The mode of treatment will depend on the grade of the lesion, clinical history, desire for further reproduction, and the experience and training of the clinician.

Conservative treatments
Electro-coagulation diathermy (ECD)

Destruction of tissue is achieved by placing a standard ECD diathermy electrode into the cervix and continuing electrode activation until all mucus has stopped bubbling. Cessation of bubbling signifies glandular destruction and completeness of the procedure. Failure rates are among the lowest of all the destructive methods.

Cryosurgery

Destruction of tissue is achieved using either N_2O or CO_2 and a double-freeze technique. This simple technique requires limited and inexpensive equipment and is ideally suited for under-resourced countries. Issues relating to a higher recurrence rate, particularly with larger lesions, and increasing reports of invasive cancers after such treatment, have limited its use in developed countries.

Laser surgery

Destruction of tissue uses an invisible CO_2 laser beam, guided by a second, visible laser beam. Tissue is vaporised after absorption of the laser energy, which essentially boils intracellular water. Such surgery is performed under colposcopic control and is very accurate, allowing precise tissue destruction. If the laser surgeon is expert then the surrounding retained tissue will have little or no thermal destruction and necrosis, making margins easier to interpret and allowing the cervix to heal rapidly. Failure rates are increased with an inappropriate depth of destruction, with greater than 5–7 mm depth of destruction recommended.

LEEP

LEEP is an acronym for loop electrocautery excision procedure, also known as loop excision or LLETZ (large loop excision of the transformation zone). It is now the most commonly utilised treatment for cervical dysplasia. The procedure can be performed under either local or general anaesthesia, provides a specimen for histopathological assessment, and requires little in the way of equipment apart from an electrosurgical generator, speculum, plume evacuator, and disposable LEEP electrodes. Excisions ideally should be no greater than 5–8 mm deep (Figure 24.10). The histological changes associated with CIN I, II and III are demonstrated in Figure 24.11 A–C.

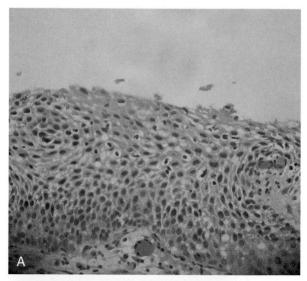

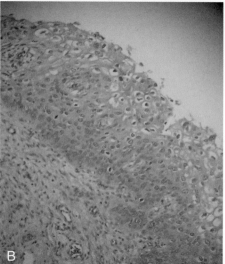

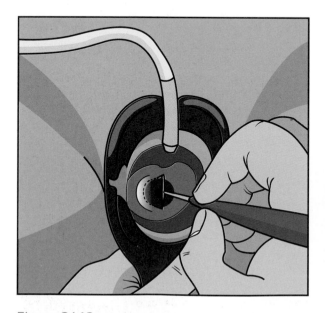

Figure 24.10
Loop electrode excision procedure (LEEP).

(Adapted from: Lawson HW. Cervical Cancer Screening. Chapter 11, page 139, figure 11-19.)

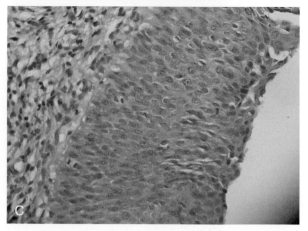

Figure 24.11 A–C
Photomicrographs of histological changes denoting CIN I, II, III.

Cold knife cone biopsy

Cold knife cone biopsy is the traditional and now largely antiquated method of excision, utilised almost exclusively for patients with adenocarcinoma in-situ (AIS). The procedure is more traumatic to the cervix than the other destructive or excisional procedures, requires a general anaesthetic, and has a greater risk of bleeding and pregnancy-related complications.

Definitive treatments — hysterectomy

The above ablative and excisional procedures are conservative surgical procedures used in patients desirous of retaining their reproductive potential. Where this is not a concern, in older patients or in patients with concomitant gynaecological pathology, hysterectomy by any route may be considered. It is important to allow for appropriate pathological examination of the cervix if this treatment is undertaken, and procedures where the cervix is damaged (e.g. morcellation performed vaginally or laparoscopically) are inappropriate.

POST-TREATMENT SURVEILLANCE

Following treatment, patients are seen at 4–6 months later for a Pap test with or without colposcopy, and again at 12 months post-treatment for a Pap test, colposcopy and HPV DNA testing. Once two sets of tests (Pap smear and HPV test) are negative on two consecutive 12-monthly occasions, the woman may return to the usual 2-yearly screening interval. If the follow-up Pap smear shows a high-grade change, then the patient should be referred for colposcopy. If the Pap smear shows only low-grade change or the HPV test is positive, then the tests should be repeated each year — there is no need to refer back to the gynaecologist for colposcopy (See treatment and follow-up algorithm — Figure 24.12).

PROGNOSIS AFTER TREATMENT

From original studies and summarised in a Cochrane review, there is no clear evidence to show superiority of any of the cervical abnormality treatment techniques in terms of treatment failure or operative morbidity. Pooled failure rates for the different treatment modalities are shown in Table 24.6. Recurrence risk is higher among women aged 30 years and older, those with human papillomavirus types 16 or 18 and those having had prior treatment.

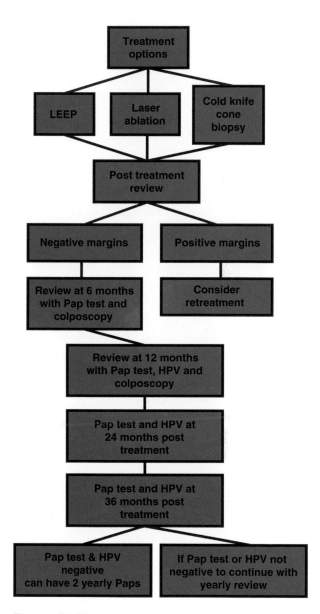

Figure 24.12
Treatment and follow-up algorithm.
(Image courtesy of author.)

OBSTETRIC OUTCOMES

Analysis of outcomes following treatment of a cervical abnormality is both confusing and controversial. It must be recognised that preterm labour (PTL), preterm delivery (PTD) and preterm premature rupture of membranes (PPROM) occur in patients who have not undergone cervical treatment. Indeed many risk factors for patients developing cervical dysplasia (e.g. smoking) are also risk factors for PTL

Table 24.6 Conservative treatment for cervical intraepithelial neoplasia

Method	Failures (%)
Electrocoagulation	2.7
Cryosurgery	8.7
Laser	5.6
Cold coagulator	6.8
LEEP	4.3

and PTD. It is therefore difficult to fully appraise this relationship; however in a recent meta-analysis there did not appear to be an increased risk of adverse pregnancy outcome with LEEP, cryotherapy or laser ablation. Cold knife cone biopsy was associated with a significantly increased risk of perinatal mortality, PTD, extreme PTD and low birth weight. As is often the case, risk must be weighed against benefit and the most important factor is to not over-treat lesions that may resolve spontaneously.

REFERENCE

1 Franco E, Harper D. Vaccination against human Papillomavirus infection: a new paradigm in cervical cancer control. Vaccine 2005;23:2388–94.

FURTHER READING

Arbyn M, Bergeron C, Klinkhamer P, et al. Liquid compared with conventional cervical cytology: a systematic review and meta-analysis. Obstet Gynecol 2008;111(1):167–77.

Arbyn M, Kyrgiou M, Simoens C, et al. Perinatal mortality and other severe adverse pregnancy outcomes associated with treatment of cervical intraepithelial neoplasia: meta-analysis. BMJ 2008;337:a1284.

Australian Institute of Health and Welfare. Cervical screening in Australia 2006–7 Cancer series no. 47. Cat. no. CAN 43. Canberra: AIHW; 2009.

Carter JR, Ding Z, Rose BR. HPV infection and cervical disease: a review. Aust N Z J Obstet Gynaecol 2011;51(2):103–8.

Chen H-C, Schiffman M, Lin C-Y, et al. Persistence of type-specific human Papillomavirus infection and increased long-term risk of cervical cancer. J Natl Cancer Inst 2011;103(18):1387–96.

Ding Z, Jiang C, Shore T, et al. Outcome of cervical intraepithelial neoplasia 2 diagnosed by punch biopsy in 131 women. J Obstet Gynaecol Res 2011;37(7):754–61.

Einstein M, Baron M, Levin M, et al. Comparison of the immunogenicity and safety of Cervarix and Gardasil human Papillomavirus (HPV) cervical cancer vaccines in healthy women aged 18–45 years. Human Vaccines 2009;5(10):1–15.

Martin-Hirsch PP, Paraskevaidis E, Bryant A, et al. Surgery for cervical intraepithelial neoplasia. Cochrane Database Syst Rev 2010;(6):CD001318.

Munoz N, Bosch FX, de Sanjose S, et al. Epidemiologic classification of human papillomavirus types associated with cervical cancer. N Engl J Med 2003;348(6):518–27.

Rao A, Pather S, Dalrymple C, et al. The role of HPV testing in patients with possible high-grade cervical cytology. Journal of Obstetrics and Gynaecology Research 2009;35(3):503–6.

Reid R, Stanhope CR, Herschman BR, et al. Genital warts and cervical cancer. IV. A colposcopic index for differentiating subclinical Papillomaviral infection from cervical intraepithelial neoplasia. Am J Obstet Gynecol 1984;149(8):815–23.

Schlecht NF, Platt RW, Duarte-Franco E, et al. Human papillomavirus infection and time to progression and regression of cervical intraepithelial neoplasia. J Natl Cancer Inst 2003;95(17):1336–43.

Slade BA, Leidel L, Vellozzi C, et al. Postlicensure safety surveillance for quadrivalent human Papillomavirus recombinant vaccine. JAMA 2009;302(7):750–7.

Vesco KK, Whitlock EP, Eder M, et al. Risk factors and other epidemiologic considerations for cervical cancer screening: a narrative review for the U.S. Preventive Services Task Force. Ann Intern Med 2011;155(10):698–705.

MCQS

Select the correct answer.

1   Which of the following is correct regarding genital HPV infection?

    A   It is an uncommon infection, particularly in developed countries.
    B   It is usually sexually transmitted.
    C   Smoking is not an important cofactor in the development of cervical cancer.
    D   The transformation zone is always located on the ectocervix.
    E   There are approximately 50 types of HPV.

2   Which of the following is correct regarding current cervical cancer screening?

    A   Pap test screening is indicated in women aged between 18 and 70 years.
    B   The Pap test is a very accurate test.
    C   The Pap test is used to diagnose cervical cancer.
    D   HPV testing is approved for screening for cervical cancer.
    E   In Australia, Pap test screening should occur annually.

3   Which of the following is correct regarding cervical cancer development?

    A   All CIN lesions require treatment.
    B   The progression of CIN III to cervical cancer is rapid, occurring in 2–5 years.
    C   Most low-grade lesions resolve without treatment.
    D   Colposcopy is indicated for all Pap test abnormalities.
    E   A high-grade lesion in pregnancy should be treated prior to delivery.

4   Which if the following is correct regarding treatment and follow-up of CIN?

    A   Cone biopsy is the most commonly used treatment option.
    B   There is no increased risk of adverse pregnancy outcome with treatment.
    C   HPV testing is approved for triage of patients.
    D   The advantage of an excisional treatment is that a specimen is produced.
    E   Cryotherapy has the lowest rate of recurrent CIN.

OSCE

Michelle, a 22-year-old woman, sees you for a routine Pap smear. What are the important factors that you need to elicit from history in regards to establishing risk factors for a Pap smear abnormality?

The result of her Pap test has predicted a 'high-grade squamous intraepithelial lesion — HGSIL'. Describe this result with Michelle and outline the likely management for her at this time.

Chapter 25

Cervical cancer

Jonathan Carter

KEY POINTS

Cervical cancer deaths are uncommon in Australia.

Once diagnosed, involvement of a specialist in gynaecological oncology is mandatory.

Staging is clinical and follows a FIGO classification system.

INTRODUCTION

In 2007 there were 46 349 new cancer cases affecting women in Australia. Of these, cervical cancer accounted for 739 (1.5%) cases. Of the 17 322 deaths, 208 (1.2%) were from cervical cancer. Over the last 3–4 decades, the incidence and mortality from cervical cancer has been declining, and it is of interest that this decline commenced before the commencement of the National Cervical Screening Program (Figure 25.1). Much of this decline in incidence relates to reduction in squamous cancers of the cervix, as the incidence of the mixed and pure adenocarcinoma has remained relatively unchanged. Chapter 24 on cervical screening describes the pathological basis for development of cervical cancer and the importance of screening in this country and globally.

HISTOLOGICAL TYPES

There are a number of histological types of cervical cancer but approximately 80% are squamous cell.

Most of the remainder are adenocarcinoma. A number of rare histologic subtypes account for a small fraction of invasive cervical cancers (Box 25.1).

GROWTH PATTERN

The gross appearance of cervical cancer is quite variable. Tumours may have an exophytic or endophytic growth pattern. The exophytic type usually arises from the ectocervix and grows into a large polypoid mass. When tumours arise from within the endocervix, progressive tumour growth results in increasing distention of the cervix and formation of the classic 'barrel shaped' tumour. Tumours may be infiltrating, showing little external abnormality but having substantial growth beneath the surface of the cervix. Ulcerating lesions may also occur, resulting in large tumour craters.

PRESENTATION

Patients with early stage disease will often be asymptomatic, their disease being diagnosed after an abnormal smear. Symptoms that may occur in early stage cervical cancer include vaginal discharge and abnormal vaginal bleeding that may be postcoital, intermenstrual, cause cycle irregularity or, uncommonly, postmenopausal bleeding.

In addition to the above symptoms, patients with late-stage disease may have symptoms related to the extent and location of disease. Pelvic or back pain may occur with metastatic disease to the bony pelvis or vertebra or as a consequence of nodal disease in that region with local infiltrative spread to the bony structures. Sciatica and neuropathic

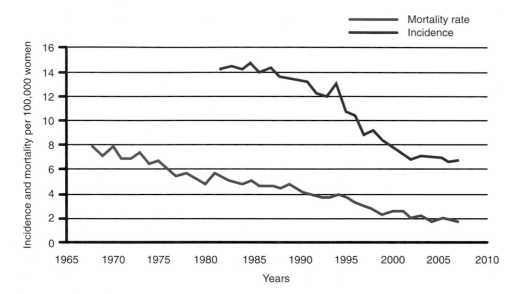

Figure 25.1
Cervical cancer incidence and mortality 1968–2007.

(Australian Institute of Health and Welfare (AIHW) 2010. ACIM (Australian Cancer Incidence and Mortality) Books. AIHW: Canberra. Australian Institute of Health and Welfare, GPO Box 570, Canberra ACT 2601)

pain occurs if there is metastatic disease to the pelvic sidewall with local infiltration of pelvic muscles and the sciatic plexus. Pelvic sidewall extension may also result in ureteric obstruction, and resultant renal failure and leg swelling may be related to either venous or lymphatic obstruction. Locally spreading disease may give rise to bladder and bowel symptoms, and in advanced disease this may be manifest as either bladder or bowel fistulae with incontinence of urine or faeces.

PATTERN OF SPREAD

The two most common spread patterns are local extension and lymphatic spread. Locally spreading disease will eventually result in extension to the vagina, parametrium laterally, bladder anteriorly and bowel posteriorly. Lymphatic spread is first to the parametrial nodes lateral to the cervix, and then to the internal iliac, obturator and external iliac nodes. Spread then occurs to the common iliac nodes and paraaortic nodes. Rarely the inguinal nodes may be involved, when disease involves the lower vagina.

While haematogenous and peritoneal spread may occur, these are most uncommon. They tend to occur in advanced stage disease and particularly with high-grade tumours of small cell or neuroendocrine types.

STAGING OF CERVICAL CANCER

The International Federation of Gynecology and Obstetrics (FIGO) is an international body whose mission is to promote the wellbeing of women and to raise the standard of practice in obstetrics and gynaecology. The FIGO Gynecologic Oncology Group reports on the results of gynaecological cancer treatment across the world. In order for the statistical information to be uniform and comparable between different centres and countries across the world, a uniform and consistent reporting system has been developed. By grouping patients into different stages according to the extent of disease detected at first presentation, outcomes can be meaningfully compared between centres across the globe.

Staging cervical cancer is unlike that for other types of gynaecological malignancies in that it is performed clinically, relying on an examination under anaesthesia, cystoscopic assessment and associated clinical investigations. Figure 25.2 illustrates the various stages of cervical malignancy.

Stage 0 comprises those cases with full-thickness involvement of the epithelium with atypical cells but with no signs of invasion into the stroma.

The diagnosis of both Stage IA1 and IA2 should be based on microscopic examination of removed

Box 25.1 Histological subtypes

Squamous cell carcinoma
- Keratinising or non-keratinising
- Verrucous
- Papillary transitional
- Lymphepithelioma-like

Other epithelial
- Adenosquamous
- Glassy cell
- Carcinomoid
- Neuroendocrine
- Small cell
- Undifferentiated

Adenocarcinoma
- Mucinous
- Endometrioid
- Clear cell
- Serous
- Mesonephric
- Well-differentiated villoglandular
- Minimal deviation (adenoma malignum)

Miscellaneous
- Melanoma
- Lymphoma
- Germ-cell type

tissue, preferably a cone biopsy, which must include the entire lesion. The depth of invasion should not be >5 mm taken from the base of the epithelial surface or the glandular components from which it originates. The second dimension — the horizontal spread — must not exceed 7 mm. Lymph vascular space involvement (LVSI) should not alter the staging but should be specifically recorded because it may affect future treatment decisions. Larger lesions should be staged as IB. As a rule, as it is impossible to clinically estimate if a cancer of the cervix has extended to the corpus, knowledge of corpus extension should not alter the assigned stage.

A patient with a tumour fixed to the pelvic wall by a short and indurated but not nodular parametrium should be allotted to Stage IIB. It is often impossible at clinical examination to decide whether a smooth and indurated parametrium is truly cancerous, or only inflammatory. Therefore, such cases should be placed in Stage III only if the parametrium is nodular to the pelvic wall or if the tumour itself extends to the pelvic wall.

The presence of hydronephrosis or non-functioning kidney resulting from stenosis of the ureter by cancer permits a case to be allotted to Stage III even if according to other findings the case should be allotted to Stage I or Stage II.

The presence of bullous oedema as such should not permit a case to be allotted to Stage IV. Ridges and furrows into the bladder wall should be interpreted as signs of submucosal involvement of the bladder if they remain fixed to the growth at recto-vaginal examination. Finding malignant cells in cytologic washings from the urinary bladder requires further histological confirmation in order to be considered for Stage IVA (Table 25.1).

PROGNOSTIC FACTORS FOR LYMPH NODE METASTASES
The risk of lymph node metastases increases with increasing stage of disease, depth of cervical invasion, infiltration of the parametrium, the presence of lymph vascular space invasion, increasing tumour grade and increasing tumour volume. Table 25.2 reports data on the risk of pelvic and paraaortic lymph node metastases according to the FIGO stage of disease.

MANAGEMENT
Management involves:
1 confirmation of the diagnosis
2 assigning a FIGO stage
3 determining spread
4 assigning treatment.

Confirmation of diagnosis
While a Pap smear may predict or suggest an invasive cancer, the diagnosis of cervical cancer must be made by cervical biopsy. A diagnostic biopsy must contain sufficient stroma to allow the pathologist to ascertain the depth of invasion. When a tumour is clinically evident, an incisional biopsy is usually sufficient. However for occult disease or when the biopsy only shows intraepithelial neoplasia or superficial invasion, a cold knife cone biopsy, aiming at excision of the lesion, is indicated.

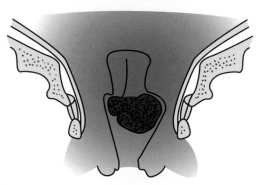

A Stage 1B: a bulbous, exophytic cervix.

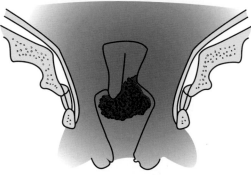

B Stage IIA: carcinoma extending into the left vaginal vault.

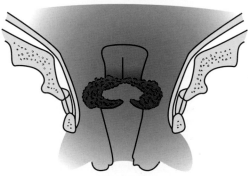

C Stage IIB: parametrium involved on both sides, but carcinoma has not invaded pelvic side wall; endocervical crater.

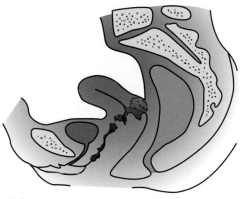

D Stage IIIA: submucosal involvement of anterior vaginal wall and small, papillomatous nodule in its lower third.

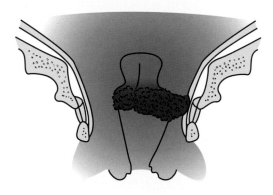

E Stage IIIB: parametrium involved on both sides at left, carcinoma has invaded pelvic wall.

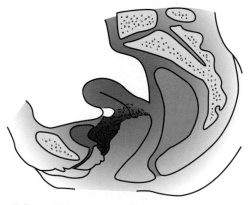

F Stage IVA: involvement of bladder.

Figure 25.2
FIGO staging.

(Adapted from: Jhingran A, Levenback C: Malignant Diseases of the Cervix. Microinvasive and invasive carcinoma: diagnosis and management. Page 765. Figure 29-10. From Petterson F, Bjorkholm E: Staging and reporting of cervical carcinoma. Semin Oncol 1982;9:289.)

Table 25.1 FIGO staging	
Stage	**Criteria**
Stage 0	**Carcinoma in situ**
Stage I	**The carcinoma is strictly confined to the cervix (extension to the corpus would be disregarded)**
IA	Invasive carcinoma which can be diagnosed only by microscopy, with deepest invasion <5 mm and largest extension <7 mm
IA1	Measured stromal invasion <3.0 mm in depth and extension of <7.0 mm
IA2	Measured stromal invasion of >3.0 mm and not >5.0 mm with an extension of not >7.0 mm
IB	Clinically visible lesions limited to the cervix uteri or preclinical cancers greater than stage IA*
IB1	Clinically visible lesions <4.0 cm in greatest dimension
IB2	Clinically visible lesion >4.0 cm in greatest dimension
Stage II	**Cervical carcinoma invades beyond the uterus, but not to the pelvic wall or to the lower third of the vagina**
IIA	Without parametrial invasion
IIA1	Clinically visible lesions <4.0 cm in greatest dimension
IIA2	Clinically visible lesion >4.0 cm in greatest dimension
IIB	With obvious parametrial invasion
Stage III	**The tumour extends to the pelvic wall and/or involves lower third of the vagina and/or causes hydronephrosis or non-functioning kidney****
IIIA	Tumour involves lower third of the vagina, with no extension to the pelvic wall
IIIB	Extension to the pelvic wall and/or hydronephrosis or non-functioning kidney
Stage IV	**The carcinoma has extended beyond the true pelvis or has involved (biopsy proven) the mucosa of the bladder or rectum. Bullous oedema does not permit a case to be allotted to stage IV**
IVA	Spread of the growth to adjacent organs
IVB	Spread to distant organs

*All macroscopically visible lesions — even with superficial invasion — are allotted to stage IB carcinomas. Invasion is limited to a measured stromal invasion with a maximal depth of 5.00 mm and a horizontal extension of not >7.00 mm. Depth of invasion should not be >5.00 mm taken from the base of the epithelium of the original tissue — superficial or glandular. The depth of invasion should always be reported in mm, even in those cases with 'early (minimal) stromal invasion' (≈1 mm).

**The involvement of vascular/lymphatic spaces should not change the stage allotment.

Table 25.2 Stage and rate of lymph node metastases

Stage	Positive pelvic nodes (%)	Positive paraaortic nodes (%)
IA1 (<3 mm)	1	0
IA2 (3–5 mm)	5	1
IB	15	2
IIA	25	10
IIB	30	20
III	45	30
IV	55	40

Assigning a FIGO stage

Since staging is clinical, an expert should perform the assessment and assign the correct stage. Only repeated examinations will allow this skill to be reliable and, given the relatively small number of cases in this country, referral to a gynaecological oncologist is mandatory. The staging must not be changed because of subsequent findings. When there is doubt as to which stage is appropriate for a given case, the earlier stage is assigned. In evaluating cervical cancer staging, only the following examinations are permitted:

1 inspection
2 palpation
3 colposcopy
4 endocervical curettage
5 hysteroscopy
6 cystoscopy
7 proctoscopy
8 intravenous urography
9 X-ray of lungs and skeleton.

Findings from additional other examinations, such as lymphangiography, arteriography, venography, laparoscopy, ultrasound, CT and MRI, are of value for planning therapy but may not be used in the clinical staging.

Determining spread

There is poor correlation between vaginal pelvic examination findings and true cervical cancer spread determined surgically. Despite the assignment of a FIGO stage, most clinicians with access to modern radiological imaging will attempt to define the true extent of disease with an abdominal–pelvic ultrasound, CT, MRI or positron emission tomography (PET), either alone or in combination. The sensitivity for CT scan in detecting positive malignant pelvic lymph nodes is 25%, and for paraaortic lymph nodes it is 34%. While PET scan may be more accurate than CT it is more expensive, and access to PET scanning is limited. PET scanning has a sensitivity of 86%; specificity of 94%, and overall accuracy of 92%. Lymphangiogram was the previous standard but is no longer performed.

Apart from the PET scan, which is a functional scan, all other imaging modalities rely on assigning positivity of lymph nodes by size criteria. However not all enlarged lymph nodes are enlarged due to cancer, with many being large due to inflammation, infection or fat infiltration. In addition, normal-size nodes may contain cancer but will not be identified and hence those positive nodes will not be detected.

For the reasons outlined above, some centres undertake formal surgical staging of their patients with cervical cancer. It must be remembered that findings from surgical staging do not change the assigned FIGO stage, but the most accurate way of defining the true extent of disease is by undertaking a formal pelvic and low paraaortic lymph node dissection and peritoneal exploration. Proponents of surgical staging would also argue that a surgical procedure removes enlarged, hypoxic and potentially radio-resistant tumour; diagnoses unsuspected peritoneal spread; enables ovarian transposition out of the intended radiation field; and ultimately allows the tailoring of radiation fields to the true extent of disease and not the implied extent as assumed from imaging. Arguments against surgical staging include the additional surgical morbidity imposed with its associated costs, and the delay such surgery would impose on the initiation of radiation therapy.

Assigning treatment

Generally, stage determines treatment. Early stage disease (Stage I–IIA) may be treated with either surgery or chemoradiation, with similar outcomes for both modalities. Locally advanced disease (Stage IIB–IVA) is treated with primary chemoradiation.

Table 25.3 Types of radical hysterectomy and indications

Type	Description	Indication
I	Extrafascial hysterectomy. The fascia of the cervix is removed with the uterus	Stage IA1
II	The uterine artery is ligated where it crosses over the ureter and the uterosacral and cardinal ligaments are divided midway towards their attachment to the sacrum and pelvic sidewall. The upper third of the vagina is resected	Stage IA2
III	The uterine artery is ligated at its origin. Uterosacral and cardinal ligaments are resected at their attachments to the sacrum and pelvic sidewall. The upper half of the vagina is resected	Stage IB-IIA
IV	The ureter is completely dissected from the vesicouterine ligament, the superior vesical artery is sacrificed and three-quarters of the vagina is resected	For selected anterior central recurrence where bladder preservation is possible
V	There is additional resection of a portion of the bladder or distal ureter with ureteral reimplantation into the bladder	For selected anterior central recurrence with involvement of the distal ureter or bladder

Disease with distant metastases (Stage IVB) is treated with systemic chemotherapy.

TREATMENT
Stage IA

For patients with stage IA1 disease with invasion less than 3 mm a conservative option of cone biopsy is acceptable in young patients. For older patients or those with concomitant gynaecological issues, a simple or type I hysterectomy is appropriate (Table 25.3). For deeper disease (>3 mm) or lymphovascular space invasion (LVSI), a modified or type II radical hysterectomy performed with staging lymphadenectomy may be considered.

Early stage disease (stage IB–IIA)
Primary surgery

Surgical options for patients with early stage IB–IIA disease may be either fertility-sparing or definitive. Fertility-sparing surgery involves either a cone biopsy or radical trachelectomy (+/− lymphadenectomy), leaving the uterine corpus and ovaries to potentially allow subsequent pregnancy (see Pregnancy below). Definitive surgery includes

performing either a type II or type III radical hysterectomy with lymphadenectomy (Table 25.3).

The advantage of primary surgery is that it is more likely to preserve ovarian and coital function. Current operative morbidity and mortality rates are very low, and such an approach allows for accurate assessment of disease extent as a formal staging lymphadenectomy is performed concurrently. There are fewer long-term bladder and bowel complications resulting from surgery compared to radiation therapy.

Prognostic factors after radical hysterectomy and pelvic lymphadenectomy are status of the lymph nodes, size of the primary tumour, depth of stromal invasion, the presence of LVSI, parametrial extension, the histologic cell type, and close or positive margins. Indications for adjuvant therapy after surgery include: positive nodes, close or positive margins, and microscopic parametrial involvement.

Primary radiation therapy

Primary radiation therapy (with concurrent chemotherapy) is the alternative to surgery for the management of early-stage cervical cancer. Therapy is delivered by a combination of teletherapy (external beam radiation therapy) and brachytherapy (internal radiation therapy). The most commonly used hypoxic cell sensitising chemotherapy agent used is weekly IV cisplatin.

The advantage of primary radiation therapy for early stage cervical cancer is that it avoids the risks and morbidity associated with surgery, including blood loss, need for blood transfusions and general anaesthesia. Hospitalisation is minimised and the survival rates are the same as for surgery. Disadvantages include an increased risk of bladder and bowel complications (stricture and fistulae), vaginal shortening and fibrosis, and premature ovarian failure.

A new modality of delivery of external beam, referred to as intensity modulated radiation therapy (IMRT), is in practice. Thousands of tiny, pencil like beams of radiation enter the body from different angles, allowing a much more accurate delivery of the radiation dose to the target while minimising the effects on surrounding tissues. Long-term results of this approach are awaited.

Locally advanced disease (Stage IIB–IVA)

Definitive surgery has little or no role in the treatment of locally advanced disease, due primarily to the fact that disease is unable to be resected with a tumour-free margin. Thus, primary chemoradiation therapy is the standard treatment. It is delivered as for early stage disease with concurrent chemotherapy (cisplatin), external beam and brachytherapy.

Recurrent disease

Despite optimal treatment, recurrences may occur, with 80% occurring within 2 years of primary treatment. Prognosis after recurrence will depend on the site of the recurrence and the ability to pursue potentially curative treatment. Overall prognosis is poor if curative therapy is not possible. Favourable prognostic factors include localised central recurrences, a disease-free interval of greater than 6 months from index treatment, tumour size less than 3 cm, and lack of pelvic sidewall fixation.

Potentially curative therapies include radiation therapy for those with previous surgery, and surgery for those previously irradiated. The triad of ureteric obstruction, sciatica and lower limb oedema imply pelvic sidewall involvement, and an attempt at surgical resection is unlikely to be successful. The incidence of local and distant recurrence varies according to FIGO stage (Table 25.4).

Table 25.4 Incidence of recurrence

Stage	Local (pelvic) (%)	Distant (%)
IA	<1	3
IB	10	16
IIA	17	31
IIB	23	26
III	42	39
IV	74	75

Recurrence may be suspected by abnormal symptoms or signs such as pain, bleeding, discharge, urinary or bowel symptoms, and on examination enlarged supraclavicular or groin nodes or a palpable vaginal mass. While abnormal symptoms or signs or new CT findings may suggest recurrence, the diagnosis must be confirmed by tissue biopsy.

PROGNOSTIC FACTORS FOR SURVIVAL

Survival depends on many factors. For early stage disease, tumour size greater than 3 cm, LVSI and deep cervical invasion are prognostic, while for advanced stage disease, nodal status, tumour size, age and performance status are prognostic. Survival according to FIGO stage is shown in Table 25.5.

SPECIAL CIRCUMSTANCES
Conservative management in the young patient

For patients desirous of retaining their reproductive potential, a non-standard approach of radical trachelectomy (removal of the cervix, parametrium with cuff of vagina, with or without staging lymphadenectomy), is undertaken with the uterine corpus sutured back to the top of the vagina. Indications for this approach are outlined in Box 25.2. To date, outcomes are similar to those achieved by standard therapy with a less than 5% recurrence rate and 2.5% death rate. The obstetric outcomes are interesting, since 60% of those that undergo this procedure do not attempt to conceive. Of those who do, 70% are successful in achieving conception, there is

Table 25.5 Survival by FIGO stage			
FIGO stage	1 year	2 year	5 year
IA1	99.8	99.5	98.7
IA2	98.2	97.7	95.9
IB1	98.7	95.1	88.0
IB2	94.8	87.8	78.8
IIA	94.1	85.6	68.8
IIB	93.3	80.7	64.7
IIIA	82.8	58.8	40.4
IIIB	81.5	62.2	43.3
IVA	56.1	35.6	19.5
IVB	45.8	23.9	15.0

Box 25.2 Indications for radical trachelectomy

- No clinical evidence of impaired fertility
- FIGO Stage IA2–IB
- Lesion size <2 cm
- Limited endocervical involvement at colposcopy
- No evidence of pelvic node metastasis
- Absence of vascular space invasion
- Adequate explanation of nature of the procedure to the patient.

a first trimester loss of 20% (the same as for any pregnancy); second trimester loss is 10% (higher than for other pregnancies), and there is a 20% preterm delivery rate (10% significantly preterm, which is higher than for other pregnancies).

Occult disease found on loop excision

When a diagnosis of occult cancer is made after a LLETZ or similar procedure, referral to a gynaecological oncologist and reassessment of the pathological sample by a gynaecological pathologist is appropriate. When the tissue sample has been removed in a single pass with clear and wide resection margins and invasion is less than 3 mm, conservative management with regular assessment may be appropriate. For all other specimens or where this is in doubt, cone biopsy to assess the lower cervix is recommended. Where invasion is greater than 3 mm, treatment should be as for stage IB.

Pregnancy

When cervical cancer is diagnosed during a pregnancy, the progress of disease is not altered by pregnancy. Depending on gestational age and after discussion with the patient about treatment risks, the cancer may be managed conservatively with observation or by limited excision. Definitive treatment can be undertaken at delivery or postpartum. A caesarean delivery would be recommended, with caesarean radical hysterectomy and pelvic lymphadenectomy the standard of care when fetal viability is reached.

Diagnosis after hysterectomy

Cervical carcinoma may be found incidentally after hysterectomy for benign disease. Management choices include further surgery with excision of the parametrium and lymphadenectomy, or chemoradiation. The decision will depend on the condition of the patient and her preference after explanation of the risks involved.

FURTHER READING

Australian Institute of Health and Welfare. Cervical screening in Australia 2006–7. Cancer series no. 47. Cat. no. CAN 43. Canberra: AIHW; 2009.

Delgado G, Bundy B, Zaino R, et al. Prospective surgical-pathologic study of disease free interval in patients with stage Ib squamous cell carcinoma of the cervix: a Gynecologic Oncology Group Study. Gynecol Oncol 1990;38:352–7.

Carter J, Fowler J, Carlson J, et al. Just how accurate is the pelvic examination? A prospective comparative study. J Reprod Med 1994;39(1):32–4.

Carter J, Carson L, Elg S, et al. Transvaginal sonography as an aid in the clinical staging of carcinoma of the cervix. J Clin Ultrasound 1992;20:283–7.

Park J, Seo S, Kang S, et al. The comparison of accuracy between PET and PET/CT for detecting lymph node metastasis in cervical cancer: prospective surgicopathologic study. J Clin Oncol 2007;25(18S):Abstract 5587.

Boughanim M, Leboulleux S, Rey A, et al. Histologic results of para-aortic lymphadenectomy in patients treated for stage IB2/II cervical cancer with negative [18F]fluorodeoxyglucose positron emission tomography scans in the para-aortic area. J Clin Oncol 2008;26(15):2558–61.

Creasman W, Zaino R, Major F, et al. Early invasive carcinoma of the cervix (3–5 mm invasion): risk factors and prognosis. A Gynecologic Oncology Group study. Am J Obstet Gynecol 1998;178:62–5.

Plante M, Gregoire J, Renaud M-C, et al. The vaginal radical trachelectomy: an update of a series of 125 cases and 106 pregnancies. Gynecologic Oncology 2011;121(2):290–7.

Carter J, Smirnova S. A personal experience with radical abdominal trachelectomy for the conservative management of invasive cervical cancer. Aust N Z J Obstet Gynaecol 2011;51(2):177–82.

Rotman M, Sedlis A, Piedmonte M, et al. A phase III randomized trial of postoperative pelvic irradiation in stage IB cervical carcinoma with poor prognostic features: follow-up of a gynecologic oncology group study. Int J Radiat Oncol Biol Phys 2006;65(1):169–76.

Sedlis A, Bundy B, Rotman M. A randomised trial of pelvic radiation therapy versus no further therapy in selected patients with stage IB carcinoma of the cervix after radical hysterectomy and pelvic lymphadenectomy. A Gynecologic Oncology Group Study. Gynecol Oncol 1999;73:177–83.

Morris M, Eifel P, Lu J, et al. Pelvic radiation with concurrent chemotherapy compared with pelvic and paraaortic radiation for high-risk cervical cancer. N Engl J Med 1999;340(15):1137–43.

Rose PG, Ali S, Watkins E, et al. Long-term follow-up of a randomized trial comparing concurrent single agent cisplatin, cisplatin-based combination chemotherapy, or hydroxyurea during pelvic irradiation for locally advanced cervical cancer: a Gynecologic Oncology Group Study. J Clin Oncol 2007;25(19):2804–10.

Carter J. Prognostic factors in advanced gynaecological cancer. In: Glare P, Nicholas A, Christakis NA, editors. Prognosis in advanced cancer. Oxford, UK: Oxford University Press; 2009.

Gien LT, Covens A. Fertility-sparing options for early stage cervical cancer. Gynecologic Oncology 2010;117(2):350–7.

MCQS

Select the correct answer.

1   Which of the following statements regarding cervical cancer is correct?

   A   The incidence of cervical cancer has been declining over the past 2–3 decades.
   B   Adenocarcinoma is the most common histological type.
   C   Cervical tumours only have an exophytic growth pattern.
   D   Patients with early-stage disease will often present with abnormal vaginal bleeding.
   E   The inguinal lymph nodes are frequently involved in cervical cancer.

2   Which of the following statements regarding staging for cervical cancer is correct?

   A   Cervical cancer, unlike other gynaecological cancers, is surgically staged.
   B   Ultrasound and CT scanning are used in assigning a FIGO stage.
   C   Lymphatic spread and local extension are the two most common spread patterns.
   D   An enlarged paraaortic lymph node on CT scan indicates stage IV disease.
   E   A PET scan should be used to define the size of nodes involved.

3   Which of the following regarding treatment for cervical cancer is correct?

   A   A radical hysterectomy does not allow preservation of ovarian and coital function.
   B   Early and/or small cancers may be treated conservatively in young women.
   C   A radical hysterectomy may involve removal of the bladder and bowel.
   D   Surgery for early stage cervical cancer has an improved survival compared to radiation therapy.
   E   Removal of the ovaries is essential for improved survival.

4   With respect to treatment of cervical cancer, which of the following is correct?

   A   Chemotherapy is usually given in conjunction with radiation therapy.
   B   The advantage of radiation therapy is it has little in the way of long-term complications.
   C   Chemotherapy is an effective treatment for advanced cervical cancer.
   D   Central pelvic recurrence after radiation is unlikely to be cured by surgery.
   E   A radical trachelectomy should be considered in a young woman with a 3 cm cervical lesion.

OSCE

Jane, a 46-year-old woman, is referred to you with a Pap smear predicting a squamous cervical cancer. What are the historical and examination features that would be important to evaluate in this patient? What further investigations are required for Jane?

Chapter 26

Uterine cancer

Yee Leung

KEY POINTS

The incidence of endometrial cancer is increasing.

Postmenopausal bleeding is the most common presentation for endometrial cancer, however endometrial cancer is not the most common cause of postmenopausal bleeding.

Investigations should include (preferably transvaginal) ultrasound and histological assessment of the endometrium.

Once diagnosed, management should be in conjunction with a specialist gynaecological oncologist and is frequently surgical.

Uterine sarcomas are uncommon and are often associated with a poor outcome.

INTRODUCTION

Uterine cancer comprises two main groups: endometrial cancer, and malignancy of the myometrium or stroma — the sarcomas. Endometrial cancer is the most common gynaecologic cancer in Australia. Due to a number of factors including rising BMI among women, the rate of endometrial cancer is increasing, but it remains one type of cancer with a good prognosis, particularly when detected early. Postmenopausal bleeding (PMB) is a primary feature of this disease, and while not the most common cause of PMB, endometrial cancer is certainly the most important. The sarcomas are much less common, have a variable and often late presentation, and generally have a poor prognosis.

EPIDEMIOLOGY

In 2011 approximately 115 000 new cancer cases were registered in Australia and uterine cancer accounted for just over 2000 of these new cases. In the United States, more than 40 000 new cases of uterine cancer were diagnosed in 2005.

The incidence of endometrial cancer is increasing, with the 60–70 year age group at greatest risk. The mortality rate has been stable over the last 25 years and rises with the patient's age. As most endometrial cancers are diagnosed while the cancer is confined to the uterus, the overall 5-year survival rate is 82.1%.

There are racial and geographic variations in the incidence of endometrial cancer. The highest-risk groups are those living in more developed countries and of Caucasian background. However African-American women are more likely to die from this cancer than their Caucasian counterparts. The cause of the observed variation is unclear. Figure 26.1 indicates uterine cancer incidence and mortality rates.

The risk of developing endometrial cancer by age 75 is 1 in 69. Obesity is a recognised risk factor, and is thought to be due to higher circulating levels of insulin-like growth factor 1 (IGF-1) and endogenous oestrogen from synthesis in peripheral

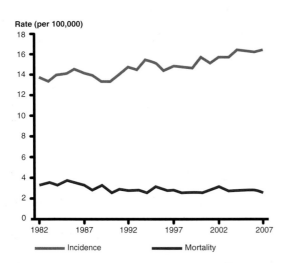

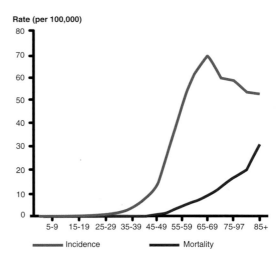

Uterine cancer incidence and mortality rates[b] 1982–2007

Uterine cancer incidence and mortality rates[c] by age at diagnosis, 2007

(a) The estimates were based on incidence/mortality data for 1998 to 2007.

(b) The rates were age-standardised to the Australian population as at 30 June 2001 and are expressed per 100,000 population.

(c) The rates shown are age-specific rates.

Figure 26.1
Uterine cancer incidence and mortality rates.

(AIHW Australian Cancer Database; AIHW National Mortality Database)

adipose tissue. It is estimated that women with a BMI >25 have a 2–3-fold increased risk of endometrial cancer, and this may be a contributing factor for the rising incidence of uterine cancer in Australia. These and other risk factors are summarised in Table 26.1.

The oral contraceptive pill offers a protective effect against endometrial cancer. Greater protection is observed with a longer duration of OCP use and among nulliparous women.

A detailed family history can be informative in women with endometrial cancer. Patients with a germ-line mutation (hereditary non-polyposis colorectal cancer or Lynch syndrome) have a lifetime risk of 16–54% for endometrial cancer, 12–48% for colorectal cancer and 1–24% for ovarian cancer. The mean age of presentation for this genetic type of endometrial cancer is 47 years, but the majority of these cases occur after the age of 40. Counselling for the risk of other cancers in the same woman and advice for family members is appropriate.

CLINICAL PRESENTATION
Endometrial cancer is more likely to occur in the postmenopausal woman. The typical presentation is PMB or an abnormal discharge. Occasionally

endometrial cancer may be suspected in an asymptomatic woman found to have abnormal glandular cells on routine Pap smear, or at the time of a hysterectomy for a prolapse.

In the premenopausal woman, a history of abnormal vaginal bleeding (intermenstrual bleeding, menorrhagia, cycle irregularity) may be the presenting complaint for an endometrial cancer. However, endometrial cancer is not a common diagnosis in a premenopausal woman, with 90% of new cases of endometrial cancer diagnosed in women 50 years and older.

In premenopausal women, a high index of suspicion should be adopted in patients with a history of PCOS. PCOS may be associated with obesity, insulin resistance and a hyper-oestrogenic state. The clinical significance of PCOS is the development of endometrial hyperplasia from the relative excess of circulating oestrogens. The presence of endometrial hyperplasia with cytological atypia may indicate a higher risk of progression to or the presence of concurrent endometrial cancer. The diagnosis of atypical endometrial hyperplasia (AEH) on endometrial biopsy is associated with a high inter-observer variability, and should be treated with caution given that cancer may coexist. This finding should always

Table 26.1 Risk factors for endometrial cancer

Factors influencing risk	Estimated relative risk
Old age	2–3
Caucasian	2
Nulliparity	3
History of infertility	2–3
Early age of menarche	1.5–3
Late age of menopause	2–3
Polycystic ovarian syndrome (PCOS)	>5
Obesity	2–5
Long-term combined oral contraceptive use	0.3–0.5
Cigarette smoking	0.5
Long-term unopposed oestrogen use	10–20
Long-term tamoxifen use	3–7
Hereditary non-polyposis colorectal cancer (HNPCC)	16–54% lifetime risk

Table adapted from Gershenson DM, McGuire WP, Gore M, Quinn MA, Thomas G, editors. *Gynecologic cancer: controversies in management.* 3rd ed. London/US: Elsevier Health Sciences: 2004.

raise the suspicion of a malignancy, with specialist review (both gynaecological oncologist and/or gynaecological pathologist) recommended.

Clinical presentations of endometrial cancer can be summarised as:
• postmenopausal bleeding
• abnormal vaginal bleeding (intermenstrual bleeding, menorrhagia, cycle irregularity, postcoital bleeding)
• incidental finding at hysterectomy
• incidental finding on Pap smear
• presence of distant metastases (pulmonary metastases).

DIAGNOSIS

There is no evidence that screening by pelvic or transvaginal ultrasound or endometrial sampling reduces the mortality from endometrial cancer in the asymptomatic general population, and such screening cannot be recommended. The use of ultrasound to screen asymptomatic women on tamoxifen is associated with a 1% positive predictive value for cancer, and therefore routine screening in this population is not recommended. Figure 26.2 demonstrates a transvaginal ultrasound of a woman with postmenopausal bleeding and an undiagnosed intrauterine polyp. In Figure 26.3, a hysteroscopic view of a malignancy of the endometrium can be seen.

Women with a proven or suspected germ-line mutation (Lynch syndrome/HNPCC) are at high risk. Families with Lynch syndrome are at risk of colorectal, endometrial and ovarian cancer. The American Cancer Society recommends these patients should consider annual endometrial sampling from the age of 35 years, but the estimated cumulative risk for endometrial cancer before the age of 40 in this group is less than 2%. The patient needs to be informed of the risks associated with endometrial sampling (unable to complete the procedure, insufficient sample obtained, pain, bleeding, uterine perforation, and infection of the endometrium). A postmenopausal woman with asymptomatic endometrial thickening (defined as >5 mm) does not require endometrial sampling. However each patient should be assessed on an individual basis, with risk factors, family history and patient concerns considered.

The use of ultrasound in conjunction with the clinical information can triage patients into low- and high-risk groups. It is important to recognise that the diagnosis of endometrial cancer can only be made histologically, and not on an ultrasound. Tissue may be obtained by an outpatient endometrial sample (pipelle) or under anaesthetic using cervical dilatation and endometrial curettage, with or without a hysteroscopy.

When the diagnosis of endometrial cancer has been confirmed, the principles of management of a patient with a newly diagnosed cancer should be followed:

1 Confirmation of diagnosis. Review of the histopathology by a gynaecological pathologist at a multidisciplinary clinico-pathological meeting is recommended.

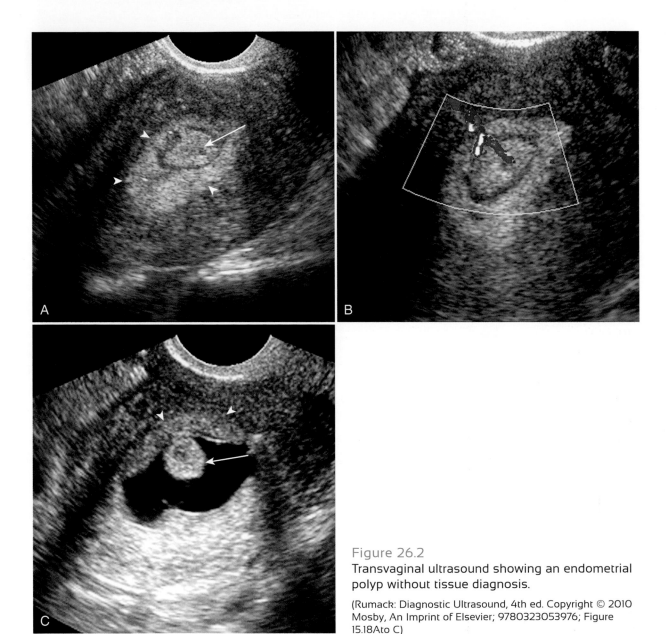

Figure 26.2
Transvaginal ultrasound showing an endometrial polyp without tissue diagnosis.

(Rumack: Diagnostic Ultrasound, 4th ed. Copyright © 2010 Mosby, An Imprint of Elsevier; 9780323053976; Figure 15.18A to C)

2 Investigate for evidence of spread. Endometrial cancer typically spreads locally to the cervix and vagina, through the myometrium, into the parametrium and adnexa and via the lymphatics to loco-regional lymph nodes (pelvic and paraaortic). In higher risk subtypes, transperitoneal (parietal peritoneum, omentum) and haematogenous (pulmonary, liver parenchyma, bone) metastases can also occur. Locally advanced uterine cancers can invade the bladder and the bowel. The metastatic screen should therefore include imaging of the chest (chest X-ray or CT), abdomen and pelvis (CT or MRI) to exclude pulmonary metastases and assess for retroperitoneal lymphadenopathy. It is important to ensure that treatment is not unduly delayed as a result of organising these tests. Pelvic MRI may assist preoperative assessment of myoinvasion, particularly in the younger woman considering fertility preservation.

3 Cancer staging attempts to categorise the extent of cancer with reference to the primary site and whether the cancer has spread beyond the primary site. Staging may be clinical (when one cannot remove the primary or the metastases) or surgical (according to

the final histopathological assessment of all surgical specimens). Endometrial cancer is surgically staged, using the International Federation of Gynecology and Obstetrics (FIGO) 2009 system. Figure 26.4 shows the FIGO staging for endometrial cancer.

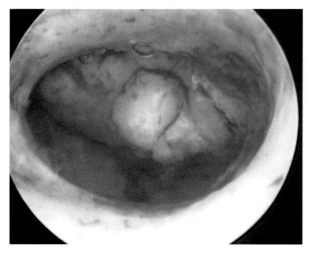

Figure 26.3
Hysteroscopic view of vascular polyp with irregular surface highly suspicious of endometrial cancer.

(Courtesy of Dr Yee Leung.)

HISTOLOGIC TYPES

Uterine cancer includes those arising in the endometrial lining (endometrial carcinoma) — these make up about 95% of all uterine cancers — and those arising in the uterine stroma or myometrial cells (uterine sarcomas).

Although endometrial cancer is associated with a good prognosis, there is a wide spectrum of subtypes within this group that are associated with a greater potential for progression and may have worse clinical outcomes. Endometrioid and mucinous adenocarcinomas are generally associated with a better prognosis than the other subtypes. (See Table 26.2.) Endometrial cancers can also display a mixed pattern of subtypes.

Endometrial cancers are also graded histologically using light microscopy according to the architectural appearance and an assessment of the nuclear morphology. Grade 1 and 2 (well-differentiated and moderately differentiated) cancers have a better prognosis than Grade 3 cancers. There is significant inter-observer variability in assessing tumour grade, and a specialist gynaecological pathologist is recommended.

This difference in clinical outcomes with different clinical presentations and tumour grades was

Stage I*	Tumour confined to the corpus uteri
IA*	No or less than half myometrial invasion
IB*	Invasion equal to or more than half of the myometrium
Stage II*	Tumour invades cervical stroma, but does not extend beyond the uterus**
Stage III*	Local and/or regional spread of the tumour
IIIA*	Tumour invades the serosa of the corpus uteri and/or adnexa#
IIIB*	Vaginal and/or parametrial involvement#
IIIC*	Metastases to pelvic and/or paraaortic lymph nodes#
IIIC1*	Positive pelvic nodes
IIIC2*	Positive paraaortic lymph nodes with or without positive pelvic lymph nodes
Stage IV*	Tumour invades bladder and/or bowel mucosa, and/or distant metastases
IVA*	Tumour invasion of bladder and/or bowel mucosa
IVB*	Distant metastases, including intraabdominal metastases and/or inguinal lymph nodes

* Either G1, G2, or G3
** Endocervical glandular involvement only should be considered at Stage I and no longer at Stage II
\# Positive cytology has to be reported separately without changing the stage

Figure 26.4
FIGO staging of endometrial carcinoma.

(FIGO website.)

Table 26.2 Histological subtypes of endometrial cancer

Histological subtypes	Prognosis
Endometrioid adenocarcinoma	Favourable
Mucinous adenocarcinoma	Favourable
Uterine papillary serous carcinoma	Poorer
Clear cell carcinoma	Poorer
Undifferentiated or de-differentiated carcinoma, including unusual neuroendocrine carcinoma	Poorer
Carcinosarcoma	Poorer

Table 26.3 Key features of type 1 and type 2 endometrial cancers

Factor assessed	Type 1	Type 2
Fertility	Anovulatory/ subfertile	No disturbance
Obesity	Present	Absent
Diabetes mellitus	Present	Absent
Background endometrium	Endometrial hyperplasia	No changes
Tumour grade	Grade 1 or 2	Grade 3
Myoinvasion	Superficial	Deep
Lymph node metastases risk	Low	High
Sensitivity to progestogens	High	Low
Associated cancers	Ovary, breast, colon	None identified
Prognosis	Favourable	Poor

Adapted from Bokhman 1983.

first observed in 1983. Endometrial cancers were categorised into two pathogenetic types — denoted types 1 and 2. The differences in these subtypes can be seen in Table 26.3.

Subsequent molecular genetic profiling has substantiated this clinical observation. Type 1 endometrial cancers tend to be oestrogen-related endometrioid adenocarcinomas, with defects in DNA-mismatch repair and mutations in PTEN, K-ras and beta-catenin. Type 2 endometrial cancers tend to be non-oestrogen-related, non-endometrioid adenocarcinomas, aneuploid and have p53 mutations.

Uterine carcinosarcomas (malignant mixed Müllerian tumours) were initially classified as a sarcoma (cancer arising from the uterine stroma). However it is becoming accepted that this poor prognostic subtype is a form of Type 2 endometrial cancer displaying epithelial mesenchymal transition. This is a process in which epithelial cells transform to assume a mesenchymal cell phenotype and acquire invasive properties. Uterine carcinosarcomas are associated with a previous exposure to pelvic radiation therapy. These tumours can present as large polypoid tumours within the endometrial cavity.

Uterine sarcomas that arise in the myometrial cells of the uterus are clinically more aggressive and are associated with a poorer prognosis. Patients with a uterine leiomyosarcoma subtype have an overall 5-year survival of 15–25%. The pattern of spread is frequently via the haematogenous route to the lungs. These sarcomas tend to occur in younger women with a median age of 50. The differential diagnosis is that of a benign myomatous uterus. The differentiation is often difficult, and in a patient with a rapidly enlarging myoma or radiological features showing necrosis or haemorrhage, a high index of suspicion should be maintained, although the diagnosis is frequently only made following removal of the uterus.

Uterine sarcomas that arise in the stroma have a variable prognosis depending on the grade of the sarcoma. These have been classified as endometrial stromal nodule, low-grade endometrial stromal sarcoma (LGESS), and high-grade endometrial stromal sarcoma (HGESS). Endometrial stromal nodules tend to be low-grade indolent tumours found incidentally in hysterectomy specimens.

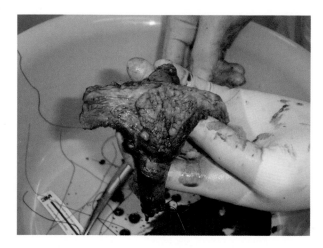

Figure 26.5
Opened hysterectomy specimen of endometrial cancer showing an enlarged uterus with extensive tumour replacing the native endometrium and infiltrating into the myometrium (deep myoinvasion).

(Courtesy of Dr Yee Leung.)

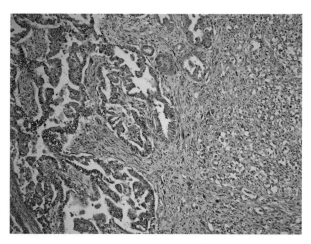

Figure 26.6
Histopathology of uterine carcinosarcoma (HE stain) showing malignant epithelial (left) and stromal elements (right).

(Reproduced with permission from Clinical Professor Colin Stewart.)

LGESS is associated with a favourable prognosis, as it tends to present at an early stage. These tumours also respond to progestogen therapy. HGESS is associated with a comparatively poorer prognosis and patients are more likely to have metastatic disease at presentation.

Figures 26.5 and 26.6 show the macroscopic and microscopic features of an endometrial cancer. The hysterectomy specimen is shown after bisection, revealing the endometrial cavity.

MANAGEMENT

The primary surgical management for endometrial cancer is to perform a total hysterectomy and bilateral salpingo-oophorectomy with or without pelvic and paraaortic lymphadenectomy. The hysterectomy may be done abdominally or laparoscopically, depending on the skill set of the surgeon; however, if the uterus is enlarged, it cannot be morcellated at the time of a laparoscopic procedure and the abdominal route is preferred in this setting. A total laparoscopic hysterectomy is associated with a significant reduction in postoperative serious adverse events and a faster recovery and an improved quality of life up to 6 months compared to a total abdominal hysterectomy for the primary surgical management of endometrial cancer.

The hysterectomy removes the primary malignant site and allows histopathological assessment of specific prognostic factors such as cancer grade, depth of myoinvasion, presence of lymphovascular invasion and cervical stromal involvement. The histopathological information obtained may be used to categorise patients with early endometrial cancer into low-risk, moderate-risk and high-risk groups for recurrent disease and prognosis.

Removal of the fallopian tubes and ovaries allows histopathological assessment for metastases or synchronous tumours of the ovaries. The presence of metastases in the adnexa will change the stage and therefore provide prognostic information. The ovaries may have:

- a primary hormone-secreting tumour resulting in high endogenous oestrogen levels (granulosa cell tumour, thecoma)
- metastases from the primary endometrial cancer in up to 5% of presumed early stage cancer
- a synchronous ovarian cancer (Lynch syndrome).

Patients with positive retroperitoneal lymph node(s) at the time of primary surgery are at high risk of recurrent disease. However the rate of lymph node metastases in low-risk endometrial cancers is only 3–5%. The role of lymphadenectomy in the management of endometrial cancer is controversial, with proponents and opponents for concurrent, routine retroperitoneal lymphadenectomy. The current data do not demonstrate any effect of lymphadenectomy on overall survival or disease-free interval. Using preoperative imaging (CT, PET, MRI) to predict myoinvasion, tumour volume and cervical involvement, as well as intraoperative assessment of the hysterectomy specimen, current research aims to identify patients at highest risk of regional lymph node metastases.

The primary surgical procedure will depend on the individual patient, tumour, and external factors to optimise outcome. There may be consideration of non-surgical management such as fertility sparing treatment in the young, nulligravid woman or women with significant comorbidities. Appropriate assessment and counselling is essential and referral to a gynaecological oncologist who is part of a multidisciplinary team is highly recommended for holistic care.

For the young woman desirous of fertility, a limited trial of progestogen, either as high-dose oral progesterone or by the progestogen intrauterine contraceptive system (Mirena) may be considered. Regular endometrial sampling is mandatory to monitor response to the therapy when conservative medical treatment is adopted. Should a hysterectomy be required due to failure of conservative medical therapy, assessment of ovarian reserve and consideration of ovarian conservation should be discussed in conjunction with a specialist unit in reproductive care.

Tumour factors requiring consideration of management approach include histologic type and association with germ-line mutations. High-risk tumour features generally require more extensive surgical staging according to the recognised pattern of spread of that histologic subtype. Lymphadenectomy provides prognostic information that will subsequently guide decision-making for postoperative adjuvant therapy. A significant risk from lymphadenectomy is irreversible leg lymphoedema that requires long-term management.

Nomograms have been developed to help predict the risk of loco-regional and distant recurrence, and overall survival. These mathematical models may help with tailoring adjuvant therapy (use of radiation with or without chemotherapy), although to date no studies have reported improved outcomes using nomograms for this purpose.

Patients presenting with advanced stage disease have a poorer prognosis despite radical surgery and adjuvant postoperative chemotherapy. Those managed in a multidisciplinary setting with a gynaecological oncologist have a statistically significant advantage in disease-specific survival compared to patients managed by a community gynaecologist (72% compared with 64%, $p < 0.001$).

FOLLOW-UP

Follow-up of cancer patients enables surveillance, and permits early detection of recurrent disease and collection of data on outcomes. There is no universally accepted follow-up protocol for patients with endometrial cancer since this is a diverse disease with a variable pattern of spread and prognosis. Overall, the risk of recurrence is 13%, but for low-risk disease the recurrence rate is only 3%. Almost all recurrences are symptomatic at diagnosis and clinical examination may detect 5–33% of recurrences; vaginal vault cytology may detect 0–4% of recurrences; and imaging/CA 125 may detect 0–21% of recurrences.

Survival following cancer recurrence is dependent on site, with disease in the vaginal vault associated with a 73% survival while distant spread has a survival of only 8%. A metastatic screen, ideally with a CT/PET scan, should be performed to exclude disease at other sites if a recurrence is diagnosed.

In 2011, the Society of Gynecologic Oncologists published evidence-based recommendations on follow-up for patients with endometrial cancer and these are listed in the further reading.

For gynaecologic cancers, psychosexual issues are very important and should be addressed and discussed by a skilled member of the multidisciplinary team. A link is provided to an online educational module that addresses these issues. When managing women with cancer, above all, it is vital to individualise the management plan to the patient, ascertain if the treatment intent is curative or palliative, and always impart an empathetic and caring approach.

FURTHER READING

Online educational module developed by Cancer Australia focusing on the psychosexual care of women affected by gynaecologic cancer. http://modules.cancerlearning.gov.au/psgc/.

Onine resource developed by Cancer Australia on endometrial cancer. http://www.canceraustralia.gov.au/search/apachesolr_search/endometrial%20cancer.

Diagnostic Guide for assessing post menopausal women with vaginal bleeding developed by Cancer Australia. http://canceraustralia.gov.au/sites/default/files/publications/ncgc-vaginal-bleeding-flowcharts-march-20111_504af02038614.pdf.

Diagnostic Guide for assessing premenopausal and perimenopausal women with abnormal vaginal bleeding developed by Cancer Australia. http://canceraustralia.gov.au/sites/default/files/publications/ncgc-vaginal-bleeding-flowcharts-march-20111_504af02038614.pdf.

AIHW, AACR & NCSG: Ian McDermid. Cancer incidence projections, Australia 2002 to 2011. Canberra: Australian Institute of Health and Welfare (AIHW), Australasian Association of Cancer Registries (AACR) and the National Cancer Strategies Group (NCSG). Canberra: AIHW; 2005.

ASTEC Writing Committee. Efficacy of systemic pelvic lymphadenectomy in endometrial cancer (MRC ASTEC trial): a randomised study. Lancet 2009;373:125–36.

Bonadona V, Bonaiti B, Olschwang S, et al. Cancer risks associated with germline mutations in MLH1, MSH2, and MSH6 genes in Lynch Syndrome. JAMA 2011;305(22):2304–10.

Creasman W. Revised FIGO staging for carcinoma of the endometrium. Int J Gynecol Obstet 2009;105:109.

Janda M, Gebski V, Brand A, et al. Quality of life after total laparoscopic hysterectomy versus total abdominal hysterectomy for stage 1 endometrial cancer (LACE): a randomised trial. Lancet Oncol 2010;11:772–80.

Kondalsamy-Chennakesavan S, Yu C, Kattan M, et al. Nomograms to predict five-year freedom from relapse and overall survival after surgery for endometrial cancer. Gynecol Oncol 2010;116(3):S7.

Leath 3rd CA, Huh WK, Hyde Jr J, et al. A multi-institutional review of outcomes of endometrial stromal sarcoma. Gynecol Oncol 2007;105(3):630–4. epub 2007 Feb 23.

May K, Dickinson HO, Kehoe S, et al. Lymphadenectomy for the management of endometrial cancer. Cochrane Database of Systematic Reviews 2010;1. Article ID CD007585.

SOGC Clinical Practice Guideline: Asymptomatic endometrial thickening. JOGC 2010;249:990–9.

Trimble CL, Kauderer J, Zaino R, et al. Concurrent endometrial carcinoma in women with a biopsy diagnosis of atypical endometrial hyperplasia: a Gynecologic Oncology Group study. Cancer 2006;106(4):812–19.

World Cancer research Fund and American Institute for Cancer Research. Food, nutrition, physical activity and prevention of cancer: a global perspective. Washington DC: AICR; 2007.

MCQS

Select the correct answer.

1   Which of the following combinations are recognised risk factors for developing endometrial cancer?

   A   obesity, nulliparity, HNPCC
   B   obesity, BRCA-1 mutation, cigarette smoking
   C   obesity, HNPCC, OCP use
   D   HNPCC, cigarette smoking, OCP use
   E   BRCA-1 mutation, OCP use, cigarette smoking

2   The standard primary surgical management of low-risk endometrial cancer is:

   A   hysterectomy only
   B   hysterectomy and bilateral salpingo-oophorectomy
   C   hysterectomy, bilateral salpingo-oophorectomy and pelvic lymphadenectomy
   D   hysterectomy, lymphadenectomy and omentectomy
   E   hysterectomy, bilateral salpingo-ophorectomy and omentectomy

3   A 60-year-old nulligravid, obese woman presents with a 4-month history of intermittent vaginal bleeding. She has been on continuous combined hormone replacement therapy since menopause 9 years ago. Pap smear performed 18 months ago was normal. Speculum examination reveals blood at the external os; otherwise the cervix appeared healthy. Which of the following is likely to arrive at the most accurate diagnosis?

   A   pipelle sampling and Pap smear
   B   Pap smear and endocervical curettage
   C   CA 125, CEA and dilation and curettage
   D   Pap smear and colposcopy
   E   hysteroscopy and endometrial biopsy

OSCE

You are seeing Georgina, a 55-year-old woman who has a 2-week history of postmenopausal bleeding. She has a history of non-insulin dependent diabetes mellitus (NIDDM) on oral hypoglycaemic medication and has a BMI of 41 kg/m^2. Her dark red vaginal bleeding is not heavy but requires several pad changes a day.

Describe the salient information on history and examination would you seek from this woman. What investigations would you recommend in this situation? Diagnosis of a Grade 1 endometrioid adenocarcinoma of the uterine corpus is confirmed on histologic review. Describe management that is likely in this setting.

Chapter 27

Cancer of the ovary

Michael Quinn

KEY POINTS

Ovarian cancer most frequently presents late in the disease course, and has a high mortality rate.

Genetics is the single most important risk factor for development of disease.

There is no adequate screening program for ovarian cancer.

Prophylactic ovarian removal is appropriate in those genetically at risk.

Investigations may include serology and imaging.

Staging is surgical and follows a FIGO classification system.

Combination surgery and chemotherapy is the mainstay of treatment of ovarian cancer.

INTRODUCTION

Cancer of the ovary occurs in approximately 1200 Australian women annually, and sadly, approximately two-thirds of these women are destined to die from the disease, a figure that has not substantially improved in the last 25 years despite the advent of more radical surgery and more effective cytotoxic chemotherapy. This mortality rate is largely due to the fact that nearly 75% of women who have ovarian cancer present with advanced disease and that although chemotherapy is effective in inducing remission, resistance to chemotherapy is extremely common. A number of strategies are currently being evaluated to try and overcome this. The peak age incidence of epithelial ovarian cancer is the sixth decade, but for germ cell tumours (chapter 22), the median age is 19 years.

AETIOLOGY OF OVARIAN CANCER AND RISK FACTORS

Most of the risk factors associated with epithelial ovarian cancer relate to ovulation, with increasing numbers of ovulations increasing risk. Conversely, lack of ovulation, as occurs for instance in multiparity, breastfeeding and prolonged use of the oral contraceptive pill, are protective against malignancy. The original pathogenetic concept was that disruption of the surface epithelium at the time of ovulation allows epithelial inclusion cysts to develop inside the ovarian substance. These tissues eventually undergo dysplastic change and subsequently malignancy develops.

This concept has recently been scrutinised and largely disproved by the startling observation that in women with inherited mutations of the BRCA-1 and 2 gene where the adnexa are removed prophylactically, at least 90% of the fimbrial ends of fallopian tubes contain serous in-situ cancers which express p53. Figure 27.1 is a series of photomicrographs of various staining patterns that highlights p53. The current hypothesis now relates to the likelihood that at the time of ovulation these in-situ cells actually implant on the ovulatory site and

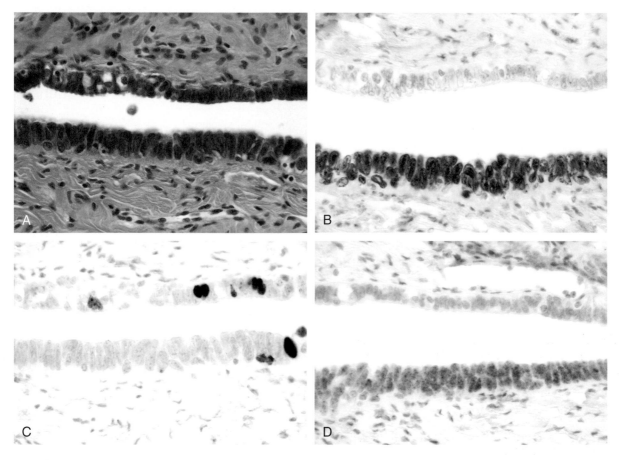

Figure 27.1
A: The p53 signature, B: haematoxylin and eosin (H&E), C: p53, and, D: H2AX.

(From Lee Y, Miron A, Drapkin R, et al. A candidate precursor to serous carcinoma that originates in the distal fallopian tube. J Pathol 2007;211:26–35, with permission. Crum: Diagnostic Gynecologic and Obstetric Pathology, 2nd ed. 9781437707649 Figure 24.18A to D Copyright © 2011 Saunders, An Imprint of Elsevier.)

become incorporated into the ovarian substance and eventually become malignant. This accounts for the development of the most common histological subtype of ovarian cancer, serous carcinoma. It is now believed that endometrioid ovarian carcinoma emanates from the endometrium spilling through the tubes into the peritoneal cavity and implanting, either becoming malignant de novo or via endometriosis formation. Clear cell ovarian cancer is thought to occur in a similar manner. Finally, mucinous ovarian cancer is considered almost certainly to derive from metastatic disease, particularly stomach, pancreas and large bowel, but also perhaps from mucinous endocervical type epithelium.

The single most important risk factor for the development of the disease is family history.

Approximately 50% of women with a BRCA-1 and 20% with a BRCA-2 mutation will eventually develop the disease. Likewise, 10% of women with hereditary non-polyposis colorectal cancer (HNPCC) will also suffer with an ovarian cancer due to mismatch repair gene defects.

For these women prophylactic bilateral salpingo-oophorectomy is recommended once childbearing is complete. With the observation however that the fallopian ends of the tubes may be important in the genesis of the disease, there will soon be studies looking at bilateral salpingectomy as an option in the premenopausal period, followed by postmenopausal oophorectomy. Figure 27.2 shows the view of ovarian cancer at laparotomy with cystic ovarian lesions seen bilaterally.

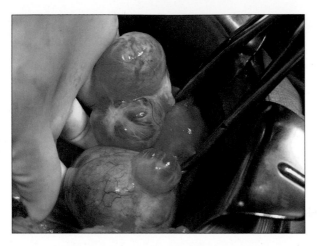

Figure 27.2
Photograph of gross stage IB ovarian cancer.
The normal uterus sits between the clamps with
both ovaries having multilocular and irregular
cystic masses.

(Bristow & Armstrong: Ovarian Cancer–Early Diagnosis and
Treatment of Cancer Series. 9781416046851; Figure 8.3
Copyright © 2009 Saunders, An Imprint of Elsevier)

Table 27.1 Most frequent presenting symptoms of ovarian cancer	
Symptom	Relative frequency
Abdominal swelling/ bloating	++++
Abdominal pain	+++
Dyspepsia	++
Urinary frequency	++
Weight change	+
Irregular bleeding	+

EPITHELIAL OVARIAN CANCERS

Traditionally epithelial ovarian cancers have been
divided into subtypes according to histology, the
most common being serous, then in descending
frequency endometrioid, mucinous, clear cell, and
Brenner. This classification has been challenged by
recent studies that use genetic arrays and have
depicted four different types of ovarian malignancy
independent of histology:

1 differentiated
2 immuno-reactive
3 mesenchymal
4 proliferative tumours.

It would appear that there is currently a transitional period of classification and tumour morphology and histology may no longer be the basis for
treatment or clinical trials, with the new genetic
tumour arrays potentially being used to assess
response to treatment and ultimately, prognosis.

CLINICAL PRESENTATION

Since the symptomatology related to ovarian malignancy is very non-specific, most women will only
present once symptoms are persistent and it is clear
that with these symptoms the disease is usually
advanced. There has been no screening test

developed to date that has been reported to reduce
the mortality of the disease, and this includes both
routine screening with ultrasound and the CA 125
level.

Table 27.1 depicts the multitude of non-specific
symptoms associated with ovarian malignancy.

With advanced disease, ascites can be a major
feature and indeed, since the tumour is usually
present throughout the peritoneal cavity involving
both parietal and visceral surfaces, obstruction of
both large and small bowel may eventuate. The
surface of the liver is commonly involved, although
rarely the liver parenchyma. Diaphragmatic disease
is frequent and pleural effusions are the most
common cause of stage IV malignancy (Table 27.2).
In Figure 27.3, CT images are shown depicting
findings of metastatic ovarian cancer as it is seen in
different body regions.

As for other types of gynaecological malignancy,
ovarian cancer has a FIGO staging system. This is
a surgical staging system that is reproduced in
Table 27.2.

MANAGEMENT

Women who present with non-specific symptoms
as outlined above should have a full history, general
abdominal and pelvic examination undertaken. Particular attention should be given to examining for
enlarged lymph nodes in the neck and groins, the
presence or absence of shifting dullness which
would denote ascites, the presence of an omental

Table 27.2 FIGO staging of ovarian cancer

Stage	Characteristics
Stage I	**Limited to the ovaries**
IA	Limited to ovary, negative washings and no surface disease
IB	Involves both ovaries, negative washings and no surface disease
IC	IA or IB with capsular rupture, ascites or positive washings
Stage II	**Involves one or both ovaries with extension to pelvis**
IIA	Extension to uterus and/or tubes
IIB	Extension to other pelvic structures
IIC	IIA or IIB associated with capsular rupture, ascites or positive washings
Stage III	**Involves one or both ovaries with disease outside pelvis or positive retroperitoneal or inguinal nodes**
IIIA	Microscopic seeding to abdominal peritoneal surfaces, negative lymph nodes
IIIB	Abdominal implants less than 2 cm, negative lymph nodes
IIIC	Abdominal implants greater than 2 cm, or positive lymph nodes
Stage IV	**Involves one or both ovaries with distant metastases or liver parenchymal disease. Pleural effusions must be confirmed with positive cytology.**

cake of tumour which is ballotable behind the umbilicus, and the presence of a 'Sister Joseph's nodule' (Figure 27.4) which is due to metastatic disease spreading along the urachus to the under surface of the umbilicus.

Pelvic examination is mandatory. Suspicious features of a mass include bilaterality, fixity in the pelvis, and nodularity in the pouch of Douglas, which is either due to malignancy or to endometriotic nodules.

Initial investigations should include an ultrasound and a blood test for tumour markers, which in the older women should include CA 125 and CEA levels and in the younger women where germ-cell tumours may exist, a raised hCG, LDH or alpha-fetoprotein will almost give a definitive diagnosis denoting the presence of a choriocarcinoma, dysgerminoma and a yolk sac tumour (endodermal sinus tumour) respectively (see chapter 22).

Features on ultrasound that are suspicious include the presence of ascites, bilaterality of tumours, solid and cystic areas within the tumour, or proliferative excrescences on the surface of the tumour.

Since the initial surgical approach is of inestimable importance to the patient, then the referring doctor should calculate a 'risk of malignancy index' (Table 27.3). Where the tumour is thought possibly to be malignant (RMI scores >200) then referral to a gynaecology oncology unit is extremely important.

PREOPERATIVE INVESTIGATIONS

If malignancy is suspected then further imaging including either a CT (Figure 27.3) or MRI scan is undertaken together with the usual preoperative investigations prior to a laparotomy, and also taking

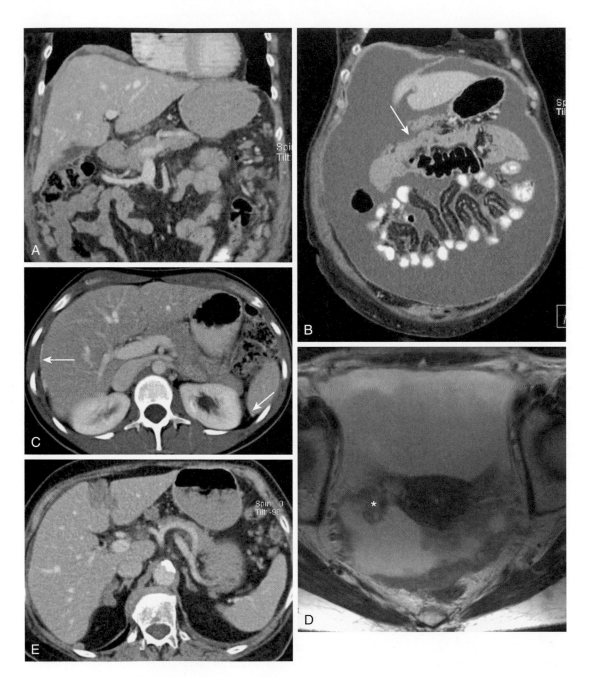

Figure 27.3
A to E: Spectrum of findings in different patients with ovarian cancer and peritoneal dissemination. Owing to ascites, diaphragmatic implants are well visualised; these may be focal along the diaphragm (A) or appear as diffuse plaque-like thickening of the parietal peritoneum (B). Broad tumour formations (arrow in B), representing omental caking adjacent to the transverse colon, are also seen. Peritoneal implants from papillary serous cancer may present as subtle calcifications (arrows in C) on the liver and splenic surfaces. Peritoneal implants encompassing the cul-de-sac can be differentiated from the small primary ovarian cancer (asterisk in D). Multiple nodular implants are demonstrated (E), including in the right posterior diaphragm, in the right liver lobe adjacent to the right adrenal gland, and along the intersegmental fissure. In addition, there are multiple small nodules along the gastrosplenic ligament and lymph nodes adjacent to the hepatic artery.

(Haaga: CT and MRI of the Whole Body, 5th ed. 9780323053754 Figure 44.38A to E Copyright © 2008 Mosby, An Imprint of Elsevier)

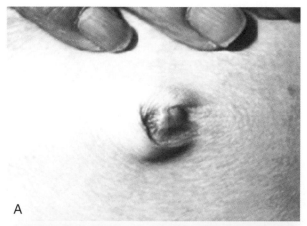

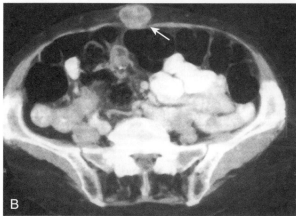

Table 27.3 Risk of malignancy index (RMI)	
Criterion	**Score**
CA 125 (A)	Absolute number
Menopausal status (B) • Premenopausal • Postmenopausal	1 3
Ultrasound features (C) • Multilocular • Solid • Bilateral • Ascites • Metastatic disease	0 Features=0 1 Feature=1 >1 Feature=3
RMI=A×B×C	

Figure 27.4

A: Sister Joseph's nodule. B: Computed tomography shows an umbilical subcutaneous nodule (arrow), which is Sister Joseph's nodule.

(Walsh: Palliative Medicine, 1st ed. 9780323056748; Figure 61.4 A and B Copyright © 2008 Saunders, An Imprint of Elsevier; A from Leow CK, Lau WY. Sister Joseph's nodule. Can J Surg 1997;40:167; B from Moll S. Images in clinical medicine. Sister Joseph's node in carcinoma of the cecum. N Engl J Med 1996;335:1568.)

into consideration the patient's medical history and any comorbidities.

SURGICAL MANAGEMENT

There are two principles that relate to surgery for epithelial ovarian cancer, the first being to stage the cancer and the second to 'debulk' the cancer (Figure 27.5). The process of debulking requires removal of disease where it has obviously spread outside of the ovary, with the aim of leaving no macroscopic visible disease. At a minimum, any tumour nodule should be reduced to less than 1 cm since it is quite

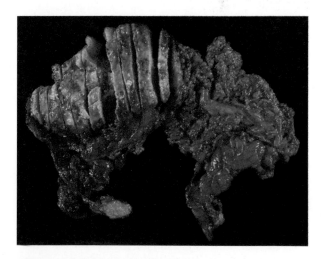

Figure 27.5

High-grade ovarian serous carcinoma involving the omentum. High-grade serous carcinoma has a strong tendency to involve the omentum, forming a 'caking' appearance. The omentum was bread-loafed to reveal the solid tumour mass.

(Bristow & Armstrong: Ovarian Cancer — Early Diagnosis and Treatment of Cancer Series. 9781416046851; Figure 2.2 Copyright © 2009 Saunders, An Imprint of Elsevier)

clear that survival is directly related to the amount of residual disease. If tumour more than 2 cm is left behind, then the chances of cure are extremely small. If no macroscopic disease is left at the end of the procedure then more than 50% of patients will live beyond 5 years. For this reason, initial surgery with a suitably trained gynaecological oncologist is preferable.

Surgery is undertaken through a vertical midline incision that allows access to the upper abdomen. At laparotomy, all peritoneal surfaces are examined for spread of tumour and the posterior peritoneum is also assessed for lymph node spread. In about 30% of cases, to effectively remove all bulk disease either a splenectomy or a bowel resection will be required. In most cases hysterectomy with removal of both tubes and ovaries is undertaken, except in a young woman in whom there is no obvious spread of disease; only one ovary is involved; and the tumour is considered to be well-differentiated on frozen section.

POSTOPERATIVE TREATMENT

Following surgery, all current management protocols include the use of six cycles of cytotoxic chemotherapy using a combination of carboplatinum and paclitaxel. If there is disease left behind, tumour response is evaluated by imaging studies. If there is no residual disease CA 125 is a useful maker to ensure the chemotherapy is being effective. Where disease is metastatic and widespread such as that seen in the lung in Figure 27.6, chemotherapy is the mainstay of management.

NEW APPROACHES

Currently, surgery in some centres involves a more aggressive approach to ensure that no residual disease is left. This may include stripping of the peritoneal surfaces of the diaphragm or indeed removal of the diaphragm itself. Other procedures such as thoracic endoscopy or pleurectomy to remove tumour nodules on the pleura, partial hepatotectomy for tumour within the substance of the liver, and even involved lymph glands around the porta hepatis are undertaken with aim of cytoreduction. Of course, such an approach is not without fairly substantial morbidity, with half the patients developing pleural effusions and a mortality rate of up to 5%. Nonetheless, increased median survivals of 5 years or longer have been observed in selected patients using this approach.

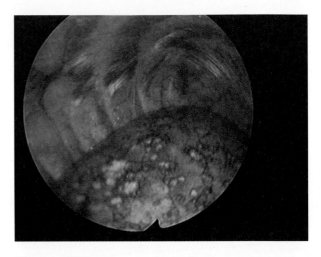

Figure 27.6
A view through the thoracoscope in a patient with multiple pulmonary metastases due to ovarian cancer (lower part of photo).

(Mason: Murray and Nadel's Textbook of Respiratory Medicine, 5th ed. 9781416047100; Figure 23.11 Copyright © 2010 Saunders, An Imprint of Elsevier)

More recently 'dose dense' cytotoxic chemotherapy has improved median survival rates. This approach requires administration of weekly intravenous paclitaxel and third weekly carboplatinum, rather than both drugs given together every 3 weeks.

Recently, intraperitoneal chemotherapy has been reported to improve median survival from this malignancy, and targeted agents based on molecular alterations detected within tumours are becoming more common. For instance, BRCA-related mutations are found to be present in about 16% of high-grade serous tumours and this allows the possibility of using such agents as poly ADP ribose polymerase (PARP) inhibitors.

Finally, it has emerged that there are two distinct types of epithelial ovarian malignancy:
1 Type 1 consisting of low-grade serous, endometrioid clear cell and mucinous tumours stemming from mutations involving such genes as KRAS, BRAF, PTEN, ERB-B2, PIK3CA and CTNNB1
2 Type 2 ovarian malignancies, which include high-grade serous, undifferentiated cancers and carcinosarcomas which are much more aggressive and widespread at presentation and are probably due to a p53 mutation in the vast majority of cases (Table 27.4).

Table 27.4 Classification of ovarian cancer

Characteristic	Type 1	Type 2
Histology	Low-grade serous Endometrioid Clear cell Mucinous	High-grade serous Undifferentiated cancer Carcinosarcomas
Origin	Borderline serous Endometriosis Transitional cells Perhaps benign tumours	Intraepithelial cancer in the fallopian tube
Clinical	Indolent Localised	Aggressive widespread
Mutations	KRAS, BRAF, PTEN, ERB-B2, PIK3CA, CTNNB1	p53

BORDERLINE EPITHELIAL TUMOURS

Approximately 15% of all ovarian tumours are of 'borderline' type. These tumours are usually of serous or mucinous type where the glandular cells are clearly neoplastic, but this does not present with invasion into the ovarian stroma. Occasionally spread outside the ovary is found, although this is uncommon and management usually involves removal of the tumours without the need for a more extensive staging approach. Unless there are invasive implants detected from borderline tumours then adjuvant treatment is not required.

FURTHER READING

http://www.ncbi.nlm.nih.gov/pubmedhealth/PMH0001891.

National Cancer Institute. http://www.cancer.gov/cancertopics/types/ovarian.

The Garvan Institute. http://www.garvan.org.au/research/our-work/cancer-ovarian?searchterm=ovarian+cancer.

The Peter McCallum Institute. http://www.petermac.org/Gynaecological?searchTerms[]=ovarian&searchTerms[]=cancer.

Kulasingam S, Havrilesky L. Health economics of screening for gynaecological cancers. Best Pract Res Clin Obstet Gynaecol 2012;26(2):163–73.

Rao A, Carter J. Ultrasound and ovarian cancer screening: is there a future? J Minim Invasive Gynecol 2011;18(1):24–30.

Thigpen T, duBois A, McAlpine J, et al. First-line therapy in ovarian cancer trials. Int J Gynecol Cancer 2011;21(4):756–62.

Winter-Roach BA, Kitchener HC, Lawrie TA. Adjuvant (post-surgery) chemotherapy for early stage epithelial ovarian cancer. Cochrane Database Syst Rev 2012;(3):CD004706. doi: 10.1002/14651858.CD004706.pub4.

Woo YL, Kyrgiou M, Bryant A, et al. Centralisation of services for gynaecological cancer. Cochrane Database Syst Rev 2012;(3):CD007945.

MCQS

Select the correct answer.

1   A 65-year-old woman presents with stage III ovarian cancer. Which of the following statements about surgical management will optimise survival?

   A   Perform radical hysterectomy, remove both ovaries and omentum.
   B   Perform debulking surgery to <1 cm and commence chemotherapy.
   C   Perform debulking surgery with no macroscopic disease.
   D   Perform debulking surgery to reduce disease to <2 cm and commence chemotherapy.
   E   Perform radical hysterectomy, remove both ovaries and omentum and commence chemotherapy.

2   A 55-year-old asymptomatic woman presents to you to discuss screening for ovarian cancer. Her paternal grandmother died from ovarian cancer at the age of 88 although there is no other first-degree relative with ovarian or breast cancer. Which of the following do you recommend?

   A   Baseline CA125 level.
   B   Referral for genetic screening for possible BRCA mutation.
   C   Reassure patient and manage expectantly.
   D   Perform pelvic ultrasound to assess RMI.
   E   Recommend prophylactic ovarian removal.

3   When considering the risk factors for the development of an epithelial ovarian cancer, which of the following statements is true?

   A   BRCA-1 carriers have a 50% lifetime risk of ovarian cancer.
   B   BRCA-2 carriers have a 50% lifetime risk of ovarian cancer.
   C   HNPCC carriers have a 50% lifetime risk of ovarian cancer.
   D   Using the OCP until menopause increases the risk of ovarian cancer.
   E   Using the OCP for 10 years increases the risk of ovarian cancer.

OSCE

Helen is a 65-year-old woman who presents with a 3-year history of increasing nausea, abdominal distension and lethargy. She has had one child, and has not had gynaecological issues before. Menopause was at 50 and she has not been on HRT. She has hypertension and had an appendicectomy. What further information will you seek on history and examination?

Helen has had increasing night sweats and weight gain of 8 kg over the last 2 months with a palpable mass in the upper abdomen and shifting dullness present. What investigations are important?

The CA 125 is 3500, the TVUS shows bilateral solid cystic mass in both ovaries with a small central uterus and ascitic fluid clearly demonstrated. The CT scan shows a large omental lesion of 8 cm and lesions on the diaphragm. There appears to be a mass at the ileocaecal junction.

What is the likely diagnosis for Helen and what management do you recommend?

MCQ ANSWERS

CHAPTER 1

1 C
2 A
3 E

CHAPTER 2

1 B
2 D
3 C
4 A

CHAPTER 3

1 D
2 B
3 E

CHAPTER 4

1 A
2 C
3 C

CHAPTER 5

1 E
2 D
3 C

CHAPTER 6

1 B
2 A
3 D

CHAPTER 7

1 E
2 D
3 D

CHAPTER 8

1 B
2 B
3 A

CHAPTER 9

1 A
2 C
3 C
4 D
5 A
6 E
7 A
8 B

CHAPTER 10

1 D
2 B
3 A
4 E

CHAPTER 11

1 D
2 A
3 C
4 E

CHAPTER 12

1 A
2 D
3 B

CHAPTER 13

1 D
2 C
3 A
4 B

CHAPTER 14

1 C
2 E
3 B

CHAPTER 15

1 E
2 B
3 A
4 A
5 C

CHAPTER 16

1 B
2 B
3 D
4 D
5 C

CHAPTER 17

1 E
2 B
3 D

CHAPTER 18

1 C
2 B
3 A

CHAPTER 19

1 B
2 B
3 C

CHAPTER 20

1 D
2 C
3 E
4 A
5 A
6 C

CHAPTER 21

1 D
2 A
3 C
4 B

CHAPTER 22

1 D
2 B
3 A

CHAPTER 23

1 E
2 C
3 B

CHAPTER 24

1 B
2 A
3 C
4 D

CHAPTER 25

1 A
2 C
3 B
4 A

CHAPTER 26

1 A
2 B
3 E

CHAPTER 27

1 B
2 C
3 A

OSCE ANSWERS

CHAPTER 2: Sexual development and puberty

Janelle, a 14-year-old female, presents to the emergency department with an acute abdomen. She has had several months of mild pain that comes and goes but is usually relieved by simple analgesia such as paracetamol and non-steroidal anti-inflammatories. This time the pain is very severe.

What are the important features on history, examination and investigation that would allow you to arrive at a diagnosis? What management would you initiate?

History

- Pain history:
  - When did it start?
  - Where is it located?
  - How severe is the pain?
  - Are there any associated features (sweating, fainting etc.)?
  - Does it radiate anywhere?
  - Describe the type of the pain in words.
  - What is the severity of the pain?
  - Has Janelle suffered pain like this previously?
  - How does the pain impact on the activities of daily living?
  - Is there any pattern to any previous episodes?
- Nausea, vomiting, diarrhoea
- Have menstrual periods started?
- Is Janelle sexually active at this time?
- Any treatments up until this time?
- Previous medical, surgical and social history
- Any medications or drug use?

Examination

- Height, weight and general appearance (Are there any features of congenital abnormality?)
- Vital signs:
  - HR
  - blood pressure
  - oxygen saturation
- Assess pubertal development:
  - breast development (Tanner staging)
  - axillary and pubic hair growth
- Abdominal examination
  - inspect the abdomen looking for scars or irregularities
  - tenderness
  - guarding/rebound
  - mass present

Investigations

- Imaging ultrasound or MRI of the abdomen and pelvis
- Consider a plain X-ray.
- FBC, EUC, CRP may all be helpful.
- β hCG to exclude pregnancy

Management

- Consultation with surgeon may be appropriate (consider appendicitis).
- Consultation with gynaecology team (if scan shows mass in the uterus or ovaries)

The best students

- May be directed to differential diagnoses with the use of imaging and test results.
- Consider the options for Müllerian tract anomalies (e.g. congenital vaginal obstruction with transverse septum).
- Consider genetic anomalies.
- Recognise the possible need for multidisciplinary management — specialist treatment required.

CHAPTER 3: Fundamentals of gynaecology: the menstrual cycle and clinical interaction

You are teaching a group of first-year medical students how to take a gynaecological history and perform a physical examination. You have 8 minutes to present your mini-tutorial. What are the important areas that you will cover?

History

- Start with the presenting issue.
- Be aware that this may not be an 'illness'.
- Be open, sensitive and non-judgmental.
- Initiate rapport with the woman and use open-ended questions where possible.
- Check your understanding of the critical issues for the woman by paraphrasing back to her.
- Take a full menstrual history — this should cover last menstrual period, her usual cycle, number of days bleeding, and problems to date.
- Onset of menarche and any problems at this time.
- Specifically ask about any pain with the cycle, non-cyclic pain and associated pain (dyspareunia, dyschesia, dysuria).
- The sensitive taking of a sexual history:
  - past pregnancies and outcomes in chronological order
  - contraceptive history
  - Pap smear history and currency
  - medical, surgical, social and medication history
  - family history (may be very important in certain situations).

Examination

- Consider a chaperone.
- Appropriate environment
- General characteristics, for example gait, pain behaviour, distress
- Assess patient comfort.
- Vital signs
- All equipment required should be within easy reach during the examination.
- Reassure the woman through examination and discussion of what you are going to do.
- Inspect the external genitalia.
- An appropriate, gentle and focused vaginal examination checking muscular tone, noting areas of tenderness or pain
- Palpate the cervix and perform a gentle bimanual examination.
- Examine the posterior compartment by palpation.
- Consider a speculum examination when needed.

The best students

- Cover all areas of history and examination thoroughly.
- Have a methodical approach to the history-taking exercise.
- Adapt to what is disclosed in the history and examination.

CHAPTER 4: Sexual activity and contraception

Amanda, a 22-year-old single university student, presents to the Student Health Service complaining of heavier, more painful, menstrual periods over the past 6 months. Amanda has been using condoms for contraception until this time but mentions that she would like to talk about alternative contraceptive methods.

What are the important features on history and examination that would be important in your decision-making? What contraceptive options are available to Amanda and what information would you need to give to her?

History

- Detailed menstrual history, including:
  - cycle length and duration of bleeding
  - how many pads or tampons used on heaviest days
  - quality and severity of period pain
  - any intermenstrual or post-coital bleeding
  - any other symptoms such as pain with intercourse, androgenic symptoms
- Previous gynaecological history including Pap smear history
- Smoking history
- General medical, surgical and medication history
- Drug use
- Full sexual history including current partner (barrier contraceptives essential if has multiple partners or new partner)
- Previous STI screens and their outcomes
- Risk-taking behaviours (binge drinking/illicit drugs/high-risk sexual practices)

Examination

- Height, weight, BMI
- Blood pressure (if thinking about starting on OCP)
- General abdominal examination
- Speculum examination, vaginal and cervical swabs or first pass urine for *Chlamydia* PCR (age-related risk)

Options and information

- The range of contraceptive options open to Amanda:
  - The OCP (non-contraceptive benefits of the COCP include a 30–80% reduction in blood loss and pelvic pain)
  - Monophasic COCPs (also allow extended use so periods may be skipped)
  - The vaginal ring (OCP in a different form)
  - Contraceptive implant, contraceptive injection and hormonal IUD
- The particular advantages and disadvantages of each of these methods as an alternative to oral contraceptive use should be explored within the context of Amanda's own individual needs and preferences.

- Some methods, such as copper IUD, are probably less suitable for Amanda since they are likely to make her periods heavier.
- Also less suitable are those methods that are less effective than condoms (diaphragm, fertility awareness).
- Apart from the medical considerations, personal and social issues such as cost, lifestyle, future plans and philosophical beliefs may all play a part in her final choice.
- Since no contraceptive method is 100% effective, it may also be worth reminding Amanda at this point of the availability and safety of emergency contraception should she need it in the future.

The best students

- Discuss when and how to take the Pill.
- Explain when she will be covered from a contraceptive perspective.
- Explain what to do if she misses a tablet(s).
- Warn her that diarrhoea, vomiting and some medications can interfere with the effectiveness of the Pill.
- Discuss side effects such as breast tenderness, nausea and irregular bleeding that are not uncommon in the first few months of use and that it may take up to three cycles before she can decide whether this Pill really suits her.
- Advise her that if she experiences any severe migraines, pains in her calf or breathlessness she should come back to discuss these as a matter of urgency.

CHAPTER 5: Sexually transmitted infections

You are working in a sexual health clinic in an Australian capital city where Sarah, a 20-year-old sales assistant, attends with a history of intermittent vaginal bleeding after sex for the past month.

What are the important points on history, examination and investigation for Sarah?

History

- Sarah's knowledge of STIs, including previous STIs and STI testing
- Safer sex knowledge and use
- The time Sarah has been sexually active
- Number of sexual partners, current partner/s (regular and casual), sex of partners (male, female, both), partners in the past 6 months
- Do any of her partners have a higher risk of sexually transmitted infections:
  - overseas travel
  - men who have sex with men
  - recreational drug use?
- Range of sexual activities
- Contraception used/possibility of pregnancy
- Vaccination history:
  - hepatitis
  - HPV
- Pap test history — last Pap test date, any history of abnormal Pap tests
- Any other symptoms, such as dysuria, dyspareunia, other irregular bleeding
- General medical, surgical, medication and social history

Examination

- Vital signs including temperature for infection
- General abdominal examination
- Genital examination, looking for signs of infection or discharge, thrush, erythema, blisters, or other localised lesions
- This is the appropriate time to take a low vaginal swab.
- Speculum examination, checking the cervix, looking for bleeding or lesions on the cervix
- A Pap smear may be taken if there is no active bleeding, with a liquid-based cytology improving the diagnosis where bleeding is present. If cervicitis is present, then the Pap smear may be deferred until this has been treated and settled.
- High vaginal and cervical swabs should be collected at this time.

Investigations

- Check a urinalysis and send off urine for MSU and first-pass *Chlamydia* and gonorrhoea PCR
- A PCR test for *Chlamydia* would be essential.
- PCR or microscopy/culture/sensitivity for gonorrhoea and other STIs
- Serological investigations for hepatitis B and C and HIV as appropriate to the history

The best students

- Arrange follow-up for the patient.
- Counsel regarding investigation and treatment for all partners.
- Know that *Chlamydia* is a notifiable disease.
- Advise her not to have unprotected sex with her partner until both have been treated.
- Discuss Pap test — further investigations could be performed at the same visit should she continue to experience any further bleeding after sex.

CHAPTER 6: Fertility

Alison and John, both aged 32, attend to see you as they are trying to conceive. What are the important features on history and examination that you need to find out from this couple? What advice would you give them about trying to conceive?

History

- When did they stop using contraception?
- What type of contraception were they using?
- What have Alison's menstrual cycles been like since cessation of contraception?
- What has her menstrual history been in the past (cyclicity, number of days bleeding)
- Is there pain associated with the menstrual cycle?
- How often are they having intercourse?
- Is the frequency of intercourse the same each month?
- How long have they been actively trying for a pregnancy?
- Have they been pregnant at all before?
- Is there any difficulty or pain with intercourse?
- Is Alison taking folic acid, and for how long?
- Has she had an antenatal screen?
- Has she had a history of STI?
- Has she had any other medical or surgical issues?
- Pap smear history
- Does Alison smoke or drink?

- Medications, drugs and allergies
- For John
  - Has he fathered a child before?
  - Does he drink or smoke?
  - Has he had a history of medical or surgical problems?
  - Has he had any testicular trauma or inguinal hernia?
  - Is there a history of mumps orchitis?
  - Has he had an STI?
  - Is he taking any medications?

Examination

- Alison: vital signs
  - BMI
  - Abdominal examination for masses, tenderness
  - External vaginal examination
  - Bimanual examination, particularly noting masses, tenderness, induration and thickening in the posterior compartment suggestive of endometriosis
  - Note size and mobility of uterus and adnexa
  - Speculum examination to assess the cervix
  - Consider swabs as indicated
- John: vital signs
  - BMI
  - Check for secondary sexual characteristics
  - External genitalia examination
  - Check for vas deferens and testicular size

Management

- Explain the normal mechanisms of fertility to John and Alison.
- Explain that it is normal to take up to 12 months to become pregnant.
- Explain monthly fecundity.
- Advise good prenatal health, including folic acid supplementation, no smoking and drinking, reduction of caffeine intake.
- Check rubella status for Alison (may recommend an antenatal screen).
- Explain the importance and timing of intercourse to maximise conception rates.
- Arrange follow-up at 12 months of trying for natural conception.
- Discuss investigations that may be performed at that time (ovulatory studies with midluteal serum progesterone, tubal assessment, semen analysis).

The best students

- Take a chronological and thorough history of both partners.
- Specifically focus on symptoms that may cause subfertility (PID, endometriosis, testicular trauma).
- Ask about lifestyle factors that may diminish fertility.
- Examine appropriately and thoroughly and know both partners need examination.
- Give appropriate counselling as to the normal length of time to become pregnant.
- In the absence of any abnormalities will not recommend immediate investigation/referral without an adequate trial of normal conception.
- Check folic acid intake and rubella status.
- Compile a list of simple investigations at 12 months if conception has not occurred.

CHAPTER 7: Problems of fertility

Polly is a 28-year-old woman who comes to see you as she is trying to conceive. She has a cycle that is variable with bleeding that lasts 4–7 days and recurs at an interval of 28–90 days. What are the further important features on history and examination that you need to collect? What investigations may be helpful in this setting?

History

- First day of last menstrual period imperative as she may be currently pregnant
- How long has she been trying for a pregnancy?
- Is this the normal pattern of her cycle?
- What contraception were Polly and her partner using prior to trying to conceive?
- A full menstrual history at this time including pain with the cycle, heaviness of menstruation, previous cycle abnormalities
- Associated symptoms such as hair growth, weight gain or loss
- Any change in visual pattern or sense of smell?
- Exercise patterns
- Has she ever been pregnant before?
- Are there any sexual difficulties?
- What is the frequency of intercourse?
- Post-coital or intermenstrual bleeding
- Pap smear history
- Past history of STI
- Past medical history — particularly diabetes
- Surgical history
- Medications and allergies
- Alcohol and cigarette intake

Examination

- Vital signs
- BMI
- General examination including signs of acne and its distribution, hair growth and distribution
- Thyroid examination
- Abdominal examination for masses, central adiposity, tenderness
- External genital examination
- Bimanual examination for uterine size, mobility and signs of localised tenderness, adnexal masses
- Speculum examination

Investigations

- TSH
- Prolactin
- Oestrogen and progesterone
- Day 2 FSH and LH
- SHBG, testosterone, FAI
- Insulin levels
- Transvaginal ultrasound
- Recommend partner to seek advice regarding semen analysis

The best students

- Take a thorough history and examination considering multiple causes of oligomenorrhoea.
- Recognise that PCOS is a common cause of oligomenorrhoea.
- Discuss other hormonal influences on the cycle (hyperprolactinaemia, CNS disease, anorexia or significant weight loss).
- Discuss the implication of PCOS for fertility and future health risk.
- Discuss options for fertility in ovulation and the risks associated with these treatments.

CHAPTER 8: Chronic pelvic pain

Jane is a 22-year-old woman with a 7-year history of chronic pelvic pain. She is presenting to you for the first time today.

What are the features on history and examination that you wish to address with Jane? What investigations and management are important?

History

- Thorough and chronological history of the pain
- Age of menarche and pain from this onset
- Menstrual history and relationship of pain to periods
- Other pain symptoms such as dysuria, dyschesia, dyspareunia, non-menstrual pelvic pain
- Use of medications to date and their effect on the pain
- Sexual history, risk factors for PID, contraception
- Plans for pregnancy
- Medical, surgical and psychiatric history
- Orthopaedic and postural problems (e.g. scoliosis, leg length issues)
- Medication and allergies

Examination

- General appearance as she enters the room, signs of mobility issues, distresses with pain at the current time
- Check vital signs
- BMI calculation
- General examination, including abdominal and musculoskeletal examination. Include the abdomen and make sure that the genital examination is not the first time that you touch the patient.
- Pelvic examination: start with the external genitalia, observe for signs of irritation or localised trauma (such as perineal tearing), discharge, bleeding, check for localised dermatoses
- Take appropriate specimens for pathology if indicated.
- Bimanual pelvic examination, checking for posterior compartment tenderness over the uterosacral ligaments or nodularity in this area
- Consider the indication for a speculum examination and the increased diagnostic capacity over a bimanual examination.

Investigations

- Transvaginal ultrasound
- *Chlamydia* swab and other STI screen as indicated on history
- Exclusion of pregnancy with β hCG

Management

- Management should be in conjunction with patient and may include any of the following:
  - Simple analgesics
  - OCP
  - Progestogens in various forms
  - Laparoscopy (note invasive nature, risk from surgery, and hospitalisation). Will allow a diagnosis.
  - Consideration of other medical options should be second-line until first-line treatments have been attempted, due to side effects of second-line treatments.
- Side effects, duration of activity and limitations of pregnancy should be considered for the medical treatments and limitations of surgery.

The best students

- Outline a thorough chronological history of the pain.
- Consider both menstrual and non-menstrual pain issues.
- Consider the impact of the pelvic pain on day-to-day functioning (bladder, bowels, intercourse, relationship, fertility, psychological state).
- Are thorough in considering aetiology of pelvic pain.
- Discuss the methods of investigating and managing pelvic pain after discussion with the patient and consideration of empiric treatments without definitive diagnosis.
- Understand the limitations of the various investigations for pelvic pain.
- Recognise that there are likely multiple factors involved in a 7-year history of pain and consider collaboration with other specialists.
- Identify the decision/concern for fertility and the timing of any fertility plans and the impact that treatment may have on these plans.

CHAPTER 10: Problems in early pregnancy

Joanne, a 23-year-old woman, presents with lower abdominal pain and some per vaginam spotting of dark blood. Her vital signs are normal with pulse rate 85 beats/min, BP 118/70 and temperature 36.8°C. She performed a home urine pregnancy test, which was positive.

What are the important features to be elicited from the history and examination? What further investigations and possible management will be required?

History

- Characteristics of the pain and its onset
- Precipitants for pain or bleeding including recent intercourse
- Menstrual history and usual pattern for bleeding
- Date of last menstrual period to give an estimate of gestational age
- Contraceptive use, particularly the presence of an IUD or long-acting progestogen that may increase the risk of ectopic pregnancy
- Past obstetric history, including any previous pregnancies and their outcomes
- Past pelvic infection, abdominal surgery or PID that may increase the risk of ectopic pregnancy
- Smoking, which may increase the risk of both ectopic pregnancy and miscarriage
- Pap smear history

Examination

- General appearance: assess for pallor and signs of clinical shock.
- Abdominal examination for site of tenderness, presence of guarding or rebound tenderness
- Speculum examination to examine cervix for local causes of bleeding and to assess if it is open or closed
- Examine for presence of products of conception in the canal and remove these if present.
- Bimanual examination to assess for the size of the uterus and presence of any adnexal masses or localising signs of pain

Investigations

- FBC
- Blood group
- Quantitative serum βhCG
- Transvaginal ultrasound

Management

- Will depend on diagnosis of ectopic pregnancy or miscarriage variant
- Expectant, medical and surgical options are available in both situations.

The best students

- Recognise the differentiating features on history, examination and investigation for miscarriage and ectopic pregnancy.
- Give options and outcomes for conservative, medical and surgical management of miscarriage and ectopic pregnancy.
- Arrange admission or appropriate follow-up depending on the scenario set by the examiner.
- Give anti-D to any Rh-negative patient.
- Counsel regarding future pregnancies.
- Recommend when to become pregnant after either miscarriage or ectopic pregnancy.

CHAPTER 11: Antenatal care

You are a general practitioner. Anne is 30 years old and is trying to get pregnant. She has regular menstrual cycles. She has type 1 diabetes and comes to you for advice. What factors do you want to know about her and how will you advise her?

History

- Gynaecological and obstetric history:
  - how long has she been trying for a pregnancy, has she ever been pregnant before? When was her last Pap smear? Is she taking periconceptual vitamins?
- Medical history:
  - how long has she had diabetes, how is it managed?

Examination

- Weight, height and hence BMI
- Blood pressure, cardiovascular and eye examination.

Investigations

- Booking blood, including:
  - blood group and antibodies
  - FBC
  - rubella, hepatitis B, hepatitis C, HIV
  - her immunity to chickenpox should be defined.
- Since Anne is diabetic an assessment of her diabetic control should be made with an HbA1c.

Management

- Advise Anne to take vitamins, in particular folic acid.
- Refer her for preconceptual counselling to an obstetric physician or diabetes physician to manage diabetes for pregnancy.
- Ensure her Pap smear is up to date.
- Advise her to ensure she has a good diet and healthy lifestyle.
- This pregnancy will need to be managed by doctors and midwives in combination. Anne will need to be seen in a clinic that manages diabetes in pregnancy. Her pregnancy should be accurately dated and she should be offered first trimester screening.
- Additional ultrasound monitoring of the growth of the fetus will be required throughout the pregnancy.
- Poorly controlled diabetes is associated with increased fetal anomalies and stillbirth. Therefore glycaemic control at conception is important.

The best students

- Assess HbA1c and glycaemic control.
- Mention the need for multidisciplinary care of the patient.

CHAPTER 12: Fetal growth and development

Ping Yin, aged 27, comes for a 30-week antenatal visit. She is highly anxious since all her friends and family have told her she looks small and must have a small baby. How do you approach the consultation and what examination would you perform?

History

- Review her medical and general history: how tall is she, what is her weight and what has been her weight gain through the pregnancy, what is her ethnic background? How big was she as a baby? Does she have any relevant medical history, e.g. a history of hypertension or autoimmune disease?
- Review the dating of her pregnancy: has her gestation been calculated accurately? Does she know her last menstrual period? Did she have a first trimester ultrasound to date the pregnancy?
- Review her 18–20 week morphology ultrasound: was the fetal growth normal at that stage and did it agree with her menstrual dates?
- Has the pregnancy progressed normally? Has there been any bleeding? Have the fetal movements been regular?

Examination

- Check her blood pressure.
- Perform a urinalysis.
- Inspect her abdomen and measure the symphysio-fundal height.
- Check the lie of the fetus and auscultate the fetal heart rate.

Investigations

- Recommend ultrasound for growth assessment and to plot centiles of fetal measurements.
- Assess the liquor volume and the placental blood flow.
- Review on a regular basis.
- Further ultrasound as needed.

Management

- Consider maternal size as a common association with a small-for-dates baby.
- If the examination findings are normal (they are), reassure.
- Plot centile growth on an appropriate growth chart and consider a repeat ultrasound if there is failure to increase size on examination.
- Routine antenatal reviews.

The best students

- Recognise that maternal characteristics are a common cause of 'small' babies.
- Take a thorough history to exclude causes of small-for-dates babies including infections, medical conditions and drugs.
- Perform an examination and recognise the importance of lie and presentation in the assessment of fetal size.
- Understand the importance of proportionality on ultrasound and the need for serial scans to determine growth restriction.
- Know that abdominal circumference is likely to be compromised first in a truly growth restricted baby.

CHAPTER 13: Infections in pregnancy

Linda Chen is a 34-year-old G1P0 who comes for her first antenatal visit at 15 weeks gestation. She brings the following antenatal screening results:

- Hb 121
- MVC 85.2
- WCC 9.5
- Plt 320
- Blood group O+ve, nil antibodies detected
- Rubella IgG 8 (>15=adequate immunity in this laboratory's reference range)
- RPR non-reactive
- HBsAg positive
- HbsAb negative
- HBeAg positive
- HbeAb negative
- HCV antibody negative
- HIV antibody negative
- MSU no growth

First trimester screen (nuchal translucency ultrasound and biochemistry): Low risk (adjusted risk Trisomy 21 1:1300, adjusted risk for Trisomy 18 1:3500, adjusted risk for Trisomy 13 1:4500). Fetal size consistent with dates.

Outline your history and examination appropriate to this case, and discuss the results, including any appropriate further investigation and management, with the patient.

History

- Check pregnancy history to date.
- Known liver disease or any history of abnormal liver function tests
- Birth/prolonged residence in area with high HBV carriage
- Known other risk factors for HBV: blood transfusion, household family member with HBV, tattoos, IVDU
- Past medical and surgical history
- Other history
- Medication/drug history
- Social history

Examination

- Vital signs and urinalysis
- Full physical examination with specific mention of checking for stigmata of liver disease (jaundice, hepatomegaly)
- Palpate for fundus, check fetal heart present.

Investigations

- Liver function tests
- HBV viral load

Management

- Expect recognition that screening results are not normal:
  - Patient is a hepatitis B carrier
  - Patient has marker of high infectivity/active disease (E antigen positive)
  - Patient has low rubella immunity
  - Discuss HBV carriage as a chronic liver disease that can lead to liver failure
  - It is a blood-borne virus, so can be transmitted from mother to child, and also spread among close household contacts or via procedures involving blood exposure
  - Refer to liver clinic/hepatologist for further discussion
  - Rubella vaccination postpartum
  - Husband and parents should also be tested (and vaccinated if HBV negative)
  - Baby will need hepatitis B vaccine and immunoglobulin after birth to prevent HBV transmission.

The best students

- Specify hepatitis B immunoglobulin and first-dose hepatitis B vaccine for baby within 12 hours of birth.
  - Mention breastfeeding is not contraindicated.
  - Remembers a rubella booster also needed.
- Will recognise risks for baby:
  - 5–10% will be born HbE antigen positive and with a high viral load; this may be decreased by maternal ingestion of antivirals but will not be zero.
- Identify ongoing management requirements for Linda:
  - Follow-up with specialist to monitor for progression of her liver disease and regarding ongoing therapy.

CHAPTER 14: Medical disorders in pregnancy

Mary is a 28-year-old primigravid woman who has been sent in for assessment at 35 weeks pregnancy with a blood pressure of 165/105 and 2+ proteinuria. What information will you seek on history and examination? What would be your expected investigation and management plan?

History

- How is she feeling at this time?
- Does she have any symptoms such as headache, visual disturbance, nausea or vomiting, or upper abdominal pain?
- Has she had any vaginal bleeding or lower abdominal pain or contractions?
- Has the baby been moving recently?
- Has she had any problems in the pregnancy until now?
- Have her antenatal visits been normal?
- Has she had issues with blood pressure to this time?
- Does she have blood pressure problems when not pregnant?
- Are there any general medical issues, particularly renal disease?
- Has she been on any medications during this pregnancy?
- Review the antenatal record for any other abnormalities during this pregnancy.

Examination

- Repeat the blood pressure.
- Check other vital signs.
- Urinalysis
- Perform an obstetric abdominal examination with lie, presentation, symphyseal–fundal height (SFH) and areas of tenderness noted.
- Check for liver enlargement or tenderness.
- Perform a neurological examination particularly checking for clonus, hyper-reflexia.
- Auscultate the heart and lungs.

Investigations

- Perform a CTG for assessment of the baby.
- Take blood for FBC, LFTs, electrolytes, urea and creatinine (EUC) and coagulation studies.
- Arrange an ultrasound for fetal growth.
- Urinary protein/creatinine ratio or 24-hour urine protein collection.

Management

- Admit to hospital for minimum day-stay monitoring.
- It is likely that this is severe pre-eclampsia and ongoing assessment, monitoring and consideration of early delivery are important.
- Multidisciplinary team involvement is optimal.
- Antihypertensives are necessary to control blood pressure and reduce maternal and fetal risks.
- Timing and mode of delivery will depend on blood pressure control, systemic maternal involvement and fetal wellbeing.

The best students

- Take a thorough history including recognition of symptoms that may reflect systemic maternal involvement.
- Ask questions that reflect fetal wellbeing and risk of abruption.
- Perform a thorough examination of the woman including neurological assessment and check lungs, liver and heart.
- Examine the abdomen and assess the infant by palpation and SFH assessment.
- Arrange appropriate and directed investigations of maternal organs, fetal assessment and severity of preeclampsia.
- Manage by admission, further assessment and recognise the severity of preeclampsia and the need for early admission.

CHAPTER 15: Labour and delivery

Angela, a 27-year-old woman who is 37+6 weeks gestation in her first ongoing pregnancy, attends the delivery suite with a 3-hour history of lower abdominal pain and a small amount of PV bleeding.

Describe how you would assess Angela on admission.

On examination you find the following:

- lie: cephalic, 2/5 palpable
- cervix 3 cm dilated, fully effaced, soft, central os. Station −2, no PV bleeding seen

Through your assessment you find that Angela has increasingly frequent and painful contractions, now spaced every 2–3 minutes. The contractions can be palpated and the uterus is relaxed between times. The fetus is appropriately grown, longitudinal lie, cephalic presentation and the head is engaged. The cervix is effaced and dilated on examination. What is your diagnosis?

History

- Details of presenting complaint:
  - Pain (is it contractile in nature, increasingly painful, increasing in frequency?)
  - Bleeding: what is the nature of the bleeding, and what amount?
  - Fetal movement
  - SRoM
- Current pregnancy:
  - Booking / dating of pregnancy
  - Course of first trimester
  - Course of second trimester
  - Has there been an ultrasound scan to confirm placental position? (not low — differential diagnosis praevia)
  - Course of third trimester
- Previous obstetric history
- Previous gynaecology history
- Medical history
  - Current medications/allergies
- Surgical history
- Social history

Examination

- Abdominal palpation
  - fundus appropriate for dates
- Vaginal examination

Investigations

- Maternal BP
- Maternal urine analysis
- Fetal heart rate/CTG

Diagnosis

- Onset of normal labour (i.e. low risk and in labour)

Management

- Expectant management
- Appropriate support/analgesia for labour
- Intermittent fetal monitoring

The best students

- Ask about the frequency and nature of the contractions.
- Define the type of bleeding.
- Ensure an ultrasound had been performed earlier to exclude placenta praevia.
- Diagnose low-risk labour.

CHAPTER 16: Obstetric emergencies

Part 1

You are called to the delivery suite. Mrs Jones, who delivered a male infant 20 minutes ago, has collapsed and is unresponsive. She is lying in a large pool of blood. Describe how you would assess and manage the situation.

- Recognise that this is an obstetric emergency and that various aspects of assessment and management are concurrent.
- Call for extra help (and define who).

Assessment

- Ask for extra history:
  - Maternal details: age; parity
- Details of this pregnancy:
  - Gestation at delivery
  - Antenatal course
  - Spontaneous / Induction of labour
  - Progress in first stage of labour
  - Progress in second stage of labour
  - ?Episiotomy / tear
  - Management of third stage
  - ?Placenta complete
  - ?Uterotonics given
- Events after placenta delivered
- Establish what analgesia has been given.

Management

- Assess state of consciousness.
- Assess haemodynamic state — (BP, HR, evidence of blood loss); direct one person for observations / record keeping.
- Resuscitate patient:
  - Establish IV access — two wide-bore cannulae
  - Send bloods for FBS, clotting profile, crossmatch
  - Replace volume with colloid/crystalloid/blood products.
- Examine to establish cause:
  - Abdominal palpation for uterine atony and to expel clots from uterus
  - Consider retained products (examine placenta and membranes)
  - Vaginal examination to assess genital trauma.

Part 2

The uterus is atonic. Describe how you would manage this situation.

Management

- Use bimanual compression to reduce loss and improve uterine tone.
- Insert urinary catheter (reduce bladder and record output).
- Pharmacology:
  - Syntocinon (bolus and infusion)
  - Ergometrine
  - Misoprostol
  - Prostaglandin f2α
- Surgery:
  - Examination under anaesthetic (systematic approach)
  - Laparotomy
  - B-Lynch suture
  - Backri/Rusch balloon
  - Uterine/internal iliac artery ligation
  - Hysterectomy

The best students

- Include anaesthetist, senior midwife and obstetric registrar in the call for help.
- Recognise risk factors such as: prolonged labour, delayed delivery of the placenta, older maternal age.
- Recognise in order the factors needed for treatment of the atonic uterus.

CHAPTER 17: Routine care of postpartum women

Miriam has just given birth to her first baby. She has been discharged home at her request the following day. She comes to see you, her GP, a week later because she thinks her bleeding may be excessive. What are the important history and examination points in helping you answer her question? How would you manage her?

History

- Review her labour and delivery.
- What sort of delivery did she have?
- Did she require an episiotomy or postpartum perineal sutures?
- Does she have pain at this time? When does the pain occur?
- How heavy is the bleeding — how many pads has she soaked?
- Does she feel well? Has she had a fever?
- How big was the baby?
- How is she feeding the baby?

Examination

- Vital signs including temperature, pulse and blood pressure
- Abdominal examination looking for uterine tenderness and involution
- Assessment of lochia and signs of endometritis (offensive lochia)
- Examination of the perineum and any sutures that are present in the perineal area
- Breast examination for signs of mastitis; check the nipples.

Investigations

- Low vaginal swab
- Full blood count

Management

- Reassure her that her symptoms are likely to be physiological.
- Check for a uterus that is contracting (involution).
- It is normal to have red bleeding at this stage, but she should not soak through more than one pad an hour.
- For women who are breastfeeding, the secretion of oxytocin will cause further contractions (afterpains).
- She can take simple analgesia for pain relief, e.g. paracetamol.
- She should keep her perineum clean by washing it every day.
- If her symptoms change she must consult medical advice, e.g. if her bleeding becomes heavier, she has a fever, or the discharge becomes offensive smelling.

The best students

- Ask how she is adjusting to motherhood. Is she sleeping?
- How is her mood?
- Is her baby settled?
- How is the baby feeding? If she is breastfeeding, does she have any problems?
- How is her bladder and bowel function: does she leak urine or faeces or flatus when she coughs or sneezes?
- Arrange for a review at 6 weeks and postpartum cervical smear if indicated.
- Refer to infant nursing program for monitoring and vaccinations as required.

CHAPTER 18: Abnormal uterine bleeding

Erin is a 35-year-old woman who presents with heavy menstrual bleeding. What are the important features on history and examination that will direct your investigations and management? What treatment options are available to Erin for her bleeding issues?

History

- How long has she had heavy bleeding?
- Bleed duration and length of intermenstrual intervals
- Volume of flow, e.g. number and type of sanitary products used and changes in the flow during menses
- Does she suffer with clots or flooding?
- Does the heaviness of her cycle interfere with her quality of life?
- Has she tried any treatments for heavy bleeding to date? What were their outcomes?
- Does she have pain or other associated symptoms with her bleeding?
- Does she have bleeding at any other time in the cycle?
- Has she noted a mass, bladder or bowel symptoms?
- Any symptoms of anaemia or thyroid disease?
- Her past obstetric history
- Plans for future pregnancies
- Contraceptive history
- Pap smear history
- General medical and surgical history
- Specifically any bleeding disorders in the family?
- Family history
- Medications and allergies.

Examination

- General examination including vital signs, BMI
- Signs of anaemia including conjunctival pallor
- Abdominal examination for masses, tenderness
- External genital examination
- Speculum examination for localised pathology or cervical pathology
- Bimanual examination for uterine size, mobility, masses, pain, localising tenderness

Investigations

- β hCG
- FBC
- Consider TFTs if appropriate
- Grey-scale (2D) transvaginal ultrasound to assess for structural abnormalities such as polyps, leiomyoma, endometrial thickening
- Consider an endometrial sampling or outpatient hysteroscopy if available.

Management

- Will depend on finding of pathology and Erin's desire for future children.
- Medical management such as NSAIDs, tranexamic acid and the OCP are all options that may be commenced.
- Localised pathology removal is appropriate if indicated.
- Endometrial ablation, hysterectomy and uterine artery embolisation should be considered as interventional options as indicated.

The best students

- Take a thorough and well-constructed history with compartmentalisation of discussion areas.
- Have thought of a variety of causes of bleeding and do not jump to a single diagnosis.
- Perform a thorough examination and look for signs of anaemia and thyroid disease.
- Investigate rationally and realise the limitations of various investigations.
- Compile a reasonable list of differential diagnoses for the patient with abnormal uterine bleeding.
- Put management options into context for specific diagnoses.
- Know risks and complications of various treatments for AUB.

CHAPTER 19: The menopause and beyond

Mary is a 56-year-old woman who presents with postmenopausal bleeding two months ago. What are the important points that you need to assess on history and examination? What investigations and management options are important for a woman with this presentation?

History

- Was this the first time she has had postmenopausal bleeding?
- Was there pain associated with the bleeding?
- When was her menopause?
- Has she had any menopausal symptoms?
- Has she been on any HRT? What other medications does she take?
- Gynaecological history and problems
- Pap smear history
- Mammogram history
- Obstetric, medical and surgical history
- Drinking and smoking history
- Family history, particularly malignancies
- Exercise and diet history

Examination

- Vital signs and BMI
- Abdominal and external genital examination
- Bimanual examination
- Speculum examination and Pap smear

Investigations

- Transvaginal ultrasound is the most important examination.

Management

- Will depend on the finding of specific pathology (e.g. polyps, endometrial thickening) or likely atrophic bleeding.
- If no pathology is evident and the endometrium is thin (<5 mm) a conservative course of action is reasonable.
- Discuss menopausal symptoms and management from local treatments (e.g. topical vaginal oestrogen for vaginal dryness) to HRT for systemic symptoms.

The best students
- Discuss weight management and regular weight-bearing exercise.
- Consider duration of HRT if started and the pros and cons of HRT.
- Describe alternatives to oestrogen and progestogen HRT.
- Give a good differential list of postmenopausal bleeding and the low likelihood of malignancy.
- Consider bone density and bone densitometry.
- Discuss breast and cervical surveillance programs.

CHAPTER 20: Incontinence

Tracey is a 36-year-old woman presenting in a primary care setting with urinary incontinence.

Take a history and list the important features on examination for Tracey and consider investigations and management options for her.

History
- Presenting issues — how long has she had the incontinence?
- When does it occur?
- Is there a stress, urge or mixed component (consider timing of incontinence, frequency, urgency, nocturia), urinary tract infections?
- Prolapse symptoms
- Bowel function
- Other gynaecological issues?
- Menstrual and obstetric history and plans for future pregnancy
- Pap smear history
- Medical and surgical history
- Medications, social and family history

Examination
- Vital signs and BMI
- Abdominal examination
- External genital examination
- Cough assessment for leakage (Valsalva manoeuvre and cough)
- Speculum examination (Simms and bivalve) for prolapse
- Digital pelvic floor examination

Investigations
- Urinalysis
- Ultrasound assessment of the pelvic floor
- Consider urodynamics.

Management
- Conservative — pelvic floor physiotherapy
- Pessary (limitations and problems)
- Medical options (stress versus urge incontinence)
- Surgical options (principles important)

The best students
- Take a thorough history with clear differentiation of types of incontinence.
- Consider risk factors for incontinence.
- Consider future pregnancy in the management plan.
- Consider quality of life for assessing severity.
- Propose balanced and focused investigations.
- Propose conservative options as a first-line treatment.
- Understand principles of pharmacotherapy for incontinence.
- Identify mixed incontinence as a confounding issue in management.
- Outline surgical principles for stress incontinence.

CHAPTER 21: Genital prolapse

Mary is a 47-year-old woman who is presenting in a primary care setting for evaluation of a vaginal bulge. What are the important features at history and on examination to determine appropriate investigations and management for this presentation?

History
- Presenting issues — how long has she noted the bulge and what symptoms does it give her?
- Urinary and bowel function, particularly frequency, urgency, leakage of urine, faeces or flatus
- Sexual concerns or dyspareunia
- Other pelvic pain
- Timing of the bulge
- Does it spontaneously reduce?
- Treatments to date
- Menstrual history
- Obstetric history including trauma during delivery
- Medical, surgical and social history
- Medications

Examination
- Vital signs and BMI
- Abdominal examination
- External genital examination at rest and with Valsalva looking for obvious signs of prolapse
- Repeat Valsalva manoeuvre with digital examination and single-bladed speculum (e.g. Simms speculum) for assessment of the prolapse
- Determine the site of prolapse within anterior, mid and posterior compartments
- Pelvic floor assessment digitally.

Investigations
- Urinalysis
- Consider translabial ultrasound.
- Recognise that urodynamic studies are unlikely to be helpful in the setting of no incontinence.

Management options
- Conservative and reassurance
- Pelvic floor physiotherapy — recognise that this will not change the prolapse, but may improve symptoms.
- Self-inserted or physician-inserted devices (pessary)
- Surgical options.

The best students

- Take a comprehensive history and know the risk factors for prolapse.
- Examine appropriately and in a logical, sequential manner.
- Offer a range of management options with the limitations and success rates for each.
- Understand the principles of types of prolapse procedures (repair, replace, remove, suspend, close) and the appropriateness of each.

CHAPTER 22: Germ cell tumours of the ovary

Justine, a 23-year-old nulligravid woman, presents with generalised abdominal distension. Describe the features in the history and examination that you wish to explore with her regarding her presentation.

History

- Onset of symptoms
- Weight loss or weight gain
- Appetite
- Bladder and bowel function
- Night sweats, malaise
- Lumps suggesting lymphadenopathy
- Gynaecological history including menarche and menstrual history (LMP essential)
- Obstetric history and sexual history including contraception and possibility of pregnancy
- Pap smear history
- Systems review
- Medical, surgical, social, medications and family history.

Examination

- General examination including BP, BMI and temperature
- Abdominal examination for masses, tenderness or ascites
- Vaginal and speculum examination for a Pap smear and swabs if specifically indicated given her young age (a *Chlamydia* cervical swab would be appropriate)
- Bimanual examination for uterine size, location or deviation, mobility, and any adnexal masses palpable

Investigations

- FBC/UEC/CA125/CA19.9/AFP/βhCG/LDH
- Ultrasound of pelvis (preferably transvaginal scan for better image quality)

Management

- If a mass was demonstrated on clinical examination and/or sonography, it requires further investigation.
- An ovarian mass of a large size, with mixed echogenicity and elevated tumour markers requires review with a specialist gynaecological oncologist.
- Surgery and histopathological assessment +/− other surgical procedures may be required.

The best students

- Will take a wide-reaching history given the general nature of the presentation.
- Consider malignancy as a possibility in this young woman.
- Localise the pathology to the pelvis.
- Determine a range of tumour markers that are helpful.
- Recognise the need for specialist help.
- Recognise that surgical intervention is helpful for diagnosis and management.
- Give differential diagnoses for an adnexal mass in a young woman.

CHAPTER 23: Gestational trophoblastic disease

Janelle is a 22-year-old woman who presents to the Early Pregnancy Assessment Service at 10 weeks with nausea and vomiting that is uncontrolled with anti-nausea agents. She has had bright red and painless bleeding.

What are the important features on history and examination that are important for this presentation? What investigations would you recommend?

History

- LMP, sure of dates?
- Menstrual history
- Any pain at all?
- Any blood tests or scans to date?
- How long has nausea been present?
- Able to tolerate any intake (risk of dehydration)?
- Associated symptoms
- Previous obstetric history
- Any medical conditions (such as thyroid disease)?
- Medications?

Examination

- Vital signs, including pulse and temperature
- Weight
- Abdominal examination for palpable mass (twins/large for gestational age uterus)
- Thyroid examination
- Speculum examination to examine os for open/closed for miscarriage variant

Investigations

- Blood group for Rhesus status
- Quantitative βhCG
- Consider thyroid function tests.
- Transvaginal ultrasound

Management

- Differentiation of threatened miscarriage and other pregnancy (ectopic, molar)
- When prompted that a molar pregnancy is likely on sonography and serology, evacuation of the uterus
- Follow-up of hCG

The best students

- Give differential list for causes of nausea, vomiting and bleeding in early pregnancy.
- Are able to differentiate partial and complete mole by investigation.
- Know the detailed follow-up for women with a molar pregnancy.
- Discuss complications from the surgical management of a molar pregnancy.
- Advise on a subsequent pregnancy.

CHAPTER 24: Cervical cancer screening

Michelle, a 22-year-old woman, sees you for a routine Pap smear. What are the important factors that you need to elicit from history in regards to establishing risk factors for a Pap smear abnormality?

The result of her Pap test has predicted a 'high-grade squamous intraepithelial lesion — HGSIL'. Describe this result with Michelle and outline the likely management for her at this time.

History

- History of previous smears, particularly interval and any abnormalities
- Menstrual cycle, particularly duration, cyclicity, intermenstrual or postmenstrual history
- Use of contraceptives including COCP
- Pregnancy history
- Sexual history including STI risk, number of partners and high-risk sexual activities
- Age at first intercourse
- Past STIs and their diagnosis and treatment
- Smoking history
- Previous vaccination to HPV

Discussion

- An explanation of 'precancer' versus 'cancer' needs to be discussed with Michelle.
- A more detailed explanation of how cervical dysplasia develops and its aetiological factors, emphasising the role of HPV and its acquisition.
- While HPV is acquired via sexual intercourse, the majority of people who have had sexual intercourse have been exposed to HPV.
- HPV exposure is not associated with infertility.
- Due to the high number of people (men and women) exposed, it is not considered an STI that requires treatment or notification (unlike *Chlamydia*, for example).
- Emphasise that it is a marker of 'normal sexual maturity'.

Management

- An explanation of the diagnostic process that would include a colposcopy and directed biopsy should be given to Michelle.
- A detailed explanation of what a colposcopy is and the need for further testing is important.
- If the diagnosis of CIN III is confirmed by colposcopy and biopsy, then treatment options including a LEEP excision would need to be discussed.
- This would include the location of the procedure, the type of anaesthetic used and risks from the procedure.
- While CIN III can be treated, explain that there is no treatment at present for HPV infection.
- That the LEEP excision will remove the CIN III but her immune system usually will eradicate the virus in time.
- Less than 5–10% of women remain persistently HPV positive.

The best students

- Discuss risk factors for development of pre-invasive cervical disease.
- Are able to discuss the role of HPV vaccination and the implication for screening women.
- Understand the pathophysiology of the development of pre-invasive cervical disease.
- Outline the natural history of low-grade and high-grade changes predicted on a Pap smear.
- Discuss the management for low-grade and high-grade changes predicted on a Pap smear.

CHAPTER 25: Cervical cancer

Jane, a 46-year-old woman, is referred to you with a Pap smear predicting a squamous cervical cancer. What are the historical and examination features that would be important to evaluate in this patient? What further investigations are required for Jane?

History

- History of previous smears, particularly interval and any abnormalities
- Menstrual cycle, particularly duration, cyclicity, intermenstrual or postmenstrual bleeding
- Use of contraceptives including COCP
- Pregnancy history and desire for any future pregnancy
- Sexual history including STI risk, number of partners and high-risk sexual activities
- Age at first intercourse
- Past STIs and their diagnosis and treatment
- Smoking history

Examination

- General examination (pulse, BP, BMI)
- Abdominal examination and examining for lymph nodes
- Abdominal examination
- Pelvic examination including speculum examination — look for any gross cervical lesion or extension into any surrounding tissues or structures
- Indication that best examination is done by a gynaecological oncologist

Investigations

- Determination of the malignancy through colposcopy and tissue biopsy is essential.
- Once confirmed, staging of the malignancy, which is performed clinically and is best done by a gynaecological oncologist.
- Often imaging studies are performed, although these are not part of the formal staging process.
- The gynaecological oncologist is likely to arrange for a formal examination under anaesthesia, biopsy and cystoscopy.
- While you are unable to preempt these findings, it is likely based on the large size of the tumour that the patient will be offered definitive chemoradiation therapy.

The best students

- Undertake a thorough history including risk factors for cervical malignancy.
- Recognise that sensitivity is required in the taking of a sexual history.
- Examine the cervix and know that there is a staging system that is clinically based.

CHAPTER 26: Uterine cancer

You are seeing Georgina, a 55-year-old woman who has a 2-week history of postmenopausal bleeding. She has a history of non-insulin dependent diabetes mellitus (NIDDM) on oral hypoglycaemic medication and has a BMI of 41 kg/m^2. Her dark red vaginal bleeding is not heavy but requires several pad changes a day.

Describe the salient information on history and examination would you seek from this woman. What investigations would you recommend in this situation? Diagnosis of a Grade 1 endometrioid adenocarcinoma of the uterine corpus is confirmed on histologic review. Describe management that is likely in this setting.

History

- More detail on previous episodes of vaginal bleeding — timing, pain, duration, frequency, heaviness.
- Gynaecologic history (menarche, parity, menopause)
- Use of hormone therapy, other vaginal bleeding or discharge
- Pap smear history
- Past significant medical and surgical history (other cancers, particularly breast and bowel cancer history, medication history or coagulopathy history) to assess comorbidities
- Family history (particularly bowel cancer for Lynch germ-line mutations) to assess familial risks

Examination

- General examination
- BMI and vital signs
- Breast examination
- Lymphadenopathy
- Pelvic examination inspecting the vulva, speculum examination of the vagina and cervix to exclude other disease such as vulvar, vaginal (rare) or cervical cancer being the cause of the bleeding
- Bimanual examination to assess the uterine size and mobility, adnexa and vaginal access.

Investigations

- Pap smear should be taken while performing speculum examination.
- Endometrial sample can be considered if resources are available.
- Pelvic (preferably transvaginal) ultrasound to check the endometrial thickness and adnexa.
- Reasonable to also request baseline full blood count, renal and liver function as well as random BSL/glycosylated haemoglobin.

Management

- Further imaging may be required to determine for any metastatic spread (CXR, abdomen and pelvis CT, MRI — dependent on resource availability).
- Explain she will require a hysterectomy and bilateral salpingo-oophorectomy.
- Explain that the expected hospitalisation and convalescence period will depend on how this procedure is performed (laparotomy or laparoscopic).
- Explain that the procedure best done by a gynaecological oncologist and multidisciplinary team.

The best students

- Take a chronological history, specifically identifying risk factors for malignancy in a post-menopausal woman.
- Propose appropriate benign and malignant conditions that may present in this manner.
- Examine the woman and perform appropriate clinical investigations including a Pap smear.
- Undertake pertinent examinations only.
- Are able to discuss the management of an endometrial malignancy when this is declared to be the diagnosis.
- Are able to manage other common causes for post-menopausal bleeding correctly.

CHAPTER 27: Cancer of the ovary

Helen is a 65-year-old woman who presents with a 3-year history of increasing nausea, abdominal distension and lethargy. She has had one child, and has not had gynaecological issues before. Menopause was at 50 and she has not been on HRT. She has hypertension and had an appendicectomy. What further information will you seek on history and examination?

Helen has had increasing night sweats and weight gain of 8 kg over the last 2 months with a palpable mass in the upper abdomen and shifting dullness present. What investigations are important?

The CA 125 is 3500, the TVUS shows bilateral solid cystic mass in both ovaries with a small central uterus and ascitic fluid clearly demonstrated. The CT scan shows a large omental lesion of 8 cm and lesions on the diaphragm. There appears to be a mass at the ileocaecal junction.

What is the likely diagnosis for Helen and what management do you recommend?

History

- Age of menarche, use of OCP, fertility treatments
- Pap smear history
- Gastrointestinal symptoms, bowel habit, appetite change
- Urinary symptoms
- Weight gain or loss
- Night sweats
- Pain in abdomen or other body areas (bones/back etc.)
- Finding of any lumps/bumps on body

Examination

- Examination should include height/weight for BMI, general examination
- Examination for lymphadenopathy
- Abdominal examination, particularly for palpable masses, tenderness or signs of ascites (shifting dullness)
- Pelvic examination for pelvic masses

Investigations

- FBC/EUC/LFT
- CA 125, CA 19.9, CEA
- Imaging investigations should include a pelvic ultrasound (transabdominal and transvaginal) and abdomino-pelvic CT as initial investigations.

Management

- The RMI is >10 000, indicating a likely malignancy, with the ovaries a likely source, although other abdominal malignancies (e.g. gastric cancer) or benign tumours are possible.
- Counselling regarding the diagnosis is mandatory and the need for further investigations and management essential.
- An ascitic tap may give cytological specimens for diagnosis.
- Referral to a gynaecological oncologist would be appropriate and further imaging of chest may be warranted.
- Management is likely to be a midline laparotomy, debulking of the ovarian masses and tumour mass, possibly including bowel resection, omentectomy and consideration of diaphragmatic stripping and adjuvant chemotherapy.

The best students

- Take an appropriate history and perform examinations consistent with the general nature of the presentation.
- Are able to identify both benign and malignant diagnoses that will be considered in the differential diagnosis list.
- Perform appropriate investigations and recognise the limitations of investigations including why screening is not indicated at this time for ovarian cancer.
- Understand the risk of malignancy index as a general indicator for cancer.
- Liaise with a gynaecologist or gynaecological oncologist for treatment.
- Recognise that surgery and adjuvant chemotherapy are likely to be needed.

Index

Page numbers followed by 'f' indicate figures, 't' indicate tables, and 'b' indicate boxes.